Poisoning

Diagnosis and Treatment

Poisoning
Diagnosis and Treatment

edited by

J. A. Vale, MD, MRCP

and

T. J. Meredith, MA, MRCP

1981

UPDATE BOOKS

LONDON · DORDRECHT · BOSTON

Available in the United Kingdom and Eire from
Update Books Ltd
33/34 Alfred Place
London WC1E 7DP
England

Available in the USA and Canada from
Kluwer Boston Inc.
Lincoln Building, 190 Old Derby Street
Hingham, Mass. 02043
USA

Available in the rest of the world from
Kluwer Academic Publishers
Group Distribution Centre
PO Box 322
3300 AH Dordrecht
The Netherlands

British Library Cataloguing in Publication Data
Poisoning.
   1. Poisoning
   I. Vale, J. A.   II. Meredith, T J
   615.9   RA1211
   ISBN 0-906141-81-8
   ISBN 0-906141-82-6 Pbk

Cover illustration provided by Mary Evans Picture Library

First Published 1981

ISBN 0 906141 81 8 (Hardback)
ISBN 0 906141 82 6 (Paperback)

Typeset and produced by R James Hall Typesetting and Book Production Services,
Harpenden, England.
Text set in IBM Press Roman, 10 pt on 12.

Printed in Great Britain by
Lowe & Brydone Printers Ltd, Thetford

Contents

Contributors

D. Barltrop, B.SC, MD, FRCP, DCH, Department of Child Health, Westminster Hospital, London.

G.M. Cochrane, B.SC, MB, MRCP, Department of Respiratory Medicine, Guy's Hospital, London.

P. Crome, MD, MRCP, Poisons Unit, Guy's Hospital, London.

R. Gardner, MB, MRCP, MRC.Psych, DPM, Department of Psychiatry, Addenbrooke's Hospital, Cambridge.

R. Goulding, B.SC, MD, FRCP, FRC.Path, Poisons Unit, Guy's Hospital, London.

M. Helliwell, MB, MRCP, Poisons Unit, Guy's Hospital, London.

G. Kazantzis, MB, Ph.D., FRCP, FSCM, FFOM, TUC Centenary Institute of Occupational Health, London School of Hygiene and Tropical Medicine.

T.J. Meredith, MA, MRCP, Poisons Unit, Guy's Hospital, London.

H.A. Reid, OBE, MD, FRCPE, FRACP, DTM & H, WHO Collaborative Centre for the Control of Antivenoms, Liverpool School of Tropical Medicine.

J. A. Vale, MD, MRCP, Poisons Unit, Guy's Hospital, London

G.N. Volans, B.SC, MD, MRCP, Poisons Unit, Guy's Hospital, London.

B. Widdop, B.SC, Ph.D, Poisons Unit, Guy's Hospital, London.

Preface

In the last decade, the incidence of acute poisoning in the developed world has risen considerably, so that hospital admissions from this cause now represent a significant part of the work load of most medical units.

The purpose of this book is to provide an up-to-date account of the diagnosis and treatment of all the clinically important poisons. Throughout the text the aim has been to emphasize the mechanisms of toxicity — wherever they are known — so that a rational approach to therapy may be devised. In addition, substantial chapters have been devoted to the psychiatric assessment of self-poisoned patients and to the role of the laboratory.

Two styles of presentation have been adopted. Certain topics are discussed in depth either because of their clinical importance or because recent data have become available concerning pathophysiology or treatment. In contrast, when subjects have been well described previously in general medical texts, for example, carbon monoxide poisoning, the discussion is far more brief and to the point. A similar style has been adopted with recently introduced drugs, where little is known about the effects in overdose. The value of certain chapters, especially those on poisonous plants and snake bites, has been enhanced by the inclusion of a large number of colour photographs. Each section or chapter includes a list of important and recent references so that the book will provide a useful introduction to original and review papers on poisoning. In addition, a summary of sources of information precedes the index.

The majority of chapters have been written by members of the Staff of the Poisons Unit, Guy's Hospital. The remaining five chapters are the work of expert collaborators from other Units and we are most grateful to them for their assistance.

As we both hold full-time clinical appointments, the preparation of the text has occupied, inevitably, many evenings and weekends. This would not have been possible but for the support of our wives, Elizabeth and Peggy, to whom we owe our thanks for their encouragement and forbearance.

Miss Joanna Brazier typed the whole of the script (several times) and produced an attractive and clear manuscript.

Our thanks are also due to the Staff of Update Publications, notably Mrs Maggie Pettifer and Miss Jemima Kallas who have been as helpful as any author or editor could wish.

Allister Vale
Tim Meredith
Guy's Hospital, London.
February 1981

Foreword

In recent years there has been increasing interest in, and awareness of, the toxicological problems of pollution, the side-effects of drugs, food additives and contaminants, the hazards of industrial processes and, most of all, self-poisoning.

There is still considerable ignorance of clinical toxicology in many countries, and misconceptions and fallacies abound regarding the treatment of poisoned patients. There are two main reasons for this. Firstly, intoxicated patients are seldom admitted to specialized units so that few physicians have sufficient experience of treating severely poisoned patients. Secondly, most books on clinical toxicology are written by non-clinicians. I am delighted that this book is an exception to the rule. It is edited and largely written by two practising clinicians from the Poisons Unit, Guy's Hospital, where an advanced and highly developed analytical service is available. It is regarded as one of the best centres in Europe.

The book rightly emphasizes the mechanisms of toxicity so that elucidation of symptoms and treatment becomes rational and is no longer, therefore, a list learned by heart. In addition, attention is given to the treatment of the patient as a whole and not just to the toxicity of the product taken and the attending symptoms and signs. Thus, there are chapters on the psychiatric assessment of self-poisoned patients and the prevention of poisoning.

Let me express the hope that the future will bring many new editions of this book in which the latest aspects of clinical toxicology may be presented and modern treatment defined.

Prof. Dr. A. N. P. Van Heijst
University of Utrecht, Holland.
*President of the European Association
of Poison Control Centres*
January 1981

Chapter 1

J. A. Vale and T. J. Meredith

Epidemiology of Poisoning in the UK

With few exceptions, poisoning is by self-administration. Murderers seldom favour this method to despatch their victims and truly accidental exposure, such as may arise from a person's work or from his environment, is rare. Admittedly mistakes can occur, but there is little doubt that most adults who swallow dangerous substances do so intentionally. In children the position is different; self-administration is the rule, but the child acts out of innocent curiosity and, unlike his elders, does not foresee the consequences.

Incidence of Acute Poisoning

In 1962, 33,600 poisoned patients were admitted to hospitals in England and Wales; 16 years later the corresponding figure was some 120,640 (Figure 1.1). These statistics, however, probably underestimate the true incidence of acute poisoning in that a large number of symptomless children, and as many as 40 per cent of adults, who present at accident and emergency departments may be sent home because they are, physically at least, only mildly poisoned. Furthermore, some patients are not referred to hospital for admission but are treated at home by their general practitioners. A more realistic estimate would be that each year in the UK some 300,000 patients ingest 'toxic' agents, either by accident in the case of children or as a parasuicidal gesture or suicidal attempt in adults.

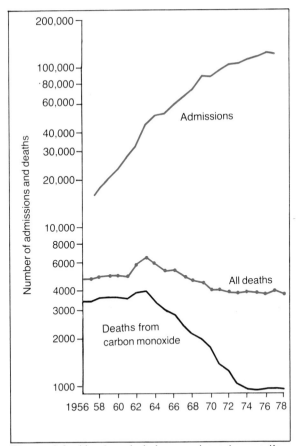

Figure 1.1. *Yearly admissions and total mortality from acute poisoning — England and Wales, 1956-1978.*

The Modern Epidemic

Acute poisoning is now so common that some have suggested it warrants the description of the 'modern epidemic'. In young adults it appears to be an almost accepted pattern of social behaviour and, as a result, it has become a major medical problem in both social and economic terms. The large number of poisoned patients admitted to hospital each year represents a significant part of the clinical work load. Indeed, in some hospitals, poisoned patients account for 20 per cent of all emergency medical admissions and one-sixth of those requiring admission to an intensive care unit. In Cambridge almost 50 per cent of acute female medical admissions between the ages of 15 and 40 years are the result of a drug overdose (Mills 1977).

Poisoning in Children

In contrast to the trend seen in adults, there has been a fall in the number of poisoned children aged less than five years admitted to hospital in the period 1971 to 1977 (Figure 1.2). There are probably two reasons for this. First, the amounts ingested by small children are often well below the lethal dose. Second, the intrinsic toxicity of the materials ingested is often not high. In addition, there is evidence that the introduction of child-resistant containers in 1976 has reduced the incidence of child poisoning with aspirin, and possibly paracetamol, though this has not influenced the overall admission rate which rose in 1977. The types of medicinal and non-medicinal poisons ingested by children are shown in Table 1.1.

Effect of Age, Sex and Time

In a three-year study conducted in the S E Thames Regional Health Authority area (Vale 1977) the incidence of acute poisoning was 2 per 1000 population per annum. As this was based on hospital admissions the true incidence is likely to be higher. The majority of patients were young (Figure 1.3) and 70 per cent were less than 36 years of age. Females outnumbered males in all age groups (female to male ratio being 1.5 : 1), except in those under 15 years of age where boys were in the majority (male to female ratio 1 : 0.87). Most patients were admitted during the summer months, at weekends and in the evening. It could therefore be argued that leisure time (and hence the opportunity for the more liberal imbibition of alcohol) predisposes to self-poisoning in adults.

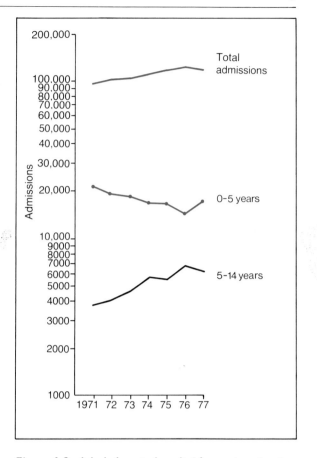

Figure 1.2. *Admissions to hospital for acute poisoning in children — England and Wales, 1971-1977.*

However, an analysis of unemployed men in Glasgow who presumably, through their misfortune, were unoccupied all day, showed that 70 per cent took an overdose after 10 p.m. (Patel 1973). About three-quarters of patients present at hospital within four hours of being poisoned, and many arrived within one hour. The majority of patients make a full physical recovery in less than 24 hours and 75 per cent are discharged from hospital within three days.

Availability of Drugs

Perhaps the most important cause for the increase in self-poisoning is the ready availability of drugs in the community, with the result that the majority of patients (and nearly all adults) are poisoned by medicinal, and often prescribed, preparations. Further evidence of the importance of availability of drugs lies in the changing pattern of drugs taken in over-dosage over the years.

Following the CURB (Campaign for the Use and Restriction of Barbiturates) campaign, most doctors have adopted a voluntary ban on the routine prescription of barbiturates (other than for the treatment of epilepsy and for use in anaesthesia), and now prescribe less toxic alternatives such as the benzodiazepines (Figure 1.4). As a result the incidence of barbiturate poisoning has fallen while that due to psychotropic drugs has increased (Figure 1.5).

Different types of poisoning tend to predominate in each age group (Figure 1.6); these patterns reflect prescribing habits and hence the availability of particular agents. Teenagers and young adults favour psychotropic agents, such as the antidepressant drugs and the benzodiazepines, whereas the elderly tend to take barbiturate and non-barbiturate hypnotics. Until recently children frequently ingested analgesics such as aspirin and paracetamol, but the introduction of child-resistant containers for these agents in 1976 has significantly, and favourably, affected the problem for salicylates at least (Craft and Sibert 1979).

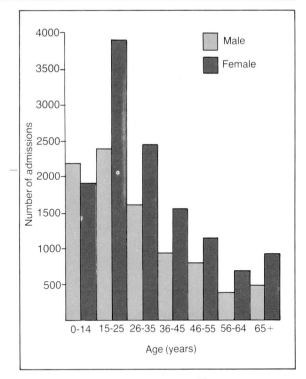

Figure 1.3. *Acute poisoning in the SE Thames RHA, 1972-1974 — age of admissions.*

Table 1.1. Deaths from poisoning in those under 10 years — England and Wales 1968–1978.

Poison	No. of deaths reported
Carbon monoxide	1066
Tricyclic antidepressants	40
Aspirin	34
Barbiturates	16
Lead	12
Digoxin	10
Iron	9
Quinine	8
'Lomotil' (atropine and diphenoxylate)	6
Orphenadrine	6
Opiates	6
Antihistamines	6
Paraquat	5
Fenfluramine	6
Petroleum products	5
Phenothiazines	3
Non-barbiturate hypnotics	3
Alkalis	2
Ethyl alcohol	2
Paracetamol	1
Miscellaneous (largely non-medicinal)	54
Total	1300

Deaths from Poisoning

The number of patients who die from acute poisoning has remained constant at about 4000 per annum in England and Wales since 1971 (Figure 1.7). It seems almost as if there lies within the population a small but numerically constant group who are intent on their own demise. This is not, of course, true of the majority of patients who take an overdose. Furthermore there is some evidence that this small group may ingest more toxic agents in greater quantities than those who intend no more than a 'cry for help'. In addition they may go to great lengths to avoid discovery and the majority of these patients, therefore, do not reach hospital alive. Indeed, less than a quarter of those patients who die from acute poisoning do so in hospital, so that the inpatient mortality is very low — approximately 0.6 per cent (Figure 1.7). Overall, females predominate in deaths from poisoning and this is particularly so in those over 45 years of age (Figure 1.8).

Carbon Monoxide Poisoning

Despite the fact that the domestic gas supply is no longer a ready source of carbon monoxide, the mortality from this cause has not fallen significantly since 1972. Indeed, the majority of deaths from poisoning in those aged less than 10 years are caused by this agent (Table 1.1). Deaths from carbon monoxide in the UK are now usually due to inefficient burners and stoves and the deliberate inhalation of exhaust fumes from motor vehicle engines.

Trends in Mortality from Poisoning

Although the total mortality from poisoning has only fallen slightly since 1972, there have been considerable changes in the individual drugs responsible for the 4000 deaths per annum. The mortality from barbiturates and non-barbiturate hypnotics has fallen, whereas the number of those dying from poisoning due to analgesics, tranquillizers and antidepressants has risen (Figure 1.9). Only the data for single-agent ingestion has been tabulated, but the pattern is similar where multiple agents are involved. The fall in mortality due to barbiturates and the increase in mortality due to tranquillizers has been paralleled by changes in prescribing habits.

Barbiturates

The majority of patients who die from barbiturate poisoning are elderly and have been supplied with the drug because they are either unwilling or reluctant to change to a less toxic alternative after a lifetime of barbiturate-induced sleep. The 50 per cent fall in the number dying from barbiturates seen between 1971 and 1978 (Figures 1.9 and 1.10) is an encouraging sign and, if present trends continue, it is probable that within five years barbiturate poisoning will no longer make a significant contribution to the total mortality from acute poisoning.

Lest it be thought that severe barbiturate poisoning is invariably fatal, it should be realized that charcoal haemoperfusion is an effective means of treatment for otherwise hopeless cases (see Chapter 8).

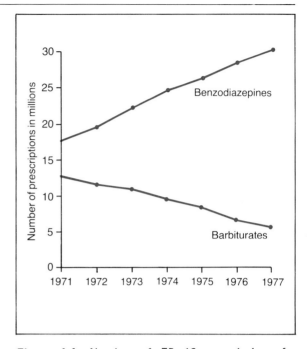

Figure 1.4. *Number of FP 10 prescriptions for barbiturates and benzodiazepines — Great Britain, 1971-1977.*

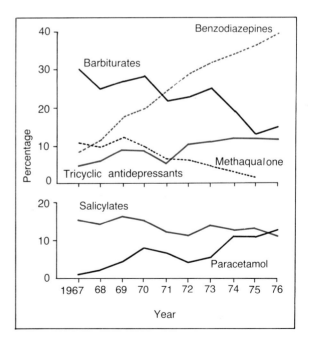

Figure 1.5. *Poison admissions to the Royal Infirmary Edinburgh 1967-1976. By kind permission of Dr A T Proudfoot and the Editor,* British Medical Journal.

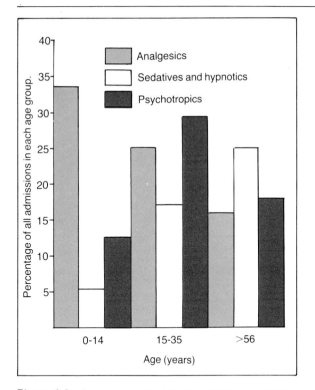

Figure 1.6. *Acute poisoning in the SE Thames RHA, 1972-1974. Types of drug ingested by different age groups.*

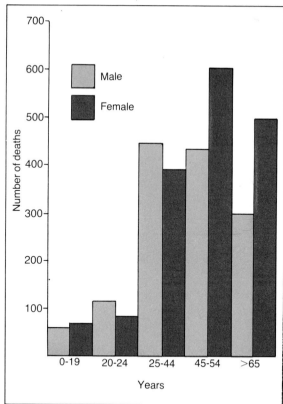

Figure 1.8. *Deaths from poisoning — England and Wales 1978 — age and sex distribution.*

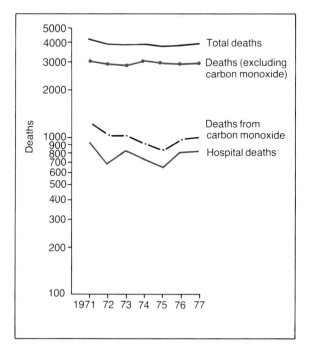

Figure 1.7. *Deaths from poisoning — England and Wales, 1971-1977.*

Antidepressants

The increase in the number of deaths from antidepressant poisoning gives cause for considerable concern; in 1978 there were 438 deaths which involved an antidepressant drug either alone or in combination. It may be that further experience will confirm the initial impression that some of the newer 'quadricyclic' antidepressants are less toxic in overdose than the 'tricyclic' antidepressants and that they may therefore be prescribed with greater safety to those who are depressed. The mortality from antidepressant poisoning in children is second only to that from carbon monoxide (Table 1.1).

Hypnotics

The fall in the number of deaths from methaqualone (112 in 1971; 18 in 1978) probably reflects the fall in popularity of this hypnotic over the last decade.

Although chlormethiazole has been advocated as a safe hypnotic in the elderly and for the treatment of withdrawal symptoms in alcoholics, it has been responsible for an increasing number of deaths (6 in 1971; 84 in 1978).

Benzodiazepines

Until recently it has been stated that 'no one ever dies from a benzodiazepine overdose'. In 1978 the Office of Population Censuses and Surveys (OPCS) officially recorded 97 patients as having died following the ingestion of benzodiazepines alone. A benzodiazepine was also involved in 192 other cases (Figure 1.11). Without doubt, other drugs and alcohol had been ingested by some of these 97 patients, but it is clearly no longer possible to claim that the mortality from this group of drugs is negligible.

Analgesics

It is significant that two out of the first five causes of death from poisoning in 1978 involved drugs which are freely available 'over the counter': aspirin and paracetamol (Table 1.2). In particular, over the last few years there has been an increase in the number of deaths from paracetamol (Figure 1.12). This may be explained by the increase in consumption of this analgesic which, in part, is probably due to education of the population by its medical advisors to believe that paracetamol has fewer side-effects than aspirin.

Deaths from 'Distalgesic' (paracetamol + dextropropoxyphene) poisoning have also risen (Figure 1.12) in line with the increasing number of prescriptions. Indeed, Distalgesic is now the most commonly prescribed analgesic in both hospital and general practice. It is probable that sensational and often misleading publicity in the press and on television has served to increase further the number of overdoses due to this drug. If a patient poisoned with Distalgesic reaches hospital alive there need not be a fatal outcome because naloxone reverses the respiratory-depressant effects of dextropropoxyphene, and oral methionine or intravenous N-acetylcysteine will reduce or abolish the hepatotoxic effects of paracetamol. Regrettably this treatment has not always been carried out, with fatal consequences.

Miscellaneous

Three further trends in poisoning are worthy of brief comment. First, 47 patients died from paraquat poisoning in 1978 and almost all of these ingested substantial quantities of the 20 per cent concentrate (Gramoxone, Dextrone). Second, 34 deaths involved β-adrenergic blocking drugs. Third, 17 people in 1978 died from cyanide poisoning so this is by no means a 'forgotten poison'.

Table 1.2. Important causes of death from poisoning — England and Wales 1978.

	Ingested alone or with ethanol	Alone and in combination with other agents
Amylobarbitone and quinalbarbitone ('Tuinal')	282	304
Tricyclic antidepressant drugs	245	395
Aspirin	215	288
Paracetamol	196	492
Amylobarbitone	140	165
Pentobarbitone	111	163
Benzodiazepines	97	192

Conclusion

The problem of poisoning is not confined to Great Britain but is common in all developed countries. For example, it has been estimated that more than five million poisonings occur every year in the USA (Meester 1977). Acute poisoning is a major medical, social and economic problem in the western world. Self-poisoning has become an established pattern of social behaviour in response to stress and, as such, must be treated with the maximum medical, psychological and social expertise.

Acknowledgements

The authors are most grateful to the Office of Population Censuses and Surveys and to the Statistical Division of the DHSS for so readily furnishing the data upon which this chapter has been based. The data are reproduced by permission of the Controller, HMSO.

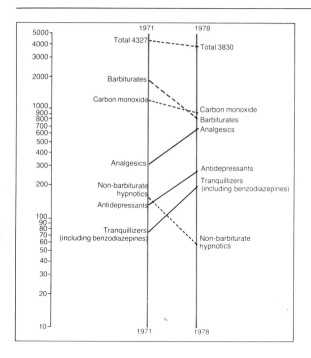

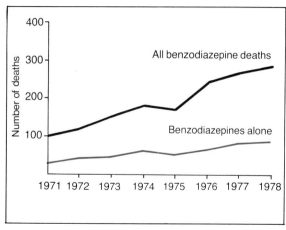

Figure 1.9. *Deaths from poisoning — England and Wales, 1971-1978 — number of deaths where a single agent was involved.*

Figure 1.11. *Deaths from benzodiazepines whether taken alone or in combination with other drugs — England and Wales, 1971-1978.*

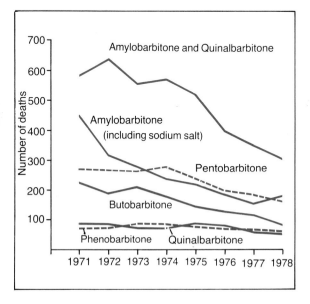

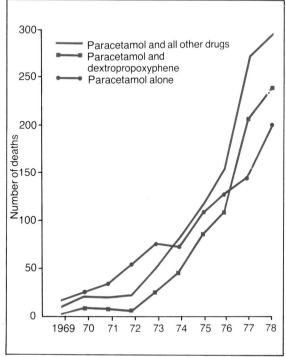

Figure 1.10. *Total deaths from named barbiturates — England and Wales, 1971-1978.*

Figure 1.12. *Deaths from paracetamol (acetaminophen) alone and in combination with other drugs — England and Wales, 1969-1978.*

References

Craft AW, Sibert JR. Preventive effect of CRC's. Pharm J 1979; 223:593.

Meester WD. Development of regional poison information and treatment centers. Acta Pharmacol Toxicol (Suppl II) 1977; 41:502–7.

Mills IH. Self-poisoning – a modern epidemic. Proc. Eur Soc Toxicol 1977; 18:11–20.

Patel AR. MD Thesis. University of Aberdeen 1973.

Proudfoot AT, Park J. Changing pattern of drugs used in self-poisoning. Br Med J 1978; 1:90–3.

Vale JA. Epidemiology of acute poisoning. Acta Pharmacol Toxicol 1977; 41:(Suppl II) 443–58.

Further Reading

Bean P. Patterns of self-poisoning. Br J Prev Soc Med 1974; 28:24–31.

Burston GR. Severe self-poisoning in Sunderland. Br Med J 1969; 1:679–81.

Collier J, Cummins TA, Hamilton M. A survey of suicidal behaviour in the Mid-Essex area. J R Coll Physicians Lond 1976; 10:381–92.

Evans JG. Deliberate self-poisoning in the Oxford area. Br J Prev Soc Med 1967; 21:97–107.

Fraser NC. Accidental poisoning deaths in British children 1958–77. Br Med J 1980; 280:1595–8.

Ghodse AH. Deliberate self-poisoning: a study in London casualty departments. Br Med J 1977; 1:805–8.

Johns MW. Self-poisoning with barbiturates in England and Wales during 1959–1974. Br Med J 1977; 1:1128–30.

Jones DIR. Self-poisoning with drugs: the past 20 years in Sheffield. Br Med J 1977; 1:28–9.

Lawson AAH, Mitchell I. Patients with acute poisoning seen in a general medical unit (1960–1971). Br Med J 1972; 4:153–6.

Krietman N (Ed). Parasuicide. London: John Wiley, 1977.

Murray JC, Campbell D, Reid JM, Telfer ABM. Severe self-poisoning: a ten-year experience in the Glasgow area. Scott Med J 1974; 19:279–85.

Smith AJ. Self-poisoning with drugs: a worsening situation. Br Med J 1972; 4:157–9.

Smith RS. An epidemiological study of self-poisoning in Penarth (South Wales). Proc R Soc Med 1974; 67:675–7.

Stewart RB, Forgnone M, May FE, Forbes J, Cluff LE. Epidemiology of acute drug intoxication: patient characteristics, drugs and medical complications: Clin Toxicol 1974; 7:513–30.

Tulloch JA. Self-poisoning: A 10-year review of patients admitted to Stracathro Hospital. Scott Med J 1972; 17:278–81.

Whelton A, Snyder DS, Walker WG. Acute toxic drug ingestions at the Johns Hopkins Hospital, 1963 through 1970. Johns Hopkins Med J 1973; 132:157–67.

Chapter 2

J. A. Vale and T. J. Meredith

Poisons Information Services

Development of Poisons Information Services

Poisons Information Services made their first appearance on a small scale in the Netherlands in 1949. Then, in 1950, the Accident Prevention Committee of the American Academy of Pediatrics undertook an enquiry into accidents in children. The completed survey showed that acute poisoning accounted for 51 per cent of accidents. As a result, the Illinois Chapter of the American Academy of Pediatrics opened an information centre in Chicago in 1963 in collaboration with the State Health Department, the State Toxicological Laboratory, various pharmaceutical interests, the American Public Health Association and seven local hospitals. So successful was this venture that a further information centre was opened in Cleveland, Ohio; other centres soon followed. There are now about 600 poison control centres in America (Crotty and Armstrong 1978).

At the instigation of the American Public Health Service a central organisation, the National Clearing House for Poison Control Centers, was formed in 1958 in Washington, D.C. by the Department of Health, Education and Welfare. State Health Departments were nominated to coordinate the poison control activities within their own territories. The staff of the Clearing House came under the direction of a doctor and pharmacist. The Clearing House issues sets of 5 x 8 in cards (16,000 are in print) which contain up-to-date information on a vast number of products that appear on the American market.

Starting in 1957, the poisons information movement in Canada developed along similar lines with a coordinating agency under the Food and Drug Directorate in Ottawa.

Benefits and Deficiencies of Poisons Information Centres

Poisons Information Centres are now found in most developed countries. Verhulst and Crotty (1971) and Goulding (1975) have assessed the advantages of such centres. The British experience has been reviewed by Goulding (1975) and is described below.

At the instigation of the Department of Health, Education and Welfare a critical evaluation of Poison Control Centres in the United States was carried out in 1972 by an independent firm of consultants. This report highlighted some of the weaknesses of the service which had been noted earlier by Crick (1968) and Lovejoy and Alpert (1970). Parochialism and local pride encourage the proliferation of poison centres. Such a movement tends to be accelerated when some central agency is ready to furnish an up-to-date index, free-of-charge, to any group undertaking to man a telephone throughout a 24-hour period.

The 1972 American report disclosed the following:

1. The majority of centres did not have their own direct telephone line.
2. There was a lack of follow-up of cases reported to the centres.
3. Only one-half of the centres kept records of their calls.
4. The majority of centres did not devote staff time to prevention activities.

Notwithstanding these deficiencies it has been estimated that between 1952 and 1969, 410,705 emergency room visits were avoided because of the telephone information provided.

The balance of international opinion at present "is toward larger national or regional centres, and away from small ones adorning practically every city in the land. Telephone lines are more expeditiously connected than qualified clinical toxicologists are trained and appointed to these duties." (Goulding 1975).

The National Poisons Information Service in the UK

In 1961, a telephone answering service was introduced in Leeds, England, which gave information to medical practitioners and others about the poisonous properties of a variety of household, agricultural and therapeutic substances. On 2 September 1963, a National Poisons Information Service was established at Guy's Hospital, London. This development owed its origin to the fourth recommendation of the Sub-Committee of the Standing Medical Advisory Committee on the emergency treatment in hospital of cases of acute poisoning (Central Health Services Council 1962). The service comprised not only the primary coordinating centre at Guy's, but also centres in Belfast, Cardiff and Edinburgh. The Republic of Ireland subsequently joined the scheme through the Jervis Street Hospital in Dublin.

The British National Poisons Information Service was established with the following functions (Ministry of Health 1963):

1. "To maintain an index of substances of common use — medicinal, veterinary, industrial, agricultural, horticultural, household, etc., showing their composition and, wherever possible, their toxicity and corrective measures in the cases of poisoning."
2. "To provide information for medical practitioners so as to facilitate treatment of cases of acute poisoning."

In contrast to many other countries, the British Poisons Information Service handles calls only from medical practitioners or their bona fide deputies, e.g. nursing officers in charge of accident and emergency departments. The reasons for this are two-fold:

1. It is considered that only a doctor 'on the spot' can adequately assess the implications of the information given in relation to the patient.
2. Some of the information on file, for example that relating to cosmetics or household products, is confidential and has been given by manufacturers

only on the understanding that it will not be released to the general public.

On the other hand, Verhulst and Crotty (1971) have argued that Poison Information Centres dealing directly with the public have the following advantages:

1. They can inform the individual that no action is necessary, or that a poisoning has occurred and a physician should be contacted. As a result, much time and expense may be saved by the patient and the number of attendances at emergency departments may be reduced.
2. They can caution against actions which are contra-indicated, e.g. the induction of vomiting when a caustic preparation has been taken.

Since the establishment of the British Poisons Information Service there has been a steady increase in the number of enquiries received each year (Figure 2.1). This rise parallels the increase in the number of patients admitted to hospital suffering from acute poisoning (Figure 2.1). In at least 90 per cent of cases the answer to an enquiry can be given immediately from the index kept at each centre. The remainder of the enquiries are referred to a physician-on-call who is ready, if this is thought desirable, to discuss the management of the patient with the doctor in charge of the patient's care.

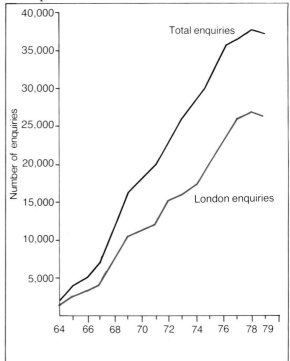

Figure 2.1. *Yearly number of enquiries received by the British Poisons Information Service.*

A feature of the National Poisons Information Service in Britain is that a brief questionnaire has been sent to every doctor telephoning one of the centres. The level of returns has been high. An analysis of the enquiries (Figure 2.2), and particularly the follow-up data on those poisoned, provides a picture of the nature of poisoning, its intensity, and of the behaviour of individual substances and products (Goulding and Volans 1980).

In this way, Mofenson and Greensher (1970) and Goulding et al. (1978) have thrown light on, for example, 'non-toxic ingestion', pointing out that numerous materials used in the home, against which accusations of toxicity have been widely levelled, are in fact virtually innocuous. Furthermore, as Goulding (1975) has reminded us, merely to answer calls from an index, or even from professional knowledge, and to neglect the clinical data that can be recovered from following up all the incidents is medically inexcusable. Such information is an indispensable part of poisons control in its widest sense for, without proceeding to direct experiments in man, human toxicological data can be accumulated which are far more relevant than the results of the most elegant experiments in animals. Furthermore, preventive and educational measures can be more efficiently designed and implemented if epidemiological data derived from the Poisons Information Centres are utilized.

Figure 2.2. *Analysis of enquiries received by the British Poisons Information Service, 1964-1979.*

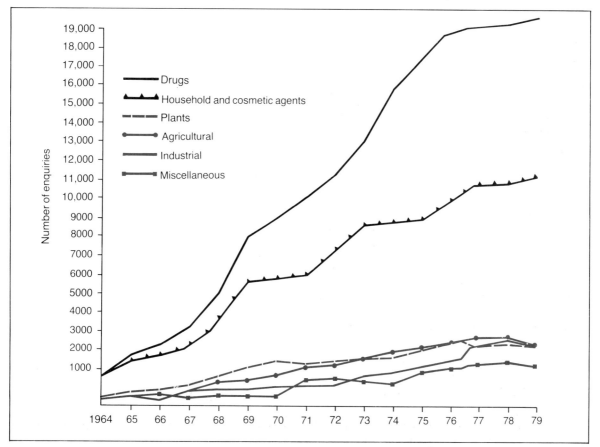

References

Central Health Services Council. Emergency Treatment in Hospital of Cases of Acute Poisoning. London: HMSO, 1962.

Crick, MFC. Poisons Information Centers. Cambridge, Mass: Bolt, Baranek and Newman, 1968, Rep No. 1579.

Crotty J, Armstrong G. National Clearing House for poison control centers. Clin Toxicol 1978; 12: 303−7.

Goulding R. Poison control centers − an essay on information and prevention. In: Essays in Toxicology, Vol 6, New York: Academic Press, 1975.

Goulding R, Ashforth GK, Jenkins H. Household products and poisoning. Br Med J 1978; 1:286−7.

Goulding R. Volans GN. Poisons information services. In: Monitoring for Drug Safety. Ed. Inman W H W. Lancaster: MTP Press, 1980.

Lovejoy Jr FH, Alpert JJ. A future direction for poison centers. Pediatr Clin North Am 1970; 17:747−53.

Ministry of Health. Poisons Information Service. Circular HM (63) 75, ECL 65/63. London: HMSO, 1963.

Mofenson HC, Greensher J. The non-toxic ingestion. Pediatr Clin 1970; 17:583−90.

Verhulst HL, Crotty JJ. Poisons information service and barbiturate poisoning. In: Acute Barbiturate Poisoning. Ed. Matthew H. Amsterdam: Excerpta Medica, 1971.

Further Reading

Pikaar SA, Van Heijst ANP. The National Poisons Information Center. Vet Hum Toxicol 1979; 21:Suppl. 76−80.

Rumack BH, Ford P, Sbarbaro J, Bryson P, Winokur M. Regionalisation of poisons centers − a rational role model. Clin Toxicol 1978; 12:367−75.

Scherz RG, Robertson WO. The history of poison control centers in the United States. Clin Toxicol 1978; 12:291−6.

Temple AR, Veltri JC. One year's experience in a regional poisons control center: the Intermountain Regional Poisons Control Center. Clin Toxicol 1978; 12:277−89.

Chapter 3

Brian Widdop

The Diagnosis of Poisoning: Use of the Laboratory

The colour plates cited in this chapter are to be found between pages 188 and 189.

Questioning the Patient

In many cases the patient, who is often only mildly poisoned, will volunteer the diagnosis. In the absence of circumstantial evidence, it should be assumed that an unconscious patient between the ages of 15 and 35 years has taken a drug overdose until proved otherwise.

Physical Signs

Skin blisters, though not pathognomonic, are found most commonly in patients who have ingested barbiturates, but they may also occur following poisoning with glutethimide, methaqualone, tricyclic antidepressants, meprobamate and carbon monoxide. It has been suggested that such blisters also occur in patients who are unconscious for other reasons. They are seen most commonly in sites where close contact between two skin surfaces has taken place, such as the interdigital clefts and inner aspects of the knees. They are seldom seen in areas of maximum pressure.

Venepuncture marks should be carefully sought. They indicate that the patient is, or has until recently, been 'mainlining' (i.e. deliberately introducing drugs intravenously). Additional signs that support a diagnosis of opiate overdose are: pin-point pupils, vomiting, depressed respiration and loss of consciousness. It must be remembered, however, that such an addict

may have taken an overdose of some other hypnotic drug, and an injection of naloxone can be diagnostic in this situation (see Chapter 5).

Use of the Laboratory

The identification and measurement of a toxic agent in the body fluids is necessary only if the diagnosis is in doubt, or where the patient's condition is serious enough to warrant consideration of active treatment in the form of either forced diuresis, haemodialysis or haemoperfusion. Not surprisingly, clinical chemistry laboratories have been reluctant to offer more than a limited analytical toxicology service since experienced analysts are scarce, the necessary equipment, when available, is often committed to routine biochemical assays and valid requests are few and intermittent. Consequently, these laboratories usually undertake analyses only for salicylates, barbiturates, iron and, more recently, paracetamol, seeing as their prime role the provision of biochemical measurements (blood gases, electrolytes, serum enzymes) to monitor physiological status. Nevertheless, investigations of a more searching nature are required from time to time and this has led to the establishment of a number of specialized laboratories such as the one at the Poisons Unit, Guy's Hospital which operates on a supraregional basis and can deal with such requests routinely.

This chapter singles out the types of poisoning incident where specific toxicological investigations are relevant. An outline of the techniques currently in vogue for the analysis of toxicological specimens is presented, and those factors which must be considered when interpreting the findings are discussed.

Application of Toxicological Analyses

Differential Diagnosis of Poisoning or Organic Disease

Newton (1974) has suggested that, in the adult patient, unconsciousness in the absence of obvious head injury is almost invariably due to drug overdose. This view has recently been challenged by Helliwell et al. (1979) who investigated a large number of cases of coma of unknown aetiology. Of the 208 patients in their survey only 108 (52 per cent) had taken an overdose of drugs. Clearly, where circumstantial evidence for poisoning is lacking, a comprehensive toxicological screen carried out in a specialized laboratory can, if positive findings ensue, obviate the need for clinical investigations such as lumbar puncture or computerized axial tomography. Conversely, negative results may help in deciding whether to instigate the above procedures.

Toxicological analyses play an analogous role in the diagnosis of brain death, particularly in patients whose primary cause of coma is known to have been drug overdose. A conference of the Medical Royal Colleges in the UK and their Faculties (1976) has emphasized the need to exclude the presence of toxic amounts of depressant drugs with prolonged activity as a cause of deep coma.

Poisoning as a means of inflicting bodily harm on others is unusual in western society, and the circumstances in which it arises are usually sufficient to arouse the suspicions of the victim (should he or she survive) or those of close friends or relatives. Regrettably, however, this form of assault is thought to be perpetrated more frequently than is realized on children, both by parents and by guardians (Rogers et al. 1976). In this context, toxicological analyses enable a diagnosis to be made and may also provide crucial evidence when legal protection is sought for the child.

Relevance to Active Management

There are few specific antidotes to poisons (Chapter 5) and the clinician is unlikely to delay their administration until his diagnosis is ratified by laboratory analyses. Poisoning with iron salts is an exception since the antidote, desferrioxamine, is a potentially toxic compound when given parenterally. In normal practice the antidote is given orally and parenteral administration is withheld until the serum iron concentration is measured. In severely intoxicated patients techniques designed to promote the elimination of the poison, such as forced diuresis, haemodialysis or charcoal haemoperfusion, may be considered (Chapter 8). Since these measures have limited application the clinician must obtain preliminary confirmation from the laboratory that a high concentration of a removable poison is present in the blood before proceeding with active treatment.

Collection of Specimens

The clinician should establish verbal contact with the laboratory, preferably with a senior analyst, before collecting and despatching any samples for analysis. By this means, the analyst is able to indicate the scope of the service available and, at the same time, give precise instructions as to the type and volume of samples required. Each sample should be placed in a separate container marked clearly with the patient's full name and the date and time of collection. A letter, or where provided a completed request form, legibly listing the name, hospital and telephone number of the clinician to be contacted with the results, should accompany the samples. It is the responsibility of the clinician to see that the samples are clearly and correctly addressed and to secure the most efficient and reliable means of transport.

Stomach Contents

After poison has been taken by mouth, vomit, gastric aspirate or lavage will contain, if collected soon enough, relatively large amounts of the poison and thus facilitate toxicological screening. Examination with the naked eye may reveal recognisable undegraded tablets or capsules and the trained analyst can discern the characteristic odours of compounds such as methyl salicylate and paraldehyde. Simple tests for detecting poisoning by iron salts, certain heavy metals (arsenic, antimony, bismuth and mercury), bromates, chlorates, nitrates and nitrites can only be applied to the stomach contents. For most purposes approximately 50 ml of sample will suffice.

Urine

Urine is far more amenable to toxicological screening than blood (see below) for three main reasons:

1. A greater volume of sample is normally available.

2. The concentration of the toxic agent is, with few exceptions, much higher in this specimen than in blood.

3. Urine often contains large amounts of drug metabolites which may be reconverted by chemical means to the parent drug or characterized separately.

Needless to say, when drugs have been self-administered intravenously, urine replaces stomach contents as the sample of choice for toxicological screening. An appropriate volume for analysis is 50 ml; this should be collected at the time of admission of the patient and preferably before the administration of any drugs as part of treatment. No preservative should be added to the sample.

Blood

Where there is little doubt as to the nature of the poison ingested the analyst will proceed to a quantitative analysis of the blood without delay. Conversely, if the diagnosis is unclear, blood samples will be reserved for future measurements once the poison has been characterized in either stomach contents or urine. This stems from the fact that most modern psychotropic drugs, in particular the tricyclic antidepressants, phenothiazines, benzodiazepines and opiate derivatives, are highly lipid-soluble and tend to be deposited predominantly in the extravascular tissues. Thus, even after acute overdose, the concentrations of these compounds in blood are so minute that they remain undetectable by simple test procedures. Comprehensive toxicological screening of blood samples is therefore feasible only in the specialized laboratory equipped with highly refined instruments.

A 10 ml sample of whole blood (preferably heparinized), or alternatively 5ml of plasma or serum, is adequate for most drug analyses. For toxic metal analyses the requirements are variable and the guidance of the analyst should be sought on every occasion.

Analytical Methods

Direct Tests on Stomach Contents and/or Urine

'Spot-tests' involve nothing more than the addition of one or two reagents to small samples of stomach contents or urine. Plate 50 illustrates the appearance of typical spot-tests. For a fuller account the reader should consult Meade et al. (1972).

Tests carried out on Sample Extracts

Direct testing of biological samples is limited to only a handful of toxic agents and, for the remainder, some means of purification away from the sample matrix is necessary before chemical characterization can be attempted. For drugs, which tend to be lipid-soluble, extraction into an organic solvent, e.g. petroleum spirit, diethyl ether or chloroform, is the most favoured procedure. Advantage is taken of the physicochemical characteristics of the compounds in order to achieve a preliminary separation. Thus, weak acids such as the barbiturates, which are predominantly unionized at an acid pH, are extracted from acidified samples. Conversely, weak bases such as the phenothiazines, tricyclic antidepressants and the opiate derivatives are extracted under alkaline conditions. The extract is then examined by one or more of the techniques described below.

Thin-layer Chromatography (TLC)

The extracts are evaporated to dryness and the residues reconstituted in a small volume (0.1 ml) of solvent. Aliquots of the concentrated extract are applied as a line of discrete spots to one end of a glass or plastic plate coated with a thin layer of silica. These spots are interspersed with small aliquots of authentic solutions of common drugs used as markers. The plate is then placed upright in a glass tank containing a small depth of a mixture of solvents. The solvent mixture soaks upwards into the silica layer, carrying with it, at varying speeds, the drugs and their metabolites. The rate of movement of the compounds is determined by their relative affinities for the silica and the solvent mixture and this in turn is dependent on their chemical structures. Thus, when the chromatographic process is terminated by removing the plate from the tank, the compounds are distributed as spots at varying distances from the base of the plate. The position of the drugs is made visible by spraying successive areas of the plate with a series of chemical reagents. The drugs are then identified on the basis of the colour produced and their positions relative to those of the authentic compounds. The appearance of a typical developed thin-layer chromatogram is shown in Plate 51.

Solvent extraction followed by thin-layer chromatographic analysis can be completed within two hours of receiving the samples. The technique is easy to perform, economical and extremely versatile since the order of separation of compounds can be altered simply by changing the nature of the developing solvent. However, interpretation of the plates can prove difficult and calls for a trained eye with considerable experience in recognising colours, spot shapes and metabolite patterns.

Ultraviolet Spectrophotometry

This technique relies on the principle that many drugs, when in solution, will absorb ultraviolet radiation. The degree of absorption depends on the chemical structure of the drug, its concentration in the solution and the wavelength of the ultraviolet light. The basic design of an ultraviolet spectrophotometer is shown in Figure 3.1. The monochromator can select from the light source an ultraviolet ray of any given wavelength ranging from 200 to 340 nm. The sample extract, usually transferred to an aqueous medium, is placed in a transparent quartz cuvette in the path of the radiation.

The amount of ultraviolet radiation which passes through the solution is measured by the photocell. Thus, by steady rotation of the monochromator it is possible to pass sequentially ultraviolet rays of all

wavelengths from 200 to 340 nm through the extract. The photocell monitors the amount of radiation absorbed at each wavelength and this is transcribed onto a recorder chart. The shape of the spectrum, the wavelength at which absorption is at a maximum and any changes brought about by changing the pH of the extract (see Figure 3.2) are all used as an aid to characterize the agent present.

Since the intensity of absorption is proportional to the concentration of the drug in the extract, the technique can be applied to the measurement of overdose levels in blood, particularly of the barbiturate drugs. A major drawback, however, is that this technique fails to distinguish which barbiturate is being measured. Since the concentrations at which different barbiturate drugs give rise to coma are variable (Table 3.1), this information is an essential factor in interpreting the results. In addition, the high incidence of multiple overdose can result in two or more drugs appearing in the same sample extract. In such a case, ultraviolet scanning can produce a composite spectrum of bewildering complexity from which neither qualitative nor quantitative information can be derived.

Table 3.1. **Plasma barbiturate concentrations associated with coma.**

Barbiturate	Plasma concentration range (mg/l)
Amylobarbitone	20—50
Barbitone	50—100
Butobarbitone	30—80
Pentobarbitone	20—50
Phenobarbitone	50—150
Quinalbarbitone	10—20

Figure 3.1. *Schematic representation of an ultraviolet spectrophotometer.*

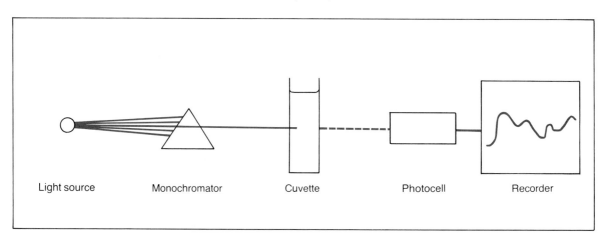

| Light source | Monochromator | Cuvette | Photocell | Recorder |

Gas–liquid Chromatography (GLC)

Gas–liquid chromatography has found great favour with analytical toxicologists since it offers a way of simultaneously separating, identifying and measuring drugs and other organic poisons. The basic design of the instrument is illustrated in Figure 3.3. A column is packed with inert granular material coated with a high boiling-point grease. This column is enclosed in an electrically heated oven which can be operated at varying temperatures up to 450°C. A stream of inert gas, usually nitrogen, is passed continually through the column in the direction indicated. The sample extract is injected, via a valve situated in the injection port, onto the column, and the drugs become partially vaporized and partially dissolved in the grease (or stationary phase). Vaporized drugs are swept along the column by the inert gas at a rate determined by their relative tendencies to dissolve in the stationary phase. Eventually the drugs emerge as discrete packages of vapour at the detector end. This is, of course, an oversimplified version of the mechanism of gas–liquid chromatographic separation.

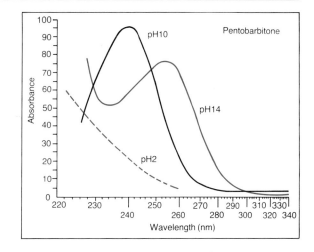

Figure 3.2. *Ultraviolet absorption spectra of a common barbiturate, pentobarbitone, at varying pH values.*

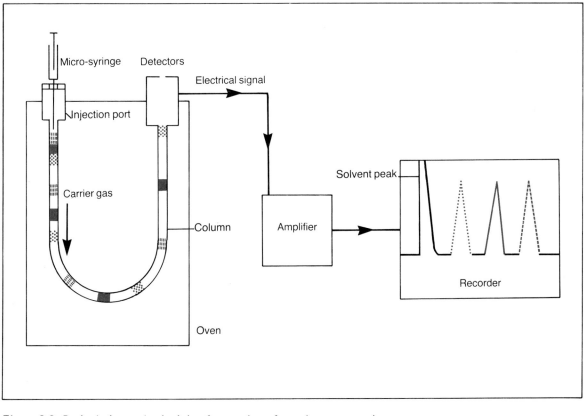

Figure 3.3. *Basic design and principle of operation of gas chromatograph.*

Nevertheless, the reader will appreciate that the major factors governing the achievement of rapid and clear cut separation of compounds are the length of the chromatographic column, the type and quantity of stationary phase, the oven temperature and the inert gas flow-rate.

The most common means of detecting the compounds is by flame-ionization. On leaving the column the inert gas is mixed with hydrogen, and either air or oxygen, and the mixture is ignited to give a continuous jet of flame. When any vaporized drug passes into the flame it is decomposed into electrically charged fragments which are collected at an electrode. This results in an electrical signal which is amplified and transmitted to a pen-recorder operating at a constant chart speed. Thus, a peak is transcribed each time a compound emerges from the column. A typical gas–liquid chromatogram is illustrated in Figure 3.4.

The use of more selective gas-chromatography detectors in toxicology laboratories has increased in recent years. Among these, the electron-capture detector, which is particularly sensitive towards halogen-containing compounds, has found wide application in the analysis of benzodiazepine drugs. The alkali-flame detector, more frequently referred to as the nitrogen detector, is highly selective for nitrogenous compounds and lends itself readily to the detection of nanogram or even picogram quantities of drugs.

The identification of compounds is based on the time they take to elute from the column following injection. This is represented on the recorder chart by the distance of the drug peak from the leading edge of the solvent peak which emerges almost immediately after injection. In practice, a compound (preferably not a drug) is incorporated into the sample extract and the elution times of any drug peaks are compared with that of this so-called internal standard.

Since the size of the drug peak can be related back to the concentration in the sample, GLC is preferably applied to blood samples, and the need to conserve the limited volume of blood available has stimulated the development of micro-extraction procedures requiring as little as 50 μl of plasma (Flanagan and Berry 1977). At present, this approach is feasible only for compounds which are readily detected in plasma by basic instrumentation, such as ethanol, methanol, barbiturates and related hypnotics. Certain benzodiazepine drugs also lend themselves to this type of plasma analysis with the aid of electron-capture detection and, in the foreseeable future, the alkali-flame (nitrogen) detector will widen still further the scope of direct plasma screening.

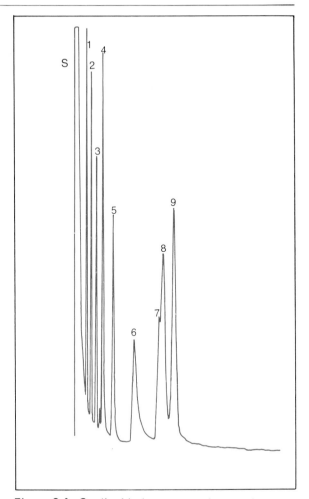

Figure 3.4. *Gas-liquid chromatograph recorder trace showing separation of various drugs and metabolites: s. solvent peak; 1. pethidine; 2. diphenhydramine; 3. methadone metabolite II; 4. methadone metabolite I; 5. methadone; 6. pentazocine; 7. codeine; 8. internal standard (tetraphenylethylene); 9. dipipanone.*

High Pressure Liquid Chromatography

High pressure liquid chromatography offers a means of separating compounds at high speeds by column chromatography. The eluting solvent is pumped against pressures of up to 5,000 psi through steel columns packed with chromatographic adsorbents, e.g. silica gel and alumina. The effluent stream passes through a detector, usually an ultraviolet spectrophotometer, and the appearance of a drug in the solvent is signalled by a recorder peak in a similar fashion to that described for GLC. Again, the size of the peak is proportional to the concentration of drug in the sample. Owing to its ability to chromatograph drugs which are non-volatile, and also polar compounds such as conjugated metabolites, it is envisaged that HPLC will eventually supplant GLC as the dominant technique in analytical toxicology.

Other Analytical Methods

Immunoassays

Radioimmunoassay. The underlying principle of radio-immunoassay is illustrated in Figure 3.5. Antibodies with a specific affinity for the drug are incubated with the sample to which a fixed quantity of radioactive drug has been added. Radioactive and cold drug compete for binding sites on the antibodies such that, at equilibrium, the relative amount of both forms bound is proportional to the concentration of cold drug in the sample. This is found by separating off the bound fraction and counting its radioactivity.

Radioimmunoassay has the inherent advantage of being able to measure with great precision substances present in concentrations so low that they defy the more conventional means of assay. Thus, compounds as diverse as cannabis, LSD, digoxin and paraquat can now be quantified in plasma.

Enzyme-Mediated Immunoassay Technique (EMIT)
The same principle of competitive binding of labelled and cold drug applies in the EMIT system (Figure 3.6). In its simplest form, i.e. for detecting drugs in urine, the marker drug is attached close to the active site of the enzyme lysozyme. A fixed quantity of this complex is incubated together with the sample, antibodies specific to the drug and a bacterial suspension. If the sample contains no drug, the antibodies bind to the enzyme-labelled drug, mask the active site of the enzyme and inactivate it. However, if drug is present, the antibodies are displaced from a proportion of the lysozyme–drug complex and the enzyme is free to degrade the bacterial suspension. This is detected by a decrease in the optical density of the solution over a fixed time interval. By modifying the type of enzyme and substrate used many drugs can now be

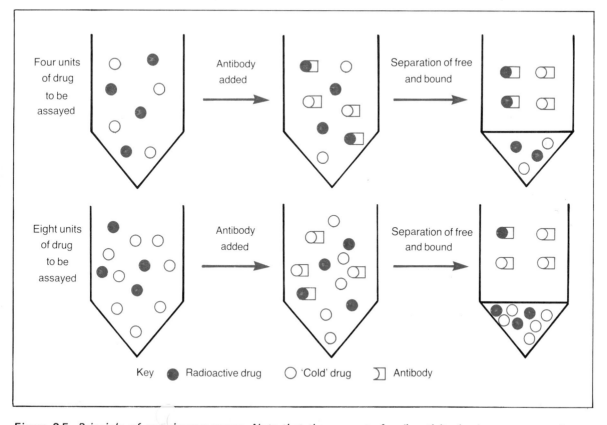

Figure 3.5. *Principle of radioimmunoassay. Note that the amount of radioactivity in the supernatant (bound fraction) is inversely proportional to the concentration of drug in the sample.*

measured in plasma by the EMIT system, and its analytical speed (approximately 1 sample per minute) makes it most suited to the handling of large batches of samples as, for example, in the monitoring of anticonvulsant therapy.

Atomic Absorption Spectrophotometry

This is the most convenient means of measuring toxic metals such as lead, mercury, cadmium and thallium. Briefly, the blood sample is introduced into a high-temperature oxyacetylene flame situated in the path of a beam of radiation. The organic matrix is combusted and the metal forms a cloud of atoms which absorbs a fraction of the radiation in proportion to the concentration of metal in the sample.

GLC-Mass-Spectrometry

GLC-mass-spectrometry is a hybrid technique which combines the chromatographic properties of GLC with the unchallenged power of characterization afforded by the mass-spectrometer. The prohibitive cost of such a system has tended to limit its availability to forensic toxicology laboratories, where the high financial outlay can be justified on the grounds that the absolute identification of a toxin may be vital evidence in a litigation procedure. With the emergence of silicon-chip technology, bringing in its wake simplification, reliability and cost deflation, it is conceivable that within a few years hospital toxicologists will no longer find this technique beyond their grasp.

Blood Assays

For reasons stated previously (see page 14), the measurement of toxic agents in blood is required in very few patients. The principal examples where this exercise can be of value are now described.

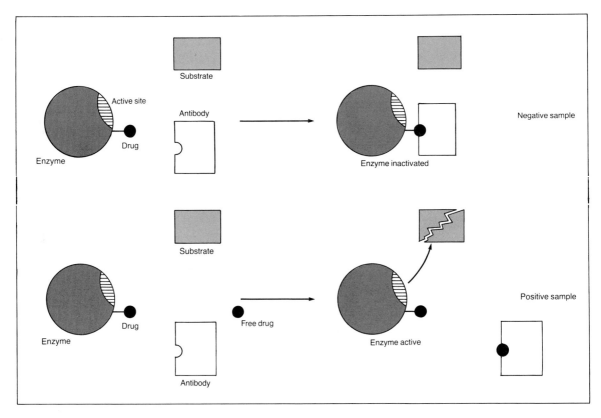

Figure 3.6. *Principle of the EMIT system.*

Salicylate

Salicylate is effectively removed by forced alkaline diuresis, but a plasma salicylate level is a prerequisite to instituting treatment. Ferric ion reagent is added to serum or plasma and the resulting purple colour is proportional to the salicylate concentration (Trinder 1954).

Paracetamol

The colorimetric method of Glyn and Kendal (1975) is adequate, although interference can arise if salicylate is also present in high concentration. The gas–liquid chromatographic method is therefore preferred. Although emergency plasma paracetamol levels are not mandatory prior to the administration of the antidotes methionine or N-acetylcysteine, they provide a useful guide to the severity of poisoning and prognosis, provided that more than four hours have elapsed since ingestion of the overdose.

Iron

The predominant victims of iron poisoning are young children who swallow pharmaceutical preparations of ferrous salts. In serious cases of iron poisoning the parenteral administration of desferrioxamine should be considered following urgent estimation of the serum iron concentration. Commercial kits based on colorimetric methods are available and these produce rapid and reliable results.

Alcohol

Ethanol is frequently taken as part of a drug 'cocktail' and can intensify the action of other depressant drugs. A blood ethanol determination conveniently distinguishes between this type of patient and the straightforward 'drunk'. In a similar fashion it provides useful information in an unconscious patient admitted with head injuries and smelling of drink. Casualty departments are now becoming equipped with devices (Alcolmeters) which give an immediate blood ethanol level by analysis of either expired air or of blood. In the laboratory, gas liquid chromatography is preferred since ethanol, methanol and other alcohols can be detected and measured with ease in a matter of minutes.

Barbiturates and Related Hypnotics

Although ultraviolet spectrophotometry is still widely used to measure barbiturate drugs, its limitations (see page 16) are profound, and gas–liquid chromatography is the method of choice (Flanagan and Berry 1977).

Paraquat

The herbicide paraquat is extremely toxic and active treatment should be instituted without delay in cases of paraquat poisoning. The measures currently advocated are drastic and a plasma paraquat measurement is a useful prognostic test which can prevent overtreatment of patients not at risk (Proudfoot et al. 1979). The most precise and sensitive method available at present is the radioimmunoassay devised by Levitt (1977).

Interpretation of Laboratory Findings

The range of toxicological tests varies enormously between laboratories and, in the event of receiving a negative result in a case where sound reasons for suspecting poisoning persist, the clinician should ascertain how far-reaching the screen has been. If the case merits a wider search for the causative agent and the local laboratory is unable to help, the aid of a specialized laboratory should be sought. It must be realised, however, that even in the most advanced laboratory no toxicological scheme of analysis is completely comprehensive.

By the same token, positive findings must be interpreted with caution. Qualitative tests can be so sensitive that they fail to distinguish between therapeutic and toxic ingestion. For example, the simple test for paracetamol will yield a clear positive in the urine for up to 24 hours after consuming one tablet of the drug. Thus, a diagnosis of poisoning might erroneously be ascribed to a patient who has taken legitimate amounts of one or more drugs and who is, in fact, a victim of organic disease. This emphasizes the value of obtaining a blood concentration measurement, where possible, for any toxic agent detected.

It is now rare to encounter patients who have ingested a single drug in overdose and the clinician should be aware that the inexperienced analyst may achieve a positive result for one of his tests and discontinue the search prematurely. This occurred, for example, in the case of a deeply unconscious patient on whom a report of moderately toxic blood concentrations of alcohol and barbiturates was returned. Unexpectedly the patient deteriorated and resuscitative measures failed. Subsequent post-mortem analysis revealed the presence of paracetamol together with an overwhelming concentration of dextropropoxyphene in the blood. It could be surmized that the outcome would have been different if the opiate antagonist, naloxone, had been administered.

A guide to the interpretation of toxicological data is given in Table 3.2. However, these figures should not be regarded as inviolable since the tolerance of individual patients to toxic ingestion is determined by factors such as previous exposure, age and state of health. Thus, a young woman presented in grade II coma with shallow respiration and normal blood pressure; her plasma at this time contained amylobarbitone at a concentration of 30 mg/l and she recovered uneventfully. In contrast, an elderly man, described as a respiratory invalid of long-standing, became hypoxic and died with a plasma amylobarbitone concentration of only 20 mg/l. The issue is further complicated when several drugs are present and synergism exists, the combined effect of the drugs being more pronounced than that due to their independent activities. The concomitant ingestion of alcohol with benzodiazepine sedatives is an increasingly common example of synergism.

Prediction of the clinical course of a drug-intoxicated patient cannot be based categorically on a single blood concentration measurement.

Table 3.2. Interpretation of toxicological data. This guide is based on data derived from the Poisons Unit at Guy's Hospital, London, and from reliable literature sources. The concentrations quoted here are approximate and take no account of factors cited in the text which may modify the individual patient's response. Particular discretion should be exercised when interpreting results in cases of multiple ingestion.

[1] All concentrations are expressed in terms of mg/l of plasma except where otherwise stated.

Classification	Therapeutic or normal levels — less than [1]	Levels associated with severe toxicity[1]
Alcohols		
Ethanol	—	3.00 g/l
Methanol	—	0.20 g/l
Analgesics		
Narcotics		
Dextropropoxyphene	0.30	1.00
Codeine	0.10	1.00
Methadone	0.10	1.00
Morphine	0.05	0.30
Pentazocine	0.20	1.00
Pethidine	0.50	2.00
Non-narcotics		
Paracetamol	20.00	200.00 (4 hours post ingestion) 70.00 (12 hours post ingestion)
Salicylate	250.00	500.00
Anticonvulsants		
Carbamazepine	10.00	50.00
Clonazepam	0.05	1.00
Ethosuximide	80.00	—
Phenytoin	20.00	40.00
Primidone	12.00	100.00
Sulthiame	12.00	30.00
Sodium valproate	80.00	—

Antidepressants

Amitriptyline (plus nortriptyline)	0.20	1.00
Clomipramine (plus norclomipramine)	0.50	1.00
Dothiepin (plus nordothiepin)	0.30	1.00
Doxepin (plus nordoxepin)	0.20	1.00
Imipramine (plus desipramine)	0.30	1.00
Mianserin	0.10	0.50
Nortriptyline	0.15	1.00
Protriptyline	0.20	1.00
Trimipramine (plus nortrimipramine)	0.30	1.00

Antihypertensives

Oxprenolol	0.20	2.00
Propranolol	0.10	2.00

Anti-inflammatories

Oxyphenylbutazone	100.00	200.00
Phenylbutazone	100.00	200.00

Antimalarials

Chloroquine	0.20	1.00
Quinine/Quinidine	5.00	10.00

Cardioactive

Digoxin	2.00	4.00
Disopyramide	3.00	8.00
Lignocaine	5.00	8.00
Mexiletine	1.50	3.00
Procainamide	8.00	16.00
Quinidine	5.00	10.00

Hypnotics

Barbiturates

Butobarbitone	10.00	80.00
Barbitone	15.00	100.00
Phenobarbitone	30.00	100.00
Other barbiturates	5.00	40.00

Non-barbiturates

Chlormethiazole	2.00	10.00 (oral dose)
Ethchlorvynol	20.00	100.00
Glutethimide	4.00	30.00
Meprobamate	10.00	40.00
Methaqualone	4.00	20.00
Trichlorethanol	10.00	50.00

Stimulants

Amphetamine	0.10	0.50
Methylamphetamine	0.05	0.30
Fenfluramine	0.20	0.50
Cocaine	0.30	3.00

Classification	Therapeutic or normal levels — less than [1]	Levels associated with severe toxicity[1]
Tranquillizers		
Benzodiazepines		
Chlordiazepoxide	1.00	5.00
Diazepam	1.00	5.00
Nordiazepam	1.50	5.00
Flunitrazepam	0.05	—
Desalkylflurazepam	0.15	0.50
Lorazepam	0.20	—
Nitrazepam	0.20	2.00
Oxazepam	1.00	5.00
Phenothiazines		
Chlorpromazine	0.10	1.00
Thioridazine	1.00	5.00
Miscellaneous		
Bromide	14.00	200.00
Dinitro-orthocresol	5.00	50.00
Ethylene glycol	—	500.00
Haloperidol	0.10	0.50
Orphenadrine	0.20	2.00
Paraquat	—	0.50 (6 hours post ingestion)
		0.25 (12 hours post ingestion)
Theophylline	20.00	40.00

Metal	Sample	Normal levels — less than [2]	Levels indicating abnormal exposure[2]
Arsenic	Blood	30.00	50.00
	Serum/plasma	20.00	50.00
	Urine	40.00	200.00
	Hair and nail	1.00	2.00
Cadmium	Blood	10.00	20.00
	Urine	10.00	20.00
Iron	Serum	1.80 mg/l	5.00 mg/l (children)
			8.00 mg/l (adults)
Lead	Blood	1.50 μmol/l (children)	4.00 μmol/l (children)
		2.00 μmol/l (adults)	5.00 μmol/l (adults)
Lithium	Serum	1.30 mmol/l	2.00 mmol/l
Mercury	Blood	15.00	40.00
	Urine	20.00	100.00
Thallium	Blood	10.00	50.00
	Urine	20.00	200.00

[2] All concentrations are expressed in terms of μg/l except where otherwise stated.

Pharmacokinetic data, e.g. plasma drug half-lives, are often derived from experimental studies in volunteers receiving single low doses. Rigid extrapolation of these data to situations where massive overdose has occurred is likely to be unrewarding since complete absorption of the drug may take many hours. The presence of other drugs which inhibit gastric emptying will serve to exacerbate delayed absorption. Serial blood concentration measurements in a deteriorating patient can prove enlightening in this context. Severely intoxicated patients presenting late after overdose are unlikely to have maintained their normal liver and renal capacities for detoxification and excretion of drugs. Again, this will mitigate the application of standard pharmacokinetic data. Patients who have been chronically exposed to stimulants of liver microsomal enzymes, e.g. alcohol and barbiturates, are particularly at risk from acute dosage with liver poisons, such as paracetamol and carbon tetrachloride, whose toxicity is mediated by metabolites.

Conclusion

From the foregoing, it is clear that toxicological investigations can be complex and far from economical in terms of time, reagents and equipment. Nevertheless, there is an unfortunate supposition on the part of many clinicians that a laboratory service exists to be used, irrespective of whether the findings will have any conceivable bearing on patient management. Nowhere is this more prevalent than in clinical toxicology, and in the specialized laboratories it has become imperative to guard against such abuse, particularly when an out-of-hours facility is provided. Protection is best contrived by interposing a clinical toxicologist (or suitable equivalent) between the laboratory staff and the clinician seeking assistance. In the author's experience this manoeuvre leads to the rejection of 9 out of 10 so-called 'urgent' requests, and thus reserves time for a concentrated and sustained investigation in cases where analytical data are essential. However, it should not be inferred from this that non-urgent samples are without value. On the contrary, careful examination of such material at leisure can be rewarding, perhaps not in an immediate sense, but certainly in the context of deriving information on the disposition, metabolism and excretion of drugs and poisons in man. Without accumulating data of this kind it is doubtful whether the treatment of poisoning will advance beyond the simple concept, albeit a worthy one, of maintaining the vital functions.

References

Conference of Medical Royal Colleges and their Faculties. Diagnosis of brain death. Br Med J 1976; 2:1187–8.

Flanagan RJ, Berry DJ. Routine analysis of barbiturates and some other hypnotic drugs in the blood plasma as an aid to the diagnosis of acute poisoning. J Chromatogr 1977; 131: 131–46.

Glynn JP, Kendal SE. Paracetamol measurement. Lancet 1975; i:1147–8.

Helliwell M, Hampel G, Sinclair E, Huggett A, Flanagan RJ. Value of emergency toxicological investigations in the differential diagnosis of coma. Br Med J 1979; 2:819–21.

Levitt T. Radioimmunoassay for paraquat. Lancet 1977; ii:358.

Meade BW, Widdop B, Blackmore DJ, Brown SS, Curry AS, Goulding R, et al. Simple tests to detect poisons. Ann Clin Biochem 1972; 9:35–46.

Newton RW. The clinician's requirements from the laboratory in the treatment of acutely poisoned patient. In: The Poisoned Patient: the Role of the Laboratory. Amsterdam: Associated Scientific Publications, 1974. Symposium 26 (new series):5–11.

Proudfoot AT, Stewart MJ, Levitt T, Widdop B. Paraquat poisoning: the significance of plasma paraquat concentrations. Lancet 1979; ii:330–2.

Rogers D. Tripp J, Bentovim A, Robinson A, Berry DJ, Goulding R. Non-accidental poisoning: an extended syndrome of child abuse. Br Med J 1976; 1:793–6.

Trinder P. Rapid determination of salicylate in biological fluids. Biochem J 1954; 57:301–3.

Further Reading

Baselt RC. Disposition of Toxic Drugs and Chemicals in Man. Vols 1 & 2. Davis, California: Biomedical Publications, 1978.

Clarke ECG (Ed). Isolation and Identification of Drugs. London: Pharmaceutical Press, 1969.

Curry AS. Advances in Forensic and Clinical Toxicology. Cleveland Ohio: CRC Press, 1972.

Curry AS. Poison Detection in Human Organs. Springfield, Illinois: Charles C. Thomas, 1976. 3rd edition.

Goulding R, Widdop B. Laboratory toxicology in the district general hospital. In: Recent Advances in Chemical Pathology. Ed. Dyke SC. Edinburgh: Churchill Livingstone, 1973: 61–72.

Porter R, O'Connor M (Eds). The Poisoned Patient: the Role of the Laboratory. Amsterdam: Associated Scientific Publications, 1974. Ciba Foundation Symposium 26 (new series).

Widdop B, Braithwaite RA. Analytical methods in clinical toxicology. Proc Eur Soc Toxicol XVIII. Amsterdam–Oxford: Excerpta Medica. 1977; 50–63.

Chapter 4

G.N. Volans

General Principles of Treatment

A review of the treatment of acute poisoning must take account of changes in the incidence of different types of poisoning, changes which in turn reflect alterations in drug prescribing, alterations in the chemicals in domestic use and the effects of publicity or fashion. Over the last decade in Great Britain barbiturate poisoning has become less frequent and its place has been taken by poisoning due to psychotropic agents such as the benzodiazepines and antidepressants. Analgesic poisoning is still common though, in the UK at least, paracetamol (acetaminophen) is now ingested as commonly as aspirin. Publicity has probably played a major role in the increased incidence of paraquat poisoning in Britain and fashion has led to widespread abuse of solvents ('sniffing').

Although some poisons require specific treatment, when all forms of acute poisoning are considered together a common pattern of basic management emerges and it is this which will be discussed in this chapter. It is logical, then, to consider the general principles of treatment in the sequence in which they should be applied.

General Principles of Treatment

To Admit or Not?

Any chemical substance is potentially a lethal poison as has been clearly demonstrated by deaths due to sodium chloride (see page 30). Nevertheless, most substances are unlikely to cause serious toxicity, at least in the amounts and in the form usually ingested. Examples of this can be seen in the ingestion of most so-called poisonous plants by children. Although the plant may contain a highly toxic chemical it is unlikely that serious poisoning will occur, either because the amount of the plant ingested is too small or because the toxin is contained within a seed which will be excreted undigested, e.g. yew berries.

Given that there is a wide variation in the inherent toxicity of chemicals it is obvious that some patients will be at serious risk of acute poisoning whilst others are at no risk at all. Therefore, it makes economic sense to avoid hospital admission for the latter. But how can the admitting doctor be expected to have a practical knowledge of the entire range of potential poisons? The answer is that he should have available for reference up-to-date information on the treatment of common acute poisonings (as provided in this book) whilst for the uncommon poisons he should be prepared to telephone one of the poisons information centres (Table 4.1) where information on toxicity,

Table 4.1 Telephone numbers of the National Poisons Information Service centres in the UK[1]

Belfast	0232 40503
Cardiff	0222 492233
Dublin	0001 745588
Edinburgh	031 229 2477
London	01 407 7600

[1] These centres share a common data base and operate 24 hours a day. In most instances the information is given by non-medical personnel, but in all cases a medical opinion is available. An analytical service is offered by the London and Edinburgh centres where patients may also be transferred for specialized treatment.

symptoms and treatment is readily available. With this backing it should be possible to determine with certainty those cases at risk of poisoning.

In children, most cases of poisoning are accidental and the majority are at no risk. They can, therefore, safely be allowed home provided the child is asymptomatic and the parents are considered responsible and capable of reporting back if any symptoms develop. Similarly accidental poisoning in adults is seldom serious and rarely requires admission. However, the same cannot be said of deliberate poisoning in adults, for in these cases the event is usually some form of 'cry for help' which should be considered in detail so that, where appropriate, social or psychiatric support can be offered in addition to any physical measures that may be required.

Proper consideration of the need for admission can save a great deal of time and money, but it is important to remember the two circumstances under which the asymptomatic patient should be admitted: first, when the onset of the symptoms of acute poisoning may be delayed for several hours (as with paracetamol and certain delayed-release drug formulations); second, to document the clinical course of patients who have ingested agents about which little is known. This will not only be in the patient's own interest but, in addition, the information gained from such cases can be made available to other clinicians.

Poisons Information Services (see Chapter 2) have an important role in the dissemination of new knowledge. To this end, a doctor who calls the Information Service in Great Britain may well receive a request for details of the treatment and the outcome of the case for which information was sought. In this way the dangers of some new drugs (e.g. disopyramide) and the safety of others (e.g. cimetidine) in acute overdosage can be established soon after the drug is marketed. The cooperation of all doctors in supplying these details is therefore essential if the Poisons Information Service is to be used to its best advantage.

Among those poisoned patients who need admission the majority will recover with no more than good supportive therapy, which varies from simple first aid to full intensive care. The more active treatments for acute poisoning naturally appeal to the doctor who wishes to feel that he is really 'doing something' for his patient. However, no procedure, even the simplest, is completely free from risk and with active treatment complications can easily outweigh the risks from poisoning. The justification for a conservative approach is easily demonstrated by the fact that in the UK only 810 patients died in hospital from acute poisoning during 1977 — a mortality of approximately 0.6 per cent.

Supportive Therapy

Respiratory Function

Respiratory function is often impaired in acute poisoning and requires immediate attention. The comatose patient is liable to obstruction of the windpipe by the tongue falling back, an event which can be prevented in the first instance by holding the jaw forward and turning the patient into the semiprone position. An oropharyngeal airway should be inserted as soon as is practical and, at this stage, it is important to consider whether ventilation is adequate. Most poisons which impair consciousness also depress respiration, a fact that may not be very obvious if the rate is normal while the depth is inadequate. It is therefore useful to measure the tidal volume and minute volume. Arterial blood gases should also be measured in all patients in grade IV coma (Table 4.2).

Apart from the CNS depressant action of the poison, respiratory function is also at risk from inhaled vomit, another reason for maintaining the semiprone, head-down position. Further risk of aspiration occurs during gastric lavage and in unconscious patients or those with respiratory depression no attempt at passing a stomach tube should be made until a cuffed endotracheal tube is in place. Oxygen should be given when indicated clinically, and especially in poisoning from carbon monoxide or irritant gases. However, oxygen is no substitute for adequate ventilation, and mechanical ventilation, if necessary, should not be delayed.

Respiratory stimulants are never indicated and are potentially dangerous. The respiratory complications of acute poisoning are discussed more fully in Chapter 7.

Shock

In acute poisoning, shock is due to expansion of the venous capacitance bed causing a relative or absolute deficiency of intravascular volume. In acute poisoning the younger patients are generally not at risk of brain or kidney damage as long as the systolic blood pressure is greater than 80 mm Hg, but in the elderly a systolic

---

Table 4.2 Grades of coma.

I	Drowsy but responds to commands
II	Unconscious but responds to minimal stimuli
III	Unconscious and responds only to maximal painful stimuli
IV	Unconscious and no response whatsoever

pressure of less than 90 mm Hg should be regarded as serious. Restoration of the blood pressure should first be attempted by means of the head-down position and the use of plasma expanders. Since the problem is usually one of increased vascular capacity, colloids (human serum albumin or hydroxyethyl starches) are more appropriate than crystalloids (dextrose and isosmolar sodium salts).

Vasoconstrictors (e.g. metaraminol and noradrenaline) are no longer recommended in acute poisoning since, in most instances, the peripheral resistance is already increased. They have little effect on the blood pressure and they do tend to decrease the blood supply to vital organs. In a few instances the newer positive inotropes, dopamine or dobutamine, may be indicated as long as fluid depletion has been adequately corrected. Of these, dopamine is perhaps to be preferred since it does not reduce renal blood flow (Editorial *British Medical Journal*, 1977).

Hypothermia

This is a common complication of acute poisoning, especially when there has been some delay before the patient is discovered. It is best treated by gradual warming in a warm moist atmosphere ($27-29°C$) with the addition of a "space blanket" to minimize heat loss.

Convulsions

These can be controlled by intravenous diazepam or intramuscular paraldehyde. However, it must be noted that these drugs further depress respiration.

Cardiac Arrhythmias

Cardiac arrhythmias in acute poisoning, e.g. with the tricyclic antidepressants, commonly respond to correction of hypoxia or acidosis. Drug therapy should be considered only in persistent, life-threatening arrhythmias since it should be remembered that the antiarrhythmic drugs may also depress myocardial function in their own right.

Gastric Aspiration and Lavage, and Emesis

If an ingested poison can be removed from the stomach before absorption takes place, the risk of poisoning can be prevented, or at least reduced. Two procedures are commonly used, namely gastric aspira-

tion and lavage, and emesis. The former is generally only practicable in hospital and is used mainly in adults. The latter is often first used before admission and may have been initiated by parents, 'first-aiders' or general practitioners. Properly used, both can be very effective but each has its own hazards and it is important to be aware of their limitations.

Gastric Aspiration and Lavage

This procedure (Table 4.3) is widely practised in accident and emergency departments and, indeed, it has been suggested that it may be over used, at least in part because of the mistaken belief that it will provide an unpleasant experience which will prevent recurrent, deliberate self-poisoning. There is no evidence to support this view, and a recent survey has suggested that at least 50 per cent of patients are being subjected to unnecessary gastric lavage (Blake and Bramble 1978). Although this report probably overstates the case (Needham 1979), there is no doubt that many of the drugs now taken in overdose are less toxic than many of those taken formerly, e.g. barbiturates.

The indications and contraindications for gastric aspiration and lavage are shown in Table 4.4. Lavage has the advantage over emesis that it can be used in the unconscious patient (providing that a cuffed endotracheal tube is in position). It can also be employed cautiously when corrosives have been ingested if there is a serious risk of corrosion lower down the GI tract, or if the risk of systemic poisoning outweighs the risk of perforation of the gut, usually

---

Table 4.3   Procedure for gastric aspiration and lavage.

1. Place the head of the patient over the end or side of the bed so that the mouth and throat are at a level lower than the larynx and trachea. (Figure 4.1)

2. Use a wide-bore tube (Jacques gauge 30) lubricated with vaseline or glycerine. In the adult, 50 cm will reach the stomach. Make sure that the tube is not in the trachea.

3. Aspirate first, then use 300 ml water for the first washing. Repeat this process at least 3 or 4 times using 300–600 ml on each occasion. Save all washings in case needed for analysis.

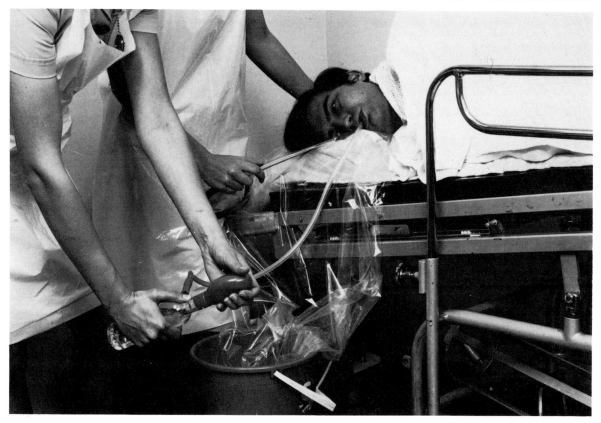

Figure 4.1. *Procedure for gastric lavage.*

the oesophagus, e.g. after ingestion of concentrated paraquat solutions. It must not be used when volatile petroleum distillates have been ingested since there is considerable risk of aspiration into the lungs and subsequent pneumonitis.

If applied correctly, clinically significant amounts of poison can be removed by gastric aspiration and lavage, but it must be noted that even in the most experienced hands there remains the risk of perforation of the oesophagus and aspiration pneumonia (Matthew et al. 1966).

At best, this technique is somewhat traumatic for both patient and staff when applied to adults. In children, however, it is little short of barbaric and it should be used only when absolutely necessary. Emesis is to be preferred in children and it has recently been suggested that emesis may be more widely applicable to adults.

Emesis

Five methods of inducing emesis merit consideration: pharyngeal stimulation, sodium chloride, copper sulphate, apomorphine and syrup of ipecacuanha.

Pharyngeal stimulation. Stimulation of the pharynx with the fingers appears to be a safe procedure in children but its efficacy is low as shown in one study where only four out of 30 children were induced to vomit by this method. When given ipecacuanha, all 30 vomited, and even the four who were successfully treated by pharyngeal stimulation vomited larger amounts (Dabbous et al. 1965). Stimulation of the pharynx is recommended for use in children outside hospital, but ipecacuanha should still be given, if indicated (Table 4.4), once the patient is in the accident and emergency department.

Table 4.4.   The correct use of gastric aspiration and lavage or emesis.

Aspiration and lavage	*Emesis*
Indications	*Indications*
1. A potentially toxic dose of poison has been ingested.	1. A potentially toxic dose of poison has been ingested.
2. Treatment can be given within four hours of ingestion (longer for salicylates and anticholinergic drugs including tricyclic antidepressants).	2. Treatment can be given within four hours of ingestion (longer for salicylates and anticholinergic drugs including tricyclic antidepressants).
3. Patient unconscious and time of ingestion not known.	
4. Cautious use if danger of systemic toxicity from corrosives, e.g. concentrated paraquat solutions or formic acid.	
Contraindications	*Contraindications*
1. Poisoning due to petroleum distillates.	1. Poisoning due to petroleum distillates.
	2. Poisoning due to anti-emetics.
	3. Poisoning due to corrosives.
	4. Impairment of consciousness.

Sodium chloride. Sodium chloride has been widely used as an emetic, but its efficacy is low and its toxicity is high. Table 4.5 lists cases where death occurred due to hypernatraemia because an excessive dose of salt was given, either at the outset or because vomiting did not occur. It can also be seen that in each case there was little risk of death from the original overdose. In view of these findings, several organizations in the UK, including the DHSS, the Chemical Industries Association and the St John's Ambulance Brigade, have made firm recommendations that the use of salt as an emetic can no longer be advised. It is likely, however, that some misinformed parents and manufacturers will continue to recommend saline emetics and it is important that a hospital doctor meeting such a case takes steps to prevent its recurrence.

Copper sulphate. The oral administration of this substance carries a risk of absorption of toxic amounts of copper and cannot be recommended.

Apomorphine. Subcutaneous or intramuscular apomorphine may cause CNS depression, and therefore is best avoided since many poisons have a similar effect.

Syrup of ipecacuanha. Syrup of ipecacuanha is the emetic of choice although its safety, efficacy and proper use needs fuller discussion.

Ipecacuanha contains several alkaloids including cephaeline and emetine (methylcephaeline) which are the active ingredients. Ipecacuanha was once used for the treatment of amoebiasis (emetine is still given, although it is cardiotoxic and is being replaced by newer, safer agents). Both cephaeline and emetine irritate the GI tract, stimulate the medullary vomiting centre and, in large doses, cause CNS depression. Ipecacuanha's safety in clinical use as an emetic derives from the small doses used and the limited time for absorption before emesis occurs.

Only one death has been recorded where syrup of ipecacuanha is thought to have been a contributing factor. In this instance a 14-month-old child was treated after chewing the leaves of an 'amaryllis plant' and died 48 hours later after repeated vomiting. Postmortem examination revealed herniation of the stomach into the chest through a congenital defect of the diaphragm (Robertson 1979). Since such defects are extremely rare and since the amaryllis could have caused the vomiting in its own right, this case does not seem to suggest a need to reconsider the use of ipecacuanha. Deaths have occurred after the accidental use of the fluid extract of ipecacuanha (which is 14 times the strength of the syrup) but that formulation is no longer normally dispensed and the problem should not arise again.

Severe, but non-fatal, CNS depression due to syrup of ipecacuanha has been described in a 23-month-old

Table 4.5. **Deaths due to the use of a saline emetic.**[1]

Age (years)	Overdose	Maximum plasma sodium (mmol/l)	Risk from overdose
74	Perphenazine Imipramine	174	Slight
35	Thioridazine	184	Slight
2	Dextropropoxyphene	189	Dextropropoxyphene not detected
23	Chlordiazepoxide	214	Slight
3	Acetylsalicylic acid	186	Plasma salicylate 270 mg/l
26	Anadin (a proprietary preparation of acetyl salicylic acid)	172	Plasma salicylate 171 mg/l
35	Acetylsalicylic acid.	200	Plasma salicylate 540 mg/l
21	Amitriptyline Chlorpromazine Diazepam Nitrazepam	227	Slight

[1] Reproduced by permission of the Editor, *Proceedings of the Royal Society of Medicine* (Goulding and Volans, 1977).

child who was given three to six times the normal dose for treatment of an anti-emetic overdose. The toxicity in this case is, of course, not unexpected and it is generally stated that all emetics are contraindicated in anti-emetic overdosage (Table 4.4). This latter statement has, however, been challenged recently in a report where ipecacuanha in normal dosage was effective in inducing emesis in 60 out of 63 cases of anti-emetic overdose (4 children, 56 adults), a result comparable to that achieved by the same authors when treating overdosage of drugs without anti-emetic properties (Manoguerra and Krenzelok 1978). However, the authors had no objective evidence that the anti-emetics had actually been ingested, i.e. detection of the drugs in vomitus, urine or plasma, and their claims are based solely on the history given by the patients. Since there are numerous reports which indicate that the history given in drug overdosage is often unreliable, more evidence is needed before a complete change is indicated in the policy for usage of syrup of ipecacuanha. Nevertheless, this report does suggest that anti-emetic overdosage may not be a total contraindication to the use of emetics. There is probably a complex dose–response relationship between the effects of the two drugs such that either action could prevail according to the levels achieved. For the moment, therefore, it may be reasonable to give the normal dose of syrup of ipecacuanha for an anti-emetic overdose but, if emesis does not occur, larger doses should not be given and lavage should be used.

Several studies have documented the efficacy of syrup of ipecacuanha as an emetic in children and it is generally agreed that the regime described in Table 4.6 will be effective in 95 to 100 per cent of cases. In adults there has been little information on the use of ipecacuanha, but recent reports have demonstrated that its efficacy is undiminished (Ilett et al. 1977; Manoguerra and Krenzelok 1978). Therefore, it seems reasonable to consider syrup of ipecacuanha for use in adults as an alternative to lavage, providing that the criteria in Table 4.4 are satisfied.

Oral Adsorbents

If a poison cannot be removed completely from the stomach by lavage or emesis there is still the possibility that an orally administered adsorbent could prevent its absorption into the blood stream. A number of substances have been recommended as general adsor-

Table 4.6. 'Syrup of ipecacuanha' dosage.

Ipecacuanha paediatric emetic draught BPC or ipecacuanha syrup (Adelaide Children's Hospital formula)

Six to eighteen months	10 ml
Older children	15 ml
Adults	30 ml

The syrup should be taken with a glass of water or fruit juice. The dose may be repeated after 20 minutes if emesis has not occurred.

bents for poisons, but currently only one, activated charcoal, merits consideration.

'Activated' charcoal consists of fine particles of low mineral content which meet British Pharmacopoeia specifications for adsorbence. Its capacity of adsorption in vitro is undeniable, but in acute poisoning in vivo its efficacy is difficult to demonstrate. In general, however, it is considered to be safe and cheap and has been recommended for a wide range of acute poisoning. It is therefore surprising that, until recently, supplies of activated charcoal for use as a poison adsorbent were not readily available and it appears to have been used infrequently in the UK.

The introduction of a new, effervescent, activated charcoal (Medicoal) has therefore stimulated a fresh interest in this treatment and its indications (Editorial, *Drug and Therapeutics Bulletin*, 1979). The following points are important:

1. Activated charcoal is an adjunct to emesis or lavage and it in no way replaces them.
2. The charcoal strongly adsorbs ipecacuanha and theoretically, certain oral 'antidotes', e.g. methionine, and it should not be given with these drugs, or at least its administration should be delayed until the ipecacuanha has been effective.
3. It is known that in order to achieve a significant reduction in absorption of the poison, charcoal must be given in a dose 5 to 10 times the estimated weight of poison.

Activated charcoal, therefore, is most likely to prove useful where small amounts of the poison produce large effects, thus: one 10 g dose of activated charcoal might adsorb forty 25 mg amitriptyline tablets but only two 500 mg paracetamol tablets. Large doses (50–100 g) of charcoal have therefore been recommended for some forms of poisoning — a recommendation made without consideration of the fact that charcoal is unpalatable and likely to be vomited back. Doses of 5 to 10 g of Medicoal are more likely to be

tolerated and should be given in a glass of water in cases where a useful amount of the poison is likely to be adsorbed. Such a situation will most commonly apply in the treatment of antidepressant overdosage but could arise with many less common overdoses of potent drugs, e.g. theophylline, phenothiazines and antihistamines.

Conclusion

In spite of the enormous number of hospital referrals for acute poisoning, many patients are at no risk and the great majority of the remainder can be successfully treated according to a general supportive policy. Advice on the risks and treatment of the less common poisons is available from the poisons information services or centres. This chapter discusses the general principles of treatment, notably the indications for hospital admission and for the use of gastric aspiration and lavage and oral activated charcoal.

References

Blake DR, Bramble MG, Evans JG. Is there excessive use of gastric lavage in the treatment of self-poisoning? Lancet 1978; ii:1362–4.

Dabbous IA, Bergman AB, Robertson WO. The ineffectiveness of mechanically induced vomiting. J Paediatr 1965; 66:952–4.

Editorial. Medicoal (effervescent activated charcoal) in the treatment of acute poisoning. Drug Ther Bull 1979; 17:2;7–8.

Editorial Dopamine in cardiac failure and shock. Br Med J 1977; 2:1563–4.

Goulding R, Volans GN. Emergency treatment of common poisons: emptying the stomach. Proc Roy Soc Med 1977; 70:766–70.

Ilett KF, Gibb SM, Unsworth RW. Syrup of ipecacuanha as an emetic in adults. Med J Aust 1977; 2:91–3.

Manoguerra AS, Krenzelok EP. Rapid emesis from high dose ipecacuanha syrup in adults and children intoxicated with antiemetics or other drugs. Am J Hosp Pharm 1978; 35: 1360–2.

Matthew H, Mackintosh TF, Tompsett SL, Cameron JC. Gastric aspiration and lavage in acute poisoning. Br Med J 1966; 1:1333–7.

Needham CD. Letter: gastric lavage for self-poisoning. Lancet 1979; i:113.

Robertson WO. Syrup of ipecacuanha associated fatality: a case report. Vet Hum Toxicol 1979; 21:87–9.

Further Reading

Clemmesen C, Nilsson E. Therapeutic trends in the treatment of barbiturate poisoning. The Scandinavian method. Clin Pharmacol Ther 1961; 2:220–9.

Driesbach RH. Handbook of Poisoning. Los Altos, California: Lange Medical Publications, 1980, 10th edition.

Matthew H, Lawson AAH. Treatment of Common Acute Poisonings. Churchill Livingstone: Edinburgh, 1979; 4th edition.

Chapter 5

T. J. Meredith and J. A. Vale

Antidotes

Supportive care is all that is required for the majority of acutely poisoned patients admitted to hospital (see Chapter 4). Specific antidotes are rarely necessary and there are few available, although in appropriate circumstances the administration of an antidote may sometimes be life-saving.

Antidotes may work in any one of a number of ways and their mechanisms of action are illustrated diagrammatically in Figure 5.1. An antidote may:

1. Interact with a poison to form an inert complex which is then subsequently excreted from the body.

2. Accelerate detoxification of a poison.

3. Reduce the rate of conversion of a poison to a more toxic compound.

4. Compete with toxic substances for essential receptor sites.

5. Block receptors through which the toxic effects of a poison are mediated.

6. By-pass the effect of a poison on the body.

Each mechanism of antidotal action will be considered in turn and the use of clinically important antidotes will be described (Table 5.1).

Inert Complex Formation

Chelating agents used in heavy metal poisoning (see Chapters 26, 27, 28) provide the best example of this form of antidotal action. The chelation of a substance usually involves the formation of a complex with a

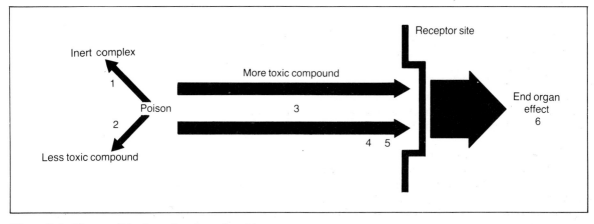

Figure 5.1. *The possible sites of action of antidotes.*

five- or six-membered ring. The incorporation of a sulphide bond in such a ring confers great stability on the chelation complex.

Dimercaprol

Dimercaprol is used in the treatment of *arsenic, mercury and gold poisoning*. The toxic activity of these metals is due to interaction with essential sulphydryl groups in enzymes. Dimercaprol possesses two sulphydryl groups and forms a stable mercaptide ring (Figure 5.2) when it interacts with one of the above metals. It is therefore able to protect and reactivate sulphydryl groups in enzyme systems. The alcohol group on the dimercaprol molecule confers water solubility and thereby enhances excretion of the complex from the body.

There is a tendency for any chelation complex to dissociate and release toxic metal ions into the circulation; for this reason it is important to maintain a constant excess of the chelating agent. Unfortunately dimercaprol is itself toxic and too great an excess may cause unpleasant side-effects such as nausea, vomiting, hypotension, tachycardia, a burning sensation in the lips, mouth and throat and a feeling of constriction in the throat, chest or hands. Side-effects occur in 50 per cent of patients at a dose of 5 mg/kg body weight, but usually subside within two hours of administration of the drug.

The usual dose of dimercaprol is 2.5 to 5 mg/kg body weight by *deep* intramuscular injection four-hourly for two days then 2.5 mg/kg body weight twice daily on the third day and once daily thereafter. The duration of therapy should depend on the clinical state and response of the patient.

Calcium Edetate

Calcium disodium edetate chelates many divalent and trivalent metal ions. Edetate itself (Figure 5.3) causes hypocalcaemic tetany when administered intravenously because of chelation of ionized calcium in the blood. The calcium salt of edetate (calcium EDTA) is therefore used as it complexes metals which have a higher affinity for the EDTA molecule than calcium.

The affinity of a metal for the edetate molecule is determined by the stability constant of the complex formed; the higher the constant the more stable the complex. A metal with a high stability constant will displace a metal with a lower stability constant (Table 5.2). Thus the stability constant of the lead complex

Table 5.1. The mechanisms of action of clinically important antidotes.

Poison	Antidote
Antidote forms an inert complex with the poison	
Arsenic, mercury, gold	Dimercaprol
Lead	Calcium disodium edetate, dimercaprol, penicillamine
Iron	Desferrioxamine
Thallium	Prussian Blue
Digoxin	Fab antibody fragments
Cyanide	Methaemoglobin, cobalt edetate, hydroxocobalamin
Cholinesterase inhibitors	Pralidoxime
Antidote accelerates the detoxification of the poison	
Cyanide	Thiosulphate
Paracetamol	Methionine, n-acetyl-cysteine
Antidote reduces the rate of conversion of the poison to a more toxic compound	
Methanol	Ethanol
Ethylene glycol	Ethanol
Antidote blocks essential receptors through which the toxic effects are mediated	
Carbon monoxide	Oxygen
Opiates	Naloxone
Antidote blocks essential receptors through which the toxic effects are mediated	
Cholinesterase inhibitors	Atropine
Antidote bypasses the effect of the poison	
Cyanide	Oxygen

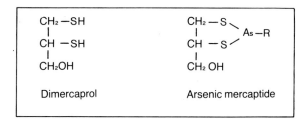

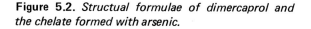

Figure 5.2. *Structual formulae of dimercaprol and the chelate formed with arsenic.*

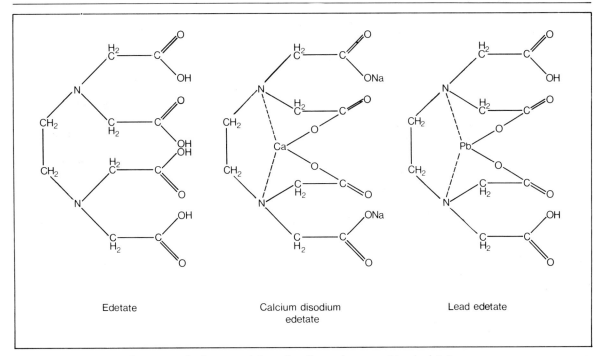

Figure 5.3. *Structural formulae of edetate, calcium disodium edetate and lead edetate.*

is 10^7 greater than that of the calcium complex and, indeed, the principal clinical role of calcium edetate lies in the treatment of *lead poisoning* (Figure 5.3).

Mercury forms a complex with EDTA which is even more stable than that formed by lead. Unfortunately this has no clinical application because mercury binds to sulphydryl groups of intracellular enzymes, and edetate, because it is ionized, penetrates cell membranes poorly.

Calcium disodium edetate (Ledclair) should be given intravenously in the treatment of lead poisoning because oral administration may enhance absorption of lead from the gut. The daily dose is 50 to 75 mg/kg by slow intravenous infusion for five days (every 2 g of EDTA should be diluted with 250 ml of normal saline). There is some evidence that the addition of dimercaprol (5 mg/kg by deep intramuscular injection hourly for 24 hours) adds to the effectiveness of the EDTA regime in the treatment of lead poisoning.

Penicillamine

Penicillamine (dimethylcysteine) is an effective chelating agent for *copper, lead, mercury and zinc.* Although cysteine is an equally effective chelating agent, it is susceptible to degradation by the enzyme cysteine desulphydrase. The addition of two methyl groups to the cysteine molecule to form dimethylcysteine (penicillamine) protects against enzyme breakdown. The principal use of penicillamine (Figure 5.4) lies in the treatment of *copper poisoning* and in Wilson's disease, where it is used to reduce the body burden of copper. It may also be used as an alternative to calcium disodium edetate in the treatment of lead poisoning.

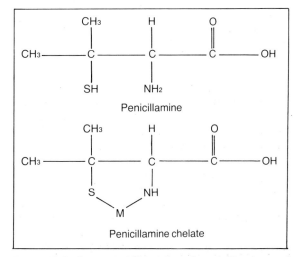

Figure 5.4. *Structural formulae of penicillamine and the penicillamine chelate.*

Table 5.2 Approximate stability constants of metal–EDTA complexes.

Metal	Log of stability constant of complex
Iron (III)	25.0
Mercury	22.0
Copper	19.0
Nickel	18.5
Lead	18.0
Zinc	16.5
Cadmium	16.5
Cobalt	16.5
Iron (II)	14.5
Manganese	14.0
CALCIUM	*11.0*
Strontium	8.5
Barium	8.0
Silver	7.5

The dose of penicillamine (Cupramine, Distamine) is 250 mg to 2 g orally each day (children 20 mg/kg body weight). In cases of acute copper poisoning, the addition of dimercaprol, in the dose specified for arsenic, mercury and gold poisoning above, may be of value.

Desferrioxamine

Desferrioxamine is the agent of choice in the treatment of *iron poisoning* (see Chapter 27). Consideration of the stability constants listed in Table 5.2 might suggest that edetate should also be effective in the treatment of iron poisoning. However, naturally occurring chelating agents, such as transferrin and ferritin, bind iron far more avidly than EDTA. Desferrioxamine (Figure 5.5) chelates iron in an octahedral complex with a stability constant of greater than 10^{30}, which enables it to remove iron from transferrin and ferritin but not from haemoglobin or cytochrome oxidase.

Prussian Blue

Thallium poisoning is rare in Great Britain but occurs more commonly in other parts of Europe where thallium is widely used as a rodenticide. The clinical features of thallium poisoning are discussed elsewhere (Chapter 26). In the body, thallium ions behave like potassium ions and move between extracellular and intracellular compartments in a similar manner.

Thallium ions are excreted, like those of potassium, through the kidneys and into the GI tract via the saliva, the bile and through the intestinal mucosa.

It is possible to sequester thallium ions in the gut and prevent reabsorption by oral administration of *Prussian Blue* — potassium ferrihexacyanoferrate (10 g.b.d.). Thallium ions are exchanged for potassium ions in the lattice of the Prussian Blue molecule and are subsequently excreted in the faeces. During treatment with Prussian Blue, plasma levels of thallium fall and urine excretion of thallium declines exponentially. In contrast, faecal excretion of thallium is detectable even when urinary excretion of the metal has ceased. Administration of Prussian Blue should therefore be continued until thallium can no longer be detected in the faeces. Thallotoxicosis is often associated with intestinal stasis and severe constipation, and for this reason a purgative (magnesium sulphate or mannitol) should be administered along with the Prussian Blue.

Gastric stasis may necessitate the use of a duodenal tube for the administration of the Prussian Blue. It is generally recommended that intravenous potassium be given to enhance excretion of thallium into the gut. Oral potassium supplements should be avoided because they are likely to interfere with the exchange between potassium and thallium ions in the gut lumen.

Digoxin-Specific Antibody Fragments

Recently advances have been made in the use of digoxin-specific antibody fragments in the treatment

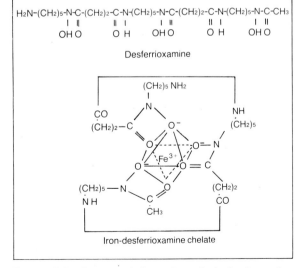

Figure 5.5. *Structural formulae of desferrioxamine and iron-desferrioxamine chelate.*

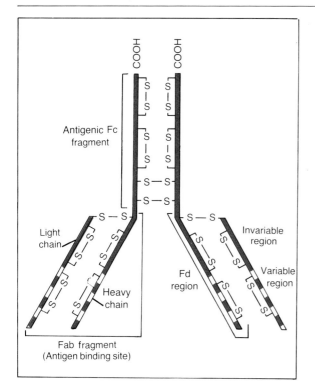

Figure 5.6. *A schematic representation of an antibody showing the two antigen-specific Fab fragments, composed of heavy and light chains, and the Fc fragment which confers antigenicity on the antibody molecule itself.*

of severe *digoxin poisoning* (see Chapter 16). These antibody fragments are not yet freely available, and in any case there are probably less than a dozen patients in the UK each year in whom the use of this treatment would be appropriate. Nevertheless, it is probable that a similar approach using specific antibody fragments will be adopted in the treatment of other forms of poisoning in the future.

In the past attempts have been made to treat experimental digoxin poisoning in animals with antibodies raised to digoxin in other species. Unfortunately, not only are whole antibodies themselves immunogenic by virtue of the presence of the Fc fragment (Figure 5.6), but they are also too large to be readily excreted in the urine. Immune degradation of the circulating antibody—digoxin complexes eventually releases large quantities of digoxin back into the circulation.

More recently, digoxin-specific Fab antibody fragments have been synthesized. They have the advantage of lacking immunogencity (no Fc fragment) and of being small enough to be excreted rapidly into the urine. Smith and his colleagues (1976) were the first to treat a patient with severe digoxin poisoning with

an infusion of Fab-fragments from digoxin-specific antibodies. A 39-year-old man ingested 22.5 mg of digoxin and developed heart block, extreme bradycardia and intractable hyperkalaemia. Sinus rhythm was restored within 10 minutes of infusion of 1100 mg of Fab and the serum free digoxin level fell from 20 ng/ml to less than 1 ng/ml within an hour of commencement of treatment.

Antidotes to Cyanide

Cyanide reversibly inhibits cellular oxidizing enzymes which contain iron in the ferric state, e.g. cytochrome oxidase. This enzyme is the terminal member of the mitochondrial electron transport chain which traps electrons liberated in the tricarboxylic acid cycle and then transfers them to mediate the formation of water from oxygen and hydrogen. In the presence of cyanide, electron transfer is blocked, the tricarboxylic acid cycle is paralyzed and cellular respiration ceases. The clinical features of cyanide poisoning are described in Chapter 29.

Thiosulphate

The principal route of detoxification of cyanide in the body is by conversion to thiocyanate (Figure 5.7) by the enzyme rhodanase. This enzyme has been isolated from beef liver and bacteria and has been used successfully to treat experimental cyanide poisoning in animals. The enzyme, however, has not been used for treatment in man. *Thiosulphate* is

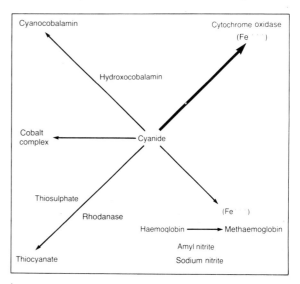

Figure 5.7. *The metabolism and detoxification of cyanide (see text).*

required for the conversion of cyanide to thiocyanate and the presence of this substance appears to be the rate-limiting factor for the reaction. Administration of thiosulphate thus increases the rate of metabolism of cyanide to a less toxic compound (Table 5.1). Unfortunately thiosulphate is not very effective when used alone because it penetrates cell membranes more slowly than cyanide and it is therefore difficult to achieve high tissue concentrations.

Amyl Nitrite and Sodium Nitrite

An alternative and more rapid way of inactivating cyanide is to convert a portion of the body's haemoglobin to methaemoglobin which contains iron in the ferric rather than the ferrous state (Figure 5.7). Almost 40 per cent of the haemoglobin in the body may be converted to methaemoglobin without illeffect. This represents about 300 g haemoglobin or 1 g iron, which theoretically should chelate 500 mg of cyanide ion. Inhalation of *amyl nitrite* has been recommended in the past to produce methaemoglobinaemia, but it is poorly tolerated and only low circulating levels of methaemoglobin may be achieved before profound hypotension occurs. Methaemoglobinemia is therefore best achieved by the intravenous administration of *sodium nitrite*.

Traditionally a combination of intravenous sodium nitrite and sodium thiosulphate is used in the treatment of cyanide poisoning. Experiments in dogs have shown that the LD_{50} for cyanide may be increased three-fold by sodium thiosulphate alone, five-fold by sodium nitrite alone and eighteen-fold by the use of the two antidotes together.

Dicobalt Edetate

Cobalt compounds (Figure 5.7) form stable inert complexes with cyanide (cobalto-cyanides and cobalticyanides). *Dicobalt edetate* (Kelocyanor) is now the treatment of choice for cyanide poisoning. It should only be administered if the diagnosis is certain because, in the absence of cyanide, the drug may cause serious side-effects including vomiting, tachycardia, hypertension, chest pain and facial and palpebral oedema. These reactions are usually self-limiting.

Hydroxocobalamin

A minor route of cyanide metabolism involves the formation of cyanocobalamin (vitamin B_{12}) from *hydroxocobalamin* (Figure 5.7). One mole of hydroxocobalamin inactivates one mole of cyanide but, on a weight-for-weight basis, 50 times more hydroxocobalamin is needed than cyanide because hydroxoco-balamin is a far larger molecule. Concentrated solutions of hydroxocobalamin are not yet freely available and use of the dilute 1 mg/ml solution employed in the treatment of pernicious anaemia is not practical. Nevertheless, patients suffering from cyanide poisoning have been treated successfully with hydroxocobalamin in France. In America, hydroxocobalamin has been used to reduce the toxicity of sodium nitroprusside infusions used to induce hypotension during surgical procedures (sodium nitroprusside is metabolized to cyanide).

Oxygen

Finally, it is possible to bypass the effect of cyanide poisoning by the administration of *oxygen* (Table 5.1). Experiments in mice using ^{14}C-labelled CO_2, to determine the switch from aerobic to anaerobic metabolism in experimental cyanide poisoning, have shown that oxygen has a synergistic antidotal action when used in combination with sodium thiosulphate and sodium nitrite. The mechanism for this is not known.

Management of Cyanide Poisoning

In summary, speed is of the essence in the treatment of cyanide poisoning. Gastric lavage should be delayed until after the administration of antidotes unless the patient is asymptomatic. Provided that the diagnosis is certain, and particularly if the patient is already unconscious, dicobalt edetate (Kelocyanor) should be given (600 mg intravenously over one minute followed by a further 300 mg if recovery does not occur within one minute). Alternatively, 10 ml of a 3 per cent solution of sodium nitrite is given intravenously over a period of two to four minutes, followed by 50 ml of a 25 per cent solution of sodium thiosulphate over 10 minutes. Oxygen therapy should also be given together with cardiorespiratory support as appropriate.

Accelerated Detoxification of the Poison

The accelerated conversion of cyanide to thiocyanate using thiosulphate has been discussed above. The use of methionine and acetylcysteine in the treatment of *paracetamol poisoning* is another example of this mode of antidotal action and is discussed in detail in Chapter 14.

Reduced Rate of Conversion to a More Toxic Compound

The clinical features of *methanol (methyl alcohol) poisoning*, which provide the best example of this form of antidotal action, are discussed in full in Chapter 19. Methanol is metabolized in the liver to formaldehyde and formic acid which, unlike the metabolites of ethanol (acetaldehyde and acetic acid) cannot be readily converted by the body to carbon dioxide (Figure 5.8).

Methyl alcohol is oxidized by human liver alcohol dehydrogenase at only one-tenth the rate of ethyl alcohol for which the enzyme has a far greater affinity. Thus it is possible to inhibit the metabolism of methanol by the concomitant administration of ethanol. The initial treatment of methyl alcohol poisoning should include gastric aspiration and lavage and the oral administration of a loading dose of ethyl alcohol followed by an intravenous infusion. The dosage regime is described on page 128.

Competition for Essential Receptor Sites

The Use of Oxygen in Carbon Monoxide Poisoning

The clinical features and general management of *carbon monoxide poisoning* are dealt with in Chapter 29, but treatment with oxygen provides a good example of an antidote competing with a poison for an essential receptor site.

Carbon monoxide (CO) combines with haemoglobin to form carboxyhaemoglobin. If carbon monoxide is inhaled, a certain number of oxygen binding sites on the haemoglobin molecule become occupied and the total oxygen-carrying capacity of the blood is reduced. This in itself results in a shift of the O_2 dissociation curve to the left, i.e. more avid oxygen binding. However, the binding of one or more CO molecules to a molecule of haemoglobin also induces an allosteric modification in the remaining oxygen binding sites. The affinity of the remaining haem

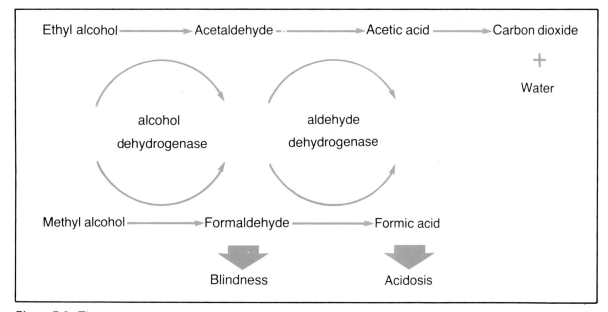

Figure 5.8. *The metabolism of ethyl alcohol and methyl alcohol. The affinity of the enzyme alcohol dehydrogenase for ethyl alcohol is far greater than that for methyl alcohol. The administration of ethyl alcohol to a patient poisoned with methyl alcohol reduces the formation of formaldehyde and formic acid by competitive inhibition of the enzyme involved.*

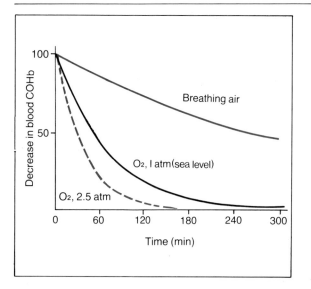

Figure 5.9. *Increasing the partial pressure of inspired oxygen accelerates the elimination of carbon monoxide, measured as the percentage of carboxy-haemoglobin in the blood.*

groups for oxygen is increased and the O_2 dissociation curve is therefore distorted as well as being shifted to the left. The degree of tissue anoxia that results is thus far greater than that which would result from simple loss of oxygen-carrying capacity.

The basis of the treatment of carbon monoxide poisoning with oxygen lies in the fact that carboxy-haemoglobin readily dissociates when the partial pressure of carbon monoxide in the alveolar air falls below that in mixed venous blood. This situation may be obtained by reducing the partial pressure of inspired carbon monoxide to zero, increasing alveolar ventilation and increasing the inspired oxygen tension. The half-life of elimination of carbon monoxide is 250 minutes when breathing room air but this is reduced to 50 minutes when 100 per cent oxygen is inspired at sea level (Figure 5.9). Hyperbaric oxygen at 2.5 atmospheres pressure further reduces the half-life to 22 minutes. In addition, hyperbaric oxygen increases the amount of oxygen dissolved in the blood and at 2 atmospheres pressure, for example, the amount of oxygen dissolved increases from 0.25 volumes per cent to 3.8 volumes per cent. However,

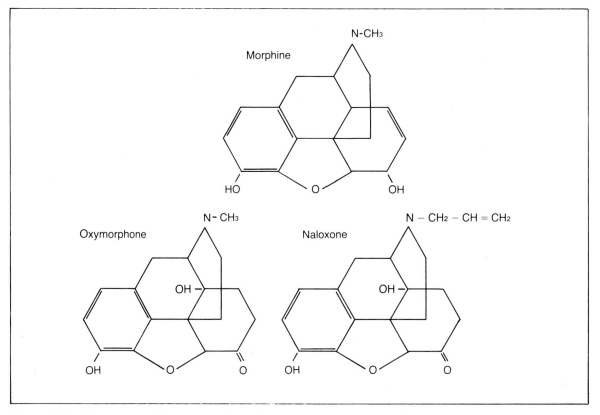

Figure 5.10. *The structural formulae of morphine, oxymorphone and naloxone. Note the similarity between morphine and the pure opiate antagonist naloxone.*

it usually takes too long to transfer a patient to a hyperbaric oxygen chamber and then to achieve full working pressure to make the use of hyperbaric oxygen practicable in cases of carbon monoxide poisoning.

It has been suggested that five to seven per cent carbon dioxide (CO_2) be added to the inspired oxygen because this further reduces the half-life of elimination of carbon monoxide at one atmosphere (sea level) to about 12 minutes. This effect of carbon dioxide is thought to be due to stimulation of alveolar ventilation and to the development of an acidaemia which promotes dissociation of carboxyhaemoglobin. However, the latter effect exacerbates the acidosis found in severe carbon monoxide poisoning and the use of added carbon dioxide as a routine measure is not recommended.

The Use of Naloxone in Opiate Poisoning

Poisoning due to *opiates and morphine derivatives* is discussed in Chapter 15. The use of partial agonists, such as nalorphine, in the treatment of opiate poisoning has been superseded by the development of the pure antagonist, naloxone. Nalorphine (N-allylnormorphine) was the first opiate antagonist to be made available for medical use but it was found to have significant disadvantages because of partial agonist activity. The most important of these disadvantages was respiratory depression. The synthesis of naloxone (N-allylnoroxymorphone) was reported in 1963, and since then it has become the opiate antagonist of choice. When the —OH group on a molecule of morphine (Figure 5.10) is substituted with an =O group, oxymorphone is formed. Oxymorphone has 10 times the analgesic activity of morphine, and when the methyl group is further substituted with an allyl group the pure antagonist naloxone results (Figure 5.10). There is now a considerable body of evidence which suggests that naloxone antagonizes the effects of opiates at stereospecific opioid receptor sites.

In man, subcutaneous doses of up to 12 mg of naloxone produce no subjective or objective changes and 24 mg causes only slight drowsiness. Oral doses of more than 1 g of naloxone have been given without ill effect. It is rapidly metabolized by the liver and for this reason it is 50 times more potent when given parenterally. One milligram of naloxone given intravenously reverses the effects of 25 mg of diamorphine. In adults, the dose of naloxone hydrochloride (Narcan) is 0.4 mg intravenously or intra-

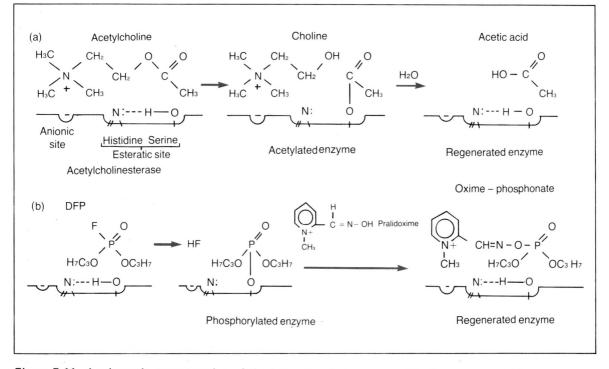

Figure 5.11. *A schematic representation of the interaction between acetylcholinesterase and (a) acetylcholine and (b) the organophosphorus compound, DFP (diisopropyl phosphorofluoridate). Pralidoxime regenerates the phosphorylated enzyme with the formation of an oxime—phosphonate complex.*

muscularly; in children, the dose is 5-10 μg (0.005 – 0.01 mg/kg body weight) intravenously or intramuscularly. These doses may be repeated if pupillary constriction and respiratory depression are not reversed within one to two minutes (the latter being assessed by respiratory rate and tidal volume). The duration of respiratory depression due to opiate drugs may sometimes exceed the duration of activity of a single dose of naloxone and, for this reason, administration of the antagonist may need to be repeated at regular intervals.

In addition to antagonizing the effects of morphine and diamorphine, naloxone also reverses the toxic effects of pethidine, apomorphine, dipipanone (Dicanol), methadone (Physeptone), dextropropoxyphene (in Distalgesic), diphenoxylate (in Lomotil), phenazocine (Narphen), pentazocine (Fortral), codeine and dihydrocodeine (DF118).

In opiate-dependent subjects, small doses of naloxone precipitate a moderate to severe withdrawal syndrome. This is very similar to that seen after abrupt withdrawal of opiates, except that the syndrome appears within minutes of administration of the antidote and subsides in about two hours.

Blockade of Receptor Sites

Organophosphorus compounds are used widely as insecticides and the clinical features and management of poisoning due to these chemicals are described in Chapter 22. The toxic effects of these compounds are due to specific inhibition of cholinesterase activity, with accumulation of acetylcholine at nicotinic and muscarinic receptor sites in autonomic ganglia, neuromuscular junctions, smooth muscle, glands and the central nervous system. Atropine blocks the effects of anticholinesterase agents at muscarinic receptor sites whereas pralidoxime reactivates phosphorylated cholinesterase enzyme and forms an inert complex with the organophosphate (Table 5.1).

The Use of Atropine in Anticholinesterase Poisoning

Muscarinic features of anticholinesterase poisoning which are inhibited by the use of *atropine* include nausea, vomiting, abdominal cramps, diarrhoea, bronchorrhoea, bronchospasm, miosis, bradycardia and involuntary micturition. Atropine sulphate should be given to adults in an initial dose of 2 mg

intravenously (intramuscularly or subcutaneously in less severely poisoned patients) followed by further 2 mg doses at five to 10 minute intervals until the clinical features of full atropinization become apparent. A dry mouth and a heart rate of 70 to 80 beats per minute are the most reliable signs. Full atropinization should be continued for two to three days and it is common for large doses of the drug to be required (25 to 50 mg atropine may be necessary in a single day). Atropine has little or no effect at autonomic ganglia and none at all at neuromuscular junctions where accumulation of acetylcholine causes weakness, and eventually paralysis, of skeletal muscles, including those responsible for respiration.

The Use of Pralidoxime in Anticholinesterase Poisoning

In order to understand the effect of *pralidoxime* on cholinesterase enzyme phosphorylated by an organophosphate it is necessary to describe the structure and function of the normal enzyme. Cholinesterase is thought to possess two active sites – an anionic site and an esteratic site these being formed by an hydroxyl group of serine and an imidazole group of histidine (Figure 5.11a). The anionic site attracts the positively charged quarternary nitrogen atom of acetylcholine, and the serine hydroxyl group interacts with the electrophilic carbon atom of the carbonyl group of the molecule. Choline is split off, leaving an acetylated enzyme, which reacts with water to produce acetic acid and the regenerated active enzyme (Figure 5.11a). The time taken for a single molecule of acetylcholine to undergo this reaction is about 80 microseconds.

Organophosphorus compounds combine with cholinesterase to produce a phosphorylated enzyme. If the alkyl groups of the organophosphate molecules are either ethyl or methyl groups, then hydrolysis of the phosphorylated enzyme will occur over a period of hours. However, if isopropyl groups are present (Figure 5.11b), hydrolysis will not occur to any significant extent and return of enzyme activity is dependent upon synthesis of new enzyme. Pralidoxime interacts with the phosphorylated enzyme to allow regeneration and, at the same time, an oxime–phosphonate complex is formed (Figure 5.11b). Ideally the pralidoxime should be given simultaneously with the atropine but, if it is not readily available, the pralidoxime should be administered as soon as possible after the atropine. Phosphorylated cholinesterase enzyme undergoes a process of 'ageing' so that, within a matter of hours, it becomes resistant to reactivation by pralidoxime. The effects of prali-doxime are most prominent at skeletal neuromuscular junctions, and muscle weakness and fasciculation should improve within 10 minutes; little effect is seen at autonomic receptor sites and almost none in the central nervous system.

The dose of pralidoxime mesylate given should be 30 mg/kg body weight either intravenously, when the rate of administration should not exceed 500 mg per minute, or intramuscularly, every 4 hours for 24 hours. If the recommended rate of intravenous adminis-tration is exceeded, pralidoxime may cause mild weak-ness, blurred vision, diplopia, dizziness, headache, nausea and tachycardia.

Experimental evidence suggests that the early addition of diazepam (10-15 mg i.m.) to the thera-peutic regime of atropine and pralidoxime affords further protection against the occurrence of seizures.

Bypass of the Effects of the Poison

This mode of antidotal action is exemplified by the use of oxygen in the treatment of *cyanide poisoning* and has been discussed on page 38.

Conclusion

Clinically important antidotes and dosage regimes are summarized in Table 5.3. However, it must be empha-sized that they represent just one part of the thera-peutic approach to a particular group of poisoned patients and the role of supportive therapy should not be forgotten.

Table 5.3.   Antidotes to toxic substances.

Toxic substance	Antidote
Carbon monoxide	Oxygen
Cholinesterase inhibitors (organo-phosphorus insecticides)	Pralidoxime mesylate (P$_2$S) 30 mg/kg body weight i.v. (should not exceed 500 mg per minute) or i.m. every four hours for 24 hours. Atropine 2 mg i.v. should also be given to produce and maintain full atropinization.
Cyanide	Dicobalt edetate (Kelocyanor) 600 mg i.v. over one minute with a further 300 mg if recovery does not occur within one minute. Alter-natively, give 10 ml of sodium nitrite (3% solution) i.v. followed by slow i.v. injection of 25 ml of a 50% solution of sodium thiosulphate.
Ethylene glycol	Ethyl alcohol (see methanol).
Heavy metals (arsenic, gold, mercury)	Dimercaprol (BAL) 2.5–5 mg/kg body weight by DEEP i.m. injection four hourly for two days; 2.5 mg/kg body weight twice daily on the third day; then once daily. Duration of therapy depends on the clinical state. [Penicillamine (see below) is also effective in mercury poisoning.]
Heavy metals (copper, mercury, zinc, lead)	Penicillamine (Cuprimine, Distamine) 250 mg–2 g orally daily (children 20 mg/kg body weight).
	Desferrioxamine mesylate (Desferal) should be given in four ways: 1. Gastric lavage using a solution of desferrioxamine (2 g in 1 litre warm water). 2. Inject 2 g (in 10 ml sterile water) i.m. 3. After gastric lavage leave 5 g (in 50 ml water) in the stomach. 4. Slow i.v. infusion 15 mg/kg/hour (maximum 80 mg/kg in 24 hours) or inject 2 g i.m. 12 hourly.

Toxic substance	Antidote
Iron	Desferrioxamine mesylate (Desferal) should be given in four ways: 1. Gastric lavage using a solution of desferrioxamine (2 g in 1 litre warm water). 2. Inject 2 g (in 10 ml sterile water) i.m. 3. After gastric lavage leave 5 g (in 50 ml water) in the stomach. 4. Slow i.v. infusion 15 mg/kg/hour (maximum 80 mg/kg in 24 hours) or inject 2 g i.m. 12 hourly.
Lead	Sodium calcium edetate (Ledclair). This preparation should not be given orally as lead absorption from the gut may be enhanced. Daily dose: 50—75 mg/kg by slow i.v. infusion (each 2 g should be diluted with 250 ml isotonic saline) for five days. There is some evidence that the addition of dimercaprol (5 mg/kg i.m. four hourly for 24 hours) adds to the effectiveness of the EDTA regime. Penicillamine, 250 mg—2 g orally daily (children 20 mg/kg body weight) may be given as an alternative to sodium calcium edetate.
Methanol	Ethyl alcohol 50 g orally stat. followed by 10—12 g/hour by i.v. infusion, which should be increased by 7—10 g/hour if haemodialysis is employed. (Maintain plasma ethanol level 1000—2000 mg/l).
Morphine and its analogues, e.g. diamorphine, pethidine (meperidine), apomorphine, codeine, dextropropoxyphene (in Distalgesic), dihydrocodeine, diphenoxylate (in Lomotil), dipipanone, methadone, pentazocine, phenazocine.	Naloxone hydrochloride (Narcan). Adults: 0.4 mg i.v. or i.m. which may be repeated. Children: 5—10 μg (0.005—0.01 mg) per kg body weight i.v. or i.m. which may be repeated.
Paracetamol	Methionine 2.5 g orally stat., then 2.5 g four-hourly for a further three doses. Total dose: 10 g methionine over 12 hours. or: N-acetylcysteine (Parvolex) 150 mg/kg i.v. over 15 minutes, then 50 mg/kg in 500 ml of 5 per cent dextrose in the next four hours and 100 mg/kg in 1000 ml of 5 per cent dextrose over the ensuing 16 hours. Total dose: 300 mg/kg over 20 hours. or: N-acetylcysteine may be given orally (Chapter 14, Table 2). N.B. The antidotes should be administered only if not more than 10 hours have elapsed from the time of ingestion of the paracetamol overdose.
Thallium	Prussian blue 10 g b.d. orally or through a stomach tube until faecal excretion of thallium has ceased.

References

Digoxin-specific Antibodies

Smith TW, Haber E, Yeatman L, Butler VP. Reversal of advanced digoxin intoxication with Fab fragments of digoxin-specific antibodies. New Engl J Med 1976; 294:797–800.

Further Reading

Chelating Agents

Anonymous. Chelating agents in medicine. Br Med J 1971; 2:270–2.

Kamerbeek HH, Rauws AG, ten Ham M, Van Heijst ANP. Prussian Blue in therapy of thallotoxicosis. Acta Med Scand 1971; 189:321–4.

Levine WG. Heavy Metal Antagonists in The Pharmacological Basis of Therapeutics. Eds. Goodman LS, Gilman A. New York: Macmillan Publishing Co Inc, 1975. 5th edition. Chapter 45, pp 912–45.

Richelmi P, Bono F, Guardia L, Ferrini B, Manzo L. Salivary levels of thallium in acute human poisoning. Arch Toxicol 1980; 43:321–5.

Stevens W, Van Peteghem C, Heyndrickx A, Barbier F. Eleven cases of thallium intoxication treated with Prussian Blue. Int J Clin Pharmacol 1974; 10:1–22.

Digoxin-specific Antibodies

Hess T, Stucki P, Barandum S, Scholtysik G, Riesen W. Treatment of a case of Ianatoside c intoxication with digoxin-specific F(ab')₂ antibody fragments. Am Heart J 1979; 98: 767–71.

Hess T, Scholtysik G, Riesen W. The effectiveness of digoxin-specific F(ab')₂ antibody fragments in the treatment of digoxin poisoning: experimental investigations in the cat. Eur J Clin Invest 1980; 10: 73–7.

Swith, TW. Treatment of advanced digitalis toxicity with specific antibodies. Eur J Clin Invest 1980; 10: 89–91.

Cyanide Poisoning

Cottrell JE, Casthely P, Brodie JD, Patel K, Klein A, Turndorf H. Prevention of nitroprusside-induced cyanide toxicity with hydroxocobalamin. New Engl J Med 1978; 298:809–11.

Evans CL. Cobalt compounds as antidotes for hydrocyanic acid. Br J Pharmacol 1964; 23:455–75.

Graham DL, Laman D, Theodore J, Robin ED. Acute cyanide poisoning complicated by lactic acidosis and pulmonary edema. Arch Intern Med 1977; 137:1051–5.

Yacoub M, Faure J, Morena H, Vincent M, Faure H. L'intoxication cyanhydrique aigue. Donnees actuelles sur le metabolisme du cyanure et le traitement par hydroxocobalamine. J Eur Toxicol 1974; 7:22–9.

Methyl Alcohol Poisoning

See Chapter 19.

Carbon Monoxide Poisoning

See Chapter 29.

Opiate Antagonists

Evans LEJ, Roscoe P, Swainson CP, Prescott LF. Treatment of drug overdosage with naloxone, a specific narcotic antagonist. Lancet 1973; i:452–5.

Foldes FF, Lunn JN, Moore J, Brown IM. N-allylnoroxymorphone: a new potent narcotic antagonist. Am J Med Sci 1963; 245:23–30.

Moore RA, Rumack BH, Conner CS, Peterson RG. Naloxone: underdosage after narcotic poisoning. Am J Dis Child 1980; 134: 156–8.

Snyder SH. Opiate receptors in the brain. New Engl J Med 1977; 296:266–71.

Anticholinesterase Poisoning

Green DM, Muir AW, Stratton JA, Inch TD. Dual mechanism of the antidotal action of atropine-like drugs in poisoning by organophosphorus anticholinesterases. J Pharm Pharmac 1977; 29:62–4.

Vale JA, Scott GW. Organophosphorus poisoning. Guy's Hosp. Reports 1974; 123:13–25.

Chapter 6

M. Helliwell

The Pathogenesis and Treatment
of Shock Due to Poisoning

Acute poisoning may be complicated by shock and, when present, this constitutes a grave threat to the survival of the patient.

The barbiturate group of drugs is the most frequent cause of shock, which is particularly likely to occur when plasma drug levels exceed 100 mg/l for 'long-acting' barbiturates and 50 mg/l for the 'medium-' and 'short-acting' barbiturates. When taken in overdose, other non-barbiturate hypnotics, such as methaqualone, glutethimide and meprobamate, also cause profound hypotension similar to that found in severe cases of barbiturate intoxication. Similarly, toxic doses of the opiate group of drugs exert a deleterious effect on the cardiovascular system by causing marked peripheral dilatation, due largely to local histamine release rather than a central effect. Alcohol causes peripheral dilatation, mainly in cutaneous vessels, but seldom causes a marked fall in blood pressure. The principal danger of alcohol lies in its ability to potentiate the cardiac and respiratory depressant effects of other drugs, particularly barbiturates and opiates. Benzodiazepine poisoning is not commonly associated with a significant fall in blood pressure. In contrast, when taken in large doses the major tranquillizers, for example chlorpromazine, may cause serious hypotension due partly to α-adrenergic receptor blockade.

Some drugs, notably the tricyclic antidepressants, give rise to cardiac arrhythmias and thereby cause cardiogenic shock. These arrhythmias are caused partly by the anticholinergic properties of these drugs and partly because the level of circulating catecholamines is increased as a result of blockade of re-uptake of noradrenaline by adrenergic neurones.

The ingestion of the combination tablet of paracetamol and dextropropoxyphene (Distalgesic) may cause severe shock due to the respiratory and cardiac depressant action of dextropropoxyphene. Both these effects, however, may be rapidly reversed by the use of intravenous naloxone.

Despite the wide number of drugs capable of adversely affecting the cardiovascular system shock occurs in less than 10 per cent of cases of acute poisoning. However, drug overdose complicated by severe hypotension is associated with a significant mortality.

Pathophysiology of Shock in Acute Poisoning

Shock occurs when inadequate blood supply and elimination of tissue metabolites leads to functional and structural disturbances in essential organs (Joseph 1976). The classic manifestations of shock are tachycardia, sweating, a cold pale skin with collapsed peripheral veins, a diminished level of consciousness, a low arterial blood pressure and oliguria. However, these features are not invariably present in shock associated with acute poisoning, particularly when barbiturate and opiate drugs are involved. Tachycardia is less common in shock caused by poisoning than in other forms of shock and the skin is often warm and dry.

The clinical features peculiar to shock due to acute poisoning led to the suggestion that hypotension in acute poisoning was due to failure of circulatory reflexes, causing a defect in both arteriolar tone and arteriolar vasoconstriction. However, a study of 15 poisoned patients by Shubin and Weil (1965) failed to support this concept. All patients were shocked, with systolic arterial pressures of less than 80 mm Hg. Haemodynamic investigations revealed that all the patients had a low cardiac output, reduced plasma volume and a high peripheral vascular resistance. The central venous pressure was either low or in the low–normal range. Treatment consisted of volume expansion and, in some instances, the use of vasopressor agents. The augmentation of plasma volume was associated with an increase in cardiac output and mean blood pressure and a fall in the peripheral vascular resistance but, despite liberal administration of fluids (up to six litres in 12 hours), there was no significant change in central venous pressure. The authors concluded that in acute poisoning there is an increase in the capacitance (venous) bed with a relative deficit of plasma volume. As a result, the venous return to the heart is reduced causing a fall in cardiac output and arterial pressure (Figure 6.1). Expansion of the vascular capacity without an accompanying increase in the circulating blood volume is now generally accepted as the major cause of shock when large doses of hypnotics and sedatives have been ingested, although other factors may be contributary. Barbiturates impair myocardial metabolism and so may precipitate congestive cardiac failure. In addition, as a result of the reduced venous tone and venous pooling, there may be escape of fluid into the extravascular space causing a reduction in the absolute plasma volume.

The Management of Shock and Patient Monitoring

Measurement of the blood pressure provides a crude but rapid indication of the patient's circulatory status, and shock may be assumed to exist when the systolic blood pressure is less than 90 mm Hg in patients older than 50 years, or less than 80 mm Hg in younger patients. However, hypotension of this order can be successfully treated in up to 80 per cent of cases simply by elevation of the lower limbs and correction of hypoxia. Should these measures prove ineffective treatment should be directed towards correction of the relative hypovolaemia by infusion of fluids (see below). In these circumstances, a central venous pressure line often becomes necessary as a guide to fluid replacement.

In circumstances when auscultation of the blood pressure proves difficult, an in-dwelling arterial line connected to a pressure transducer may be of value, and has the advantage of providing continuous readings. The arterial catheter may also be used for repeated sampling of arterial blood for blood gas determinations.

The arterial pH and lactate concentrations reflect the degree of tissue hypoxia. A fall in the systolic pressure, arterial PO_2 and pH, and a rise in the arterial

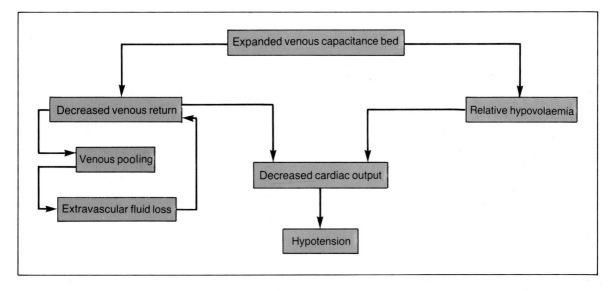

Figure 6.1. *The mechanism of hypotension in acute poisoning with barbiturate, opiate and sedative drugs.*

lactate level, indicate a poor prognosis. Changes in the core—peripheral temperature deficit provide a useful guide to the adequacy of tissue perfusion and parallel closely alterations in cardiac output. The urinary output should be measured by means of an in-dwelling vesical catheter and an hourly flow of more than 30 ml signifies satisfactory renal perfusion. Small intravenous doses of a diuretic can be given to augment urinary flow and protect against acute tubular necrosis. Continuous ECG monitoring is essential for the prompt recognition of cardiac arrhythmias.

Volume Expansion in the Treatment of Hypotension

The choice of fluid for volume expansion lies between crystalloids and colloids.

Crystalloids

Crystalloids, such as Ringer's lactate, may correct interstitial fluid loss and, by reducing the haematocrit, improve capillary blood flow. However, there are a number of disadvantages to the use of crystalloids. They are rapidly lost from the circulation into the extravascular compartment and, since shock in acute poisoning is due more to a disparity between vascular capacity and volume than to extravascular fluid loss, infusion of colloids would seem a more rational approach to treatment. Infusion of large volumes of crystalloids reduces the osmotic—hydrostatic gradient, increases lung water and has been implicated in the development of 'shock lung' in severely hypotensive patients. Nevertheless, the infusion of crystalloids may be of value in some circumstances as studies have shown that the oxygen-carrying capacity of the blood is optimal at a haematocrit of about 30 per cent (Gruber et al. 1976). Conversely, the infusion of red cells, in the absence of blood loss, may worsen tissue hypoxia by increasing blood viscosity, promoting capillary sludging and lowering oxygen transport.

Colloids

As far as colloids are concerned, albumin is too expensive for routine use and stored pooled plasma or dried plasma carry a small but definite risk of transfusion hepatitis. This hazard may be avoided by the use of purified plasma protein solutions.

There are three major alternatives to plasma preparations for volume expansion: dextrans, hydroxyethyl starches and Haemaccel.

Dextrans

Several dextran preparations are available — high molecular weight (Dextran 70) and low molecular weight (Dextran 40). In addition to antithrombotic properties, dextrans lower blood viscosity and so prevent the formation of erythrocyte aggregates that occur in the microcirculation in low flow states. However, volume replacement with large quantities of dextran may impair blood coagulation and should be limited to no more than one litre or approximately 15 ml/kg body weight. Dextran 40 increases urine viscosity and has been incriminated as a cause of acute renal failure. It should be remembered that low molecular weight dextran (Dextran 40) has powerful oncotic properties and that the transfer of extracellular fluid to the intravascular compartment may cause pulmonary oedema in patients with poor cardiac function. For these reasons, high molecular weight dextran (Dextran 70) is the preparation of choice for volume expansion in hypotensive patients.

Hydroxyethyl Starches

Hydroxyethyl starches (Hetaplas) cause similar increases in the plasma volume to dextrans, but acute renal failure due to hyperviscosity of the urine has not been described. The toxicity of hydroxyethyl starches is limited to minor coagulation abnormalities and rarely anaphylactoid reactions.

Haemaccel

Haemaccel, a degraded gelatin solution, has colloidal properties superior to those of dextran and remains in the circulation for at least four hours. It has no specific erythrocyte disaggregating effect but appears to improve microcirculatory blood flow in shocked patients by restoring blood volume and reducing blood viscosity. It also confers some protection on the kidneys by promoting an osmotic diuresis. A further advantage over dextran solutions is that Haemaccel does not interfere with subsequent typing or cross-matching of blood.

Vasoactive and Inotropic Drugs in the Treatment of Hypotension

The underlying pathology of shock in poisoned patients is a low cardiac output associated with low cardiac filling pressures. However, the presence of persistent hypotension despite adequate volume replacement (CVP 10–15 cm H_2O) suggests a failing heart, and any further elevation in cardiac filling pressures is likely to precipitate pulmonary oedema. Restoration of a normal cardiac function curve can be obtained only by the use of drugs capable of improving myocardial performance (Figure 6.2). It is mandatory, however, that these drugs should only be used in the presence of a normal circulating blood volume which may be gauged indirectly by the use of a central venous pressure line.

Alpha-adrenergic Stimulants

Alpha-adrenergic stimulants, such as metaraminol, should not be used because, in many cases, the peripheral vascular resistance is high and the use of these drugs further compromises the blood supply to essential organs. Prolonged use of metaraminol increases

Figure 6.2. *Cardiac function curves depicting normal and impaired myocardial performance in response to volume changes.*

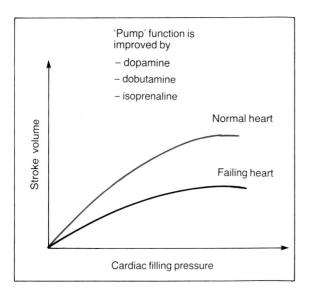

'Pump' function is improved by

– dopamine

– dobutamine

– isoprenaline

Normal heart

Failing heart

Stroke volume

Cardiac filling pressure

capillary hydrostatic pressure, causing loss of fluid into the extravascular compartment and hypovolaemia. The major hazard of metaraminol is ischaemic renal failure from vasoconstriction of the renal arteries.

Isoprenaline

Isoprenaline is a β-adrenergic agonist and, given as an infusion, increases cardiac output and reduces peripheral vascular resistance by causing arterial vasodilatation in skeletal muscle and splanchnic vessels. It should be administered only after proper fluid replacement as vasodilatation in the presence of hypovolaemia will result in a rapid fall in arterial blood pressure. Isoprenaline increases heart rate and myocardial oxygen consumption and may initiate cardiac arrhythmias. Similarly, vasodilators such as phenoxybenzamine, phentolamine and sodium nitroprusside, which dilate venous capacitance vessels, should never be administered without full replacement of any fluid deficit. When these agents are given, strict monitoring of the central venous pressure and arterial pressure is essential.

Dopamine

Dopamine, a naturally occurring precursor of noradrenaline, increases myocardial contractility by a direct action on β-adrenergic receptors and also by releasing noradrenaline from myocardial catecholamine storage sites (Goldberg 1977). Dopamine also stimulates specific dopamine receptors in the renal vasculature causing vasodilatation and thereby improving glomerular filtration and urine flow. Experimentally, dopamine reverses pooling of blood in the venous capacitance bed of dogs with endotoxic shock, and so would appear to be a suitable drug in the treatment of shock associated with acute poisoning. Its effect on myocardial oxygen consumption is less than that of isoprenaline, as heart rate is little changed. However, in large doses (greater than 20 $\mu g/kg/min$) dopamine stimulates α-adrenergic receptors, causing an increase in peripheral vascular resistance and a fall in renal blood flow. Cardiac arrhythmias are more common at these doses because of excessive β-stimulation. The combination of inotropic activity and a lack of α-adrenergic stimulation (except in high doses) makes dopamine a therapeutically attractive agent in the management of shock when fluid replacement alone has not proved effective.

Dobutamine

Dobutamine is an almost pure inotrope and has a direct action on the myocardium which is not dependent on endogenous noradrenaline release. It has little effect on blood vessels and even in high doses does not stimulate α-adrenergic receptors. The chronotropic and arrhythmogenic effects are less than those of dopamine. The comparative actions of isoprenaline, dopamine and dobutamine are shown in Table 6.1.

Treatment of the Metabolic Consequences of Shock

As a result of hypoxia and inadequate tissue perfusion in shock, aerobic metabolism is inhibited and cells begin to utilize the anaerobic pathway in order to obtain energy. Lactic acid accumulates, leading to an influx of sodium and water and causing cellular swelling. Lysosomal membranes containing hydrolytic enzymes eventually rupture and thereby increase intracellular acidosis. As the cell dies lysosomal enzymes are released and may damage adjacent cells. Circulating lysosomal enzymes are cardiotoxic and cause cardiac depression by reducing myocardial contractility and coronary blood flow. Tissue perfusion is further decreased, cellular hypoxia continues and so the cycle is propagated (Figure 6.3). The cornerstone of treatment of the metabolic abnormalities associated with shock is the restoration of a normal circulation.

Extreme acidosis decreases the responsiveness of the heart to circulating catecholamines and in some circumstances it becomes justifiable to give sodium bicarbonate to reverse the acidosis. The amount of bicarbonate required is estimated by multiplying the base deficit by the extracellular fluid volume (approximately one-third of the body weight). Thus a 70 kg man with a base deficit of 10 mEq/l will require in the order of 200 mEq bicarbonate. Half of this should be given initially at a rate of 1 to 2 mEq/min, unless rapid correction of acidosis is required because of cardiac arrhythmias.

The infusion of glucose, potassium and insulin is claimed to be beneficial in improving the metabolic derangement of shock. Although the mechanism is not clear, solutions containing glucose, potassium and insulin increase cardiac performance and appear to protect the heart from arrhythmias. Corticosteroids in large doses exert a positive inotropic effect on the myocardium and induce α-adrenergic receptor blockade, thus improving tissue perfusion. Cell damage is alleviated by the stabilization of lysosomal membranes. The use of corticosteroids in the therapy of shock from acute poisoning is poorly documented, but there is general agreement that they are ineffective in practice.

Summary

Shock may complicate poisoning caused by a variety of drugs, barbiturates being the commonest. The reduction in cardiac output and resultant hypotension are attributed to a disparity between the vascular capacity and the circulating blood volume. Initial treatment should be directed towards establishing a patent airway and the correction of hypoxia. Elevation of the lower limbs may improve hypotension but restoration of an effective plasma volume, guided by

Table 6.1. Comparison of the actions of dopamine, dobutamine and isoprenaline on the cardiovascular system.

	Effects on myocardium			Effects on blood vessels	
	Heart rate	Contractility	Potential for arrhythmias	Vasoconstriction	Vasodilatation in renal vasculature
Dopamine	+ +	+ + +	+ +	o to + + +	+ + +
Dobutamine	+	+ + +	+	o to +	o
Isoprenaline	+ + +	+ + +	+ + +	o	o

o   None
+   Slight
+ +   Moderate
+ + +   Marked

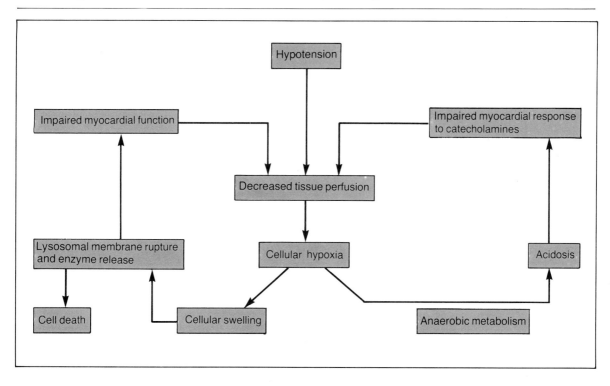

Figure 6.3. *Pathophysiology of shock.*

central venous pressure measurements, is often necessary. Of the vasoactive drugs currently in use, dopamine, and more recently dobutamine, improve cardiac output and tissue perfusion without the detrimental effects of increased peripheral vascular resistance. However, prior restoration of a normal circulating blood volume is essential.

References

Goldberg LI. Recent advances in the pharmacology of catecholamines. Intensive Care Med 1977; 3:233–6.

Gruber UF, Sturm V, Messmer K. Fluid replacement in shock. In: Shock, Clinical and Experimental Aspects. Ledingham IMcA. Ed. Amsterdam: Excerpta Medica 1976; 238–41.

Joseph SP. The management of acute hypotension. Br J Hosp Med 1976; 16:349–56.

Shubin H, Weil MH. The mechanism of shock following suicidal doses of barbiturates, narcotics and tranquillizer drugs, with observations on the effects of treatment. Am J Med 1965; 38:853–63.

Further Reading

Afifi AA, Sacks ST, Liu VY, Weil, MH, Shubin H. Accumulative prognostic index for patients with barbiturate, glutethimide and meprobamate intoxication. New Engl J Med 1971; 285; 1497–1502.

Rudowski WJ. Evaluation of modern plasma expanders and blood substitutes Br J Hosp Med 1980; 23:389–99.

Shubin H, Weil MH. Shock associated with barbiturate intoxication. J Am Med Assoc 1971; 215:263–8.

Thompson WL. Drug therapy of shock. In: Recent Advances in Clinical Pharmacology. Turner P, Shand DG. Eds. Edinburgh: Churchill Livingstone, 1978; 123–45.

Vohra J, Burrows GD. Cardiovascular complications of tricyclic antidepressant overdose. Drugs 1974; 8:432–7.

Chapter 7

G. M. Cochrane

Respiratory Complications and their Management in Self-Poisoned Patients

The majority of self-poisoning incidents are associated with the ingestion of hypnotic, sedative or psychotropic drugs which impair the level of consciousness and depress respiration. There is little information concerning the incidence of respiratory complications and death in self-poisoning. The one report which carefully analyses this problem refers only to patients severely poisoned following the ingestion of sedative drugs. Jay et al (1975) recorded a 77 per cent incidence of intubation and ventilation with nine deaths (4.6 per cent), eight of which were associated with progressive respiratory insufficiency; four of these had autopsy evidence of bacterial pneumonia. This study noted the relationship between high blood levels of drugs, hypotension, gastric aspiration and the occurrence of severe respiratory insufficiency and death.

The available data suggest that respiratory complications associated with self-poisoning may be due to one of the following:

1. A direct effect of the ingested or inhaled drugs on the respiratory system (Table 7.1).
2. Secondary effects of self-poisoning on the respiratory system (Table 7.2).
3. Problems associated with the treatment of the drug overdose (Table 7.3).

Table 7.1.   Direct effects of drug overdosage on the respiratory system.

Acute respiratory failure (e.g. barbiturates)

Pulmonary oedema due to inhalation of toxic chemicals and drugs (e.g. petroleum, arsine)

Acute pulmonary oedema with respiratory failure (e.g. aspirin, diamorphine)

Table 7.2.   Secondary effects of drug overdosage on the respiratory system.

Inhalation pneumonia

Hypostatic pneumonia

Pulmonary embolus

Progressive respiratory failure — acute respiratory distress syndrome

Table 7.3.   Respiratory complications associated with the treatment of patients with drug overdose.

Pulmonary oedema — fluid overload

Pneumothorax
- due to insertion of a central venous line
- collapse of left lung and right pneumothorax — due to intubation of the right main bronchus and positive pressure ventilation of this lung alone

Failed mechanical ventilation
- occlusion of airway
- ventilator failure or incorrect use of the ventilator

Direct Action of the Drug

Acute Respiratory Failure

Incidence

The incidence of acute respiratory failure is not known as a proportion of such deaths occur either before help is forthcoming or before admission to hospital. Furthermore, because many of these patients take a mixture of drugs, the cause of death is often difficult to determine.

Direct Action on the Respiratory Centre

Patients may die of acute respiratory failure after admission to hospital due to a direct action of the ingested drug on the respiratory centre. Such patients need not die because the respiratory failure may be corrected by intervention using either a specific antidote or supportive ventilation. Occasionally the drug, or drug combination, taken is not recognized as being a respiratory depressant. Rapid recognition of hypoventilation or an obstructed airway is important and can prevent death.

Airway Patency

The general principles of management of the airway and removal of foreign bodies have been dealt with in Chapter 4. It cannot be stressed too strongly that patency of the airway is essential in any severely poisoned patient. Secretions, or debris from vomiting, should be removed from the mouth, remembering that considerable haemorrhage may occur from the oropharyngeal lining if the epithelium is traumatized. An oropharyngeal airway should be inserted to prevent the tongue from falling backwards and occluding the airway. If a cough or gag reflex is present the airway is usually rejected rapidly, but if it is tolerated it suggests that the patient is deeply unconscious.

When the cough reflex is found to be suppressed completely a cuffed endotracheal tube should be inserted. The insertion of an endotracheal tube is not without hazards, but these usually occur either at the time of insertion or after extubation. The head should be slightly flexed during the insertion of the endotracheal tube to prevent pressure on the larynx, and the cuff should be deflated regularly for up to 10 minutes every two hours whenever possible. Intubation of the right main bronchus or right lower lobe has been reported in up to 10 per cent of severely poisoned patients requiring ventilation. Rapid recognition by both auscultation and by chest x-ray immediately after intubation will prevent collapse of the left lung or a right-sided pneumothorax.

Humidification of inspired air, with pre-warming in the case of the hypothermic patient, is essential to prevent drying of the airway and further body cooling. Careful bronchial toilet to remove secretions is necessary to prevent crusting of secretions and insidious airway obstruction.

Assessment of Adequate Ventilation

Assessment of the adequacy of ventilation remains a difficult problem: there is still no respiratory equivalent to the ECG in most hospitals. Not only is there a need to confirm adequate ventilation (movement of air in and out of the chest) but there is also the need to determine the efficiency of gas exchange. The simultaneous measurement of minute volume, respiratory rate and arterial blood gases is therefore required on admission to hospital.

Minute Volume. The minute volume may be measured easily using a Wright's spirometer, which is fitted either over the face using a closely fitting mask or by direct connection to the expiratory valve of an endotracheal tube. Although the addition of a dead space or direct facial stimulation may increase ventilation, a minute volume of less than 4 1/min. is almost always associated with respiratory depression.

Respiratory Rate. A very high respiratory rate, due to a drug-induced or metabolic acidosis, may lead to a high minute volume even though only the dead space may be ventilated. It is therefore wise to check the respiratory rate at the same time as the minute volume so that a crude index of alveolar ventilation may be calculated. Although anatomical dead space is about 150 ml, this is almost halved by the use of an endotracheal tube.

Arterial blood gases. Arterial blood gases should be measured in the deeply unconscious patient at the same time as the minute volume so that the two may then be related. It should be borne in mind that previous lung disease may lead to a greater fall in PaO_2 than would be anticipated from the minute volume. Reduced body metabolism can lead to a lower $PaCO_2$ than anticipated and there may be an even lower PaO_2 in patients with acute poisoning, especially when due to barbiturate overdose. Barbiturate poisoning is also unusual in that the respiratory rate increases initially until respiratory depression is severe and there is then a sudden fall in ventilatory rate with CO_2 retention, severe hypoxia and respiratory arrest.

Patients with respiratory depression who are known to have taken opium derivatives should be given intravenous naloxone, though this may have to be repeated because it has a comparatively short half-life, due to first pass metabolism, compared with the longer half-life of the opium alkaloids.

Frequency of assessment. Assessment of minute volume and respiratory rate should be repeated in deeply unconscious patients. The frequency of assessment should depend on the level of consciousness, the changes in minute volume and whether drugs are still being absorbed from the gut.

Ventilation Techniques

Oxygen therapy. It is impossible to give strict criteria for increasing inspired oxygen and applying intermittent positive pressure ventilation but the following approach is a useful guideline. In the presence of a reduced $PaCO_2$, but with values above 8kPa (60 mm Hg) and a $PaCO_2$ between 5.3 and 6.6 kPa (40—50 mm Hg, the inspired oxygen concentration should be increased to 24 per cent if the minute volume is above 4 litres. If after 30 minutes, repeat arterial blood gases demonstrate a persistently low PaO_2 with no rise in $PaCO_2$, 28 per cent inspired oxygen should be given. Thereafter, further incremental increases in the inspired oxygen concentration may be introduced in an attempt to raise the PaO_2 to 10.7 kPa (80 mm Hg) without increasing $PaCO_2$, and keeping the inspired oxygen concentration below 50 per cent. If this is not possible assisted ventilation should be considered.

Assisted ventilation. Assisted ventilation should be considered in any deeply unconscious patient with a minute volume below 4 litres, a PaO_2 below 8 kPa (60 mm Hg) (in the absence of a history of severe lung disease) or a $PaCO_2$ above 6.6 kPa (50 mm Hg). The purpose of assisted ventilation is to achieve near normal values for PaO_2 and $PaCO_2$, but it must be remembered that high inspired oxygen concentrations are toxic and a low $PaCO_2$ is associated with diminished cerebral blood flow. Anaesthetists are usually responsible for assisted ventilation but this does not allow the physician concerned to abdicate his reponsibility for the patient.

Ventilation Equipment

Patients are usually ventilated using a volume-cycled ventilator with facilities for warming and humidifying the inspired air, as well as those for increasing the inspired oxygen concentration. Most machines have the facility for applying positive end expiratory pressure (PEEP), a technique which stabilizes the small airways and prevents premature small airway closure, with consequent alveolar atelectasis and development of a pulmonary shunt. Positive end expiratory pressure has been shown to improve PaO_2 for any given inspired oxygen concentration and may therefore be used to avoid high inspired oxygen concentrations. PEEP may lead to decreased venous

return to the heart and a diminution in cardiac output. However, pressures of 5 to 10 cm of water do not usually lead to a significant fall in cardiac output while they can lead to substantial improvements in the PaO_2 (see below). Volume-cycled ventilators will administer a fixed tidal volume regardless of changes in compliance but an indication of changing compliance may be obtained from rising peak and mean inspiratory pressures. Increasing inspiratory pressures may be due to airflow obstruction following gastric inhalation, pulmonary oedema and pneumonia, and such changes may be the first indication of a deterioration in the patient's condition.

Inhalation of Toxic Chemicals and Drugs

Poisoning by inhalation is usually accidental rather than premeditated though the 'sniffing' of organic solvents is an exception. The effect of any such inhalation is related to the properties of the drug inhaled, whether it be a corrosive, an irritant or hot vapour. Death may occur from suffocation, or from the pharmacological properties of the vapour for example petrol (gasoline) and arsine. Many inhaled drugs cause pulmonary oedema and management then consists of supported ventilation because the effects are often only temporary.

Acute Pulmonary Oedema

Acute pulmonary oedema is usually associated with a tachypnoea and because of this patients with respiratory failure secondary to pulmonary oedema are often misdiagnosed. Many analgesics, notably aspirin in high doses, and acid (especially hydrochloric acid) fumes are associated with increased pulmonary capillary leak of filtrated serum into the interstitial space. If this leak is greater than the lymphatic drainage of the lung, which is often reduced in the presence of hypoventilation, pulmonary oedema will follow, not only with tachypnoea but also with a fall in PaO_2 and $PaCO_2$ gas tensions. In addition, cardiac output will decrease and there will be an increase in the core—peripheral temperature deficit. In these circumstances, the recognition of pulmonary oedema is sometimes difficult radiographically because upper lobe diversion is absent, as the cause is an alveolar capillary leak rather than left ventricular failure. The radiological recognition of pulmonary oedema may also be complicated when the chest x-ray is an anteroposterior film taken at a non-standardised distance in the supine position (compared with the normal erect PA film of 2 metres).

The treatment of pulmonary oedema is dealt with on page 56.

Secondary Effects of Drug Overdosage on the Respiratory System

Inhalation Pneumonia

Inhalation or aspiration of gastric contents (usually of a low pH) frequently occurs before patients arrive at hospital, but it may also occur because of active intervention following admission. Gastric aspiration is associated with a localized pneumonitis, often visible on chest x-ray, related to the position in which the patient was found (the most dependent portion of the lung being affected). Frequently severe airflow obstruction (either localized or generalized) is present and lung abscesses may occur despite antibiotic therapy. The frequency of inhalational pneumonia is considerably increased with combination drug poisoning and especially when alcohol has been ingested.

The effect of a chemical or bacterial pneumonitis associated with airflow obstruction is to reduce the PaO_2 which, in the presence of reduced respiratory drive due to sedative drugs, may lead to a critical fall in arterial oxygen saturation.

Unfortunately gastric aspiration, in some cases, follows medical intervention. Gastric lavage is indicated in certain self-poisoned patients (Chapter 4) but, in the absence of a cough reflex and in a patient who is in grade II or greater coma, this should not be performed without a cuffed endotracheal tube in situ. Frequently the endotracheal tube is removed following a stomach washout but, if it is easily tolerated, it should be left in place until assessment of ventilation is complete.

The treatment of gastric aspiration has seen many vogues, but there is evidence to suggest that the reduced PaO_2 should be dealt with in a manner as outlined above. Bronchospasm should be treated with 'asthma' size doses of steroids (4 mg/kg body weight of hydrocortisone 6-hourly for 24 hours and then 2 mg and 1 mg/kg body weight 6-hourly over the next 2 days). A broad-spectrum antibiotic such as ampicillin should be given intravenously for bacterial infection. Bronchodilator therapy with β_2 agonists such as salbutamol (albuterol), or a phosphodiesterase inhibitor such as aminophylline, may be given intravenously if bronchospasm is severe and persistent. If the pneumonia persists, as indicated by a raised temperature, a high white blood count and an abnormal chest x-ray, or if a lung abscess develops, then intravenous metronidazole should be added to the antibiotic regime. Benzylpenicillin has also been recommended by some authors in place of metronidazole in the treatment of anaerobic organisms and it has the advantage of being cheaper. In addition, postural drainage of any abscess cavity, suction and physiotherapy should be instituted.

Some workers believe that the gastric pH should be kept high in the unconscious patient to prevent some of the problems associated with aspiration and also to prevent or decrease gastric haemorrhage due to stress ulceration. This may be achieved with regular alkali medicines and/or the use of cimetidine.

Hypostatic Pneumonia

Secondary bacterial infection is common in patients with reduced levels of consciousness, though such infection is only partly caused by alveolar hypoventilation. Most hypnotic and antidepressant overdoses are associated with a diminution in the cough reflex and discoordinate breathing, with loss of normal sighing and periodic spontaneous large breaths. The basal atelectasis and sputum retention associated with this change in respiratory pattern lead to distal airway collapse and secondary bacterial invasion. Little is known about the depressant effect of hypnotics on the mucociliary escalator (the most important clearance mechanism of sputum for the distal airways). However, it is known that sleep considerably reduces clearance of particulate matter from distal airways and it is therefore assumed that sputum clearance is diminished in drug overdose, especially in those patients with reduced cough reflexes (the most important mechanism for clearing the large airways).

When patients have the clinical signs outlined above, together with radiographic changes in the lungs, broad-spectrum antibiotics should be given after blood cultures have been taken together with a urinary catheter specimen when indicated. Physiotherapy and regular turning of the patient tend to prevent hypostatic pneumonias. Bronchoscopic clearance of airways secretions has been recommended but unless there is radiological evidence of lobar collapse it is probably unhelpful.

Pulmonary Embolus

Pulmonary embolus is always a hazard in any hospitalized patient, especially when the patient is immobile. Furthermore, the practice of obtaining blood from the femoral artery for analysis of blood gases or electrolytes, especially in hypotensive patients, may lead to the development of femoral vein thrombosis. The close proximity of the femoral vein to the femoral artery means that heavy pressure applied to the arterial region can trap the femoral vein against the ischial bone. Unless, because of severe hypotension, it is absolutely essential to obtain blood from the femoral artery or vein, other vessels should be used. Arterial blood gases are easily obtained in most patients from the non-dominant radial artery and, if severe respiratory problems are envisaged, radial artery catheterization should be performed.

Progressive Respiratory Failure

Adult Respiratory Distress Syndrome (Table 7.4)

Progressive respiratory failure is a recognised cause of death in drug overdose and usually follows the development of the adult respiratory distress syndrome (ARDS). Although this syndrome has been recorded following any major assault on the human frame, it classically follows severe hypotension, especially when this is associated with gastric aspiration, orthopaedic trauma or severe drug overdose.

The syndrome consists of an event, e.g. trauma or overdose, followed 12 to 24 hours later by tachypnoea, defined as a respiratory rate of 20 to 45 per minute, increasing pulmonary infiltration on chest x-ray and falling PaO_2 tensions despite progressively increased inspired oxygen concentrations. Previously this syndrome was associated with a poor prognosis, due to progression to untreatable respiratory failure associated with a large right-to-left shunt and lungs so stiff that mechanical ventilation became impossible. Recently the prognosis has been improved considerably by early ventilation and careful management.

The mechanisms for the development of this syndrome are still disputed, but there is evidence to support a multifactorial theory once the initial assault has occurred. Severe hypotension and diminished cerebral perfusion have been shown to lead to a marked temporary rise in pulmonary venous pressure with diminished pulmonary capillary blood flow. The rise in pulmonary venous pressure may be associated with increased pulmonary capillary leak, a factor which is worse after gastric aspiration. Some workers have demonstrated a marked increase in platelet aggregation in the pulmonary capillary circulation with local thrombotic phenomena and the release of vasoactive substances which results in an increased loss of filtrated serum and leakage of albumin

Table 7.4. Clinical features of the adult respiratory distress syndrome.

Severe drug overdose 12–24 hours previously

Tachypnoea — respiratory rate greater than 25/minute

'Stiff lung' (high inspiratory pressure on ventilation)

Progressive pulmonary infiltration on chest x-ray

Falling PaO_2 despite increased concentrations of inspired oxygen (F_iO_2)

and large protein molecules. The increase in pulmonary interstitial water, as a result of this loss of fluid and protein, floods alveoli and compresses small airways. In turn, this leads to atelectasis of the dependent lung with a further fall in gas exchange. The presence of albumin in the interstitial space increases the local oncotic pressure and may lead to further increases in the net flow of fluid into the interstitial space.

Treatment of Respiratory Failure

Respiratory failure associated with the above syndrome develops rapidly and should be treated early with intermittent positive pressure ventilation with positive end expiratory pressure. The means by which PEEP is effective are not fully understood but it may prevent small airways from collapsing and, by maintaining patient airways and alveoli, increase lymphatic drainage. High inspired concentrations of oxygen are toxic as they diminish surfactant production, lead to alveolar atelectasis and, in concentrations of 60 per cent or more, lead to oxygen pneumonitis. The addition of PEEP (5 to 10 cm H_2O) is often a safer method of increasing PaO_2 than increasing the inspired oxygen concentration. Unfortunately the former is not always possible because PEEP may lead to a reduced cardiac output which is unacceptable in a patient whose cardiovascular system is already embarrassed. Moreover, high circulating blood volumes or left ventricular failure increase pulmonary interstitial volume and lead to further falls in PaO_2. Large volumes of intravenous crystalloids may therefore exacerbate the degree of respiratory failure and, at the same time, colloids may leak from the pulmonary circulation early in the syndrome and make the pulmonary oedema worse by their extravascular oncotic action. In these circumstances moderate cystalloid replacement with plasma expanders, or whole blood if the haemoglobin is reduced, is preferred.

Careful fluid balance using, where necessary, both CVP and pulmonary arterial lines with left atrial wedge pressure measurement, improves the prognosis considerably because a balance between cardiac output, left atrial filling pressures and total fluid volume load (CVP) may be determined.

Diuretics may be useful if fluid overload occurs. The use of steroids is controversial. There is evidence to support their use after inhalation, but large doses of methylprednisolone have not been shown to improve dramatically the prognosis for adult respiratory distress syndrome, and they are therefore indicated only for associated bronchospasm. As ventilation may be required for some days after respiratory failure, parenteral feeding may need to be instituted. Antibiotics should be given in the presence of purulent sputum, fever and a raised white count. Meticulous care of fluid balance, electrolyte balance and nursing of the unconscious patient are all essential and improve the prognosis. Less than 15 per cent of patients with severe progressive respiratory failure should now die.

Respiratory Complications Associated with the Treatment of Patients with Drug Overdose (Table 7.3)

Many of the complications associated with the management of the severely poisoned unconscious patient have already been mentioned but a number require further comment.

Pulmonary Oedema

Fluid overload in the absence of an adequate diuresis will lead to pulmonary oedema. In addition to the causes described earlier in this chapter, it should be remembered that, in patients with a raised blood urea, there is a tendency for an increased loss of sodium ions to occur across the capillary endothelium. This sodium leak is accompanied by water and thus, in patients with acute renal dysfunction, pulmonary oedema may occur at comparatively low left atrial pressures. In patients with acute renal failure following drug overdose, careful fluid balance (and, if necessary, the measurement of left atrial wedge pressure, cardiac output and filling pressures) helps to prevent and control pulmonary oedema.

Pneumothorax

Pneumothorax is associated with drug overdose but it is rarely an effect of the drug itself and is far more commonly a complication of therapy. Pneumothorax is associated with the inaccurate insertion of subclavian or external jugular central venous lines, with perforation of the visceral pleura. The other common iatrogenic cause of a pneumothorax is intubation of the right main bronchus, a mistake easily made when a long endotracheal tube is used in the supine patient. Intubation of the right main bronchus leads to collapse of the left lung, while positive pressure ventilation of the right main bronchus or the right lower lobe bronchus can lead to pneumothorax. Clearly, if a pneumothorax occurs and IPPV is required, both withdrawal of the endotracheal tube to the midtrachea and insertion of an underwater chest drain are required because without the latter a tension pneumothorax may easily develop.

Failed Mechanical Ventilation

The use of pressure-cycled ventilators in poisoned patients can lead to significant hypoventilation as a result of changes in lung compliance that follow the development of fluid overload or pulmonary oedema. Tidal volumes, therefore, may be reduced even though the pre-set ventilator pressure is attained. Failed ventilation may also occur as a result of an occluded airway and because of machine failure. Occlusion of the airway may follow a change in the position of the patient or because of sputum plugging the endotracheal tube. Care of the airways is just as essential when the patient is on a ventilator as when the patient is breathing spontaneously. Deaths occur when the assumption is made that attachment to a mechanical pump is a foolproof way of maintaining ventilation: this is not the case!

Sublaryngeal Stricture

A comparatively late complication of IPPV with endotracheal intubation is the development of a sublaryngeal stricture following excessive pressure of a cuffed endotracheal tube. This complication rarely occurs before three months, although acute laryngeal oedema following extubation can occur and is associated with stridor; re-intubation or even tracheostomy may be required. Previously arbitrary time limits were accepted for the period for which an endotracheal tube should remain in place, as the incidence of sublaryngeal stricture following prolonged intubation (greater than seven days) was high. However, the introduction of softer latex cuffs has diminished the need for prophylactic tracheostomy.

Patients who complain of breathlessness and who have previously had either prolonged intubation or a tracheostomy should be screened for inspiratory airways obstruction by measuring the mean inspiratory and expiratory mid-vital capacity flow rates during a maximal respiratory flow volume manoeuvre. Patients with sublaryngeal stenosis have reduced inspiratory flow rates compared with normal patients, whose expiratory flow rates are less than the inspiratory flow rates. Sublaryngeal stenosis is surgically correctable.

References

Jay SJ, Johanson WG Jr, Pierce AK. Respiratory complications of overdose with sedative drugs. Am Rev Respir Dis 1975; 112:591−8.

Further Reading

Beyer A. Shock lung. Br J Hosp Med 1979; 21:248−58.

Benowitz NL, Rosenberg J, Becker CE. Cardiopulmonary catastrophes in drug overdosed patients. Med Clin North Am 1979; 63:267−96.

Burton GG, Gee GN, Hodgkin JE. Eds. Respiratory Care − A Guide to Clinical Practice. Philadelphia: Lippincott, 1977.

Glauser FL, Miller JE, Falls R. Effects of acid aspiration on pulmonary alveolar epithelial membrane permeability. Chest 1979; 76:201−5.

Murrary HW. Antimicrobial therapy in pulmonary aspiration. Am J Med 1979; 66:188−90.

Rees PJ, Higgenbottam TW, Clark TJH. Use of a single pair of magnetometer coils to monitor breathing patterns in an intensive care unit. Thorax 1980; 35:384−88.

Shibel EM, Moser KM. Eds. Respiratory Emergencies. St. Louis: CV Mosby, 1977.

Snashall PD. Pulmonary oedema. Br J Dis Chest 1980; 74: 2−22.

Chapter 8

J. A. Vale and T. J. Meredith

Forced Diuresis, Dialysis and Haemoperfusion

The colour plates cited in this Chapter are to be found between pages 188 and 189.

The majority of poisoned patients recover with little more than nursing care though a small proportion (about 10 per cent) require intensive supportive measures to maintain vital functions. In very few patients are methods to increase drug elimination either feasible or appropriate and such measures are obviously contraindicated if specific antidotes are available. Nonetheless, "poisoned patients are often subjected to unnecessary and potentially harmful haemodialysis and forced diuresis. Unfortunately, there are few instances in which these measures have clearly been shown to reduce morbidity and mortality, and much of the information on which claims for efficacy have been based is either inadequate or invalid . . . Clinicians seeem to have an irresistible urge to carry out some form of treatment on their patients, and this is particularly so for an unconscious patient whose relatives may be clamouring for something to be done. In practice, there are few indications for the use of haemodialysis and forced diuresis to accelerate the removal of drugs in poisoned patients". (Prescott 1974). The latter statement would also apply to the use of haemoperfusion.

Inappropriate Use of Methods of Drug Elimination

Most drugs taken in overdose are extensively detoxified by the liver to produce inactive metabolites which are voided in the urine. Sometimes hepatic degradation produces active metabolites, as in the case of some of the tricyclic antidepressants and phenothiazines, but the secondary compounds are then converted to non-toxic derivatives. Under these circumstances, forced diuresis is inappropriate.

Dialysis and haemoperfusion are of little value in the treatment of patients who have ingested drugs with large volumes of distribution, such as the tricyclic antidepressants, since the plasma contains only a small proportion of the total amount of drug in the body and the rate of transfer from the tissues to the plasma is often very slow. Moreover, the amount of drug removed from the plasma is negligible compared to that eliminated by the liver.

Renal Excretion of Poisons

The two main ways in which unchanged poisons are handled by the kidneys are as follows:

1. *Passive glomerular filtration.* Only that fraction of a drug which is non-protein-bound is filtered in this way.

2. *Passive tubular diffusion.* Drugs may also be eliminated by passive diffusion across the epithelium of the tubule into the lumen. Theoretically this process can occur in both directions. However, as water is progressively reabsorbed from the tubular fluid as it passes distally, a favourable concentration gradient is created for the reabsorption of dissolved substances back into the bloodstream.

Forced Diuresis

Rationale

Most drugs are weak electrolytes which, at the physiological pH, exist partly as undissociated molecules.

The extent of ionization is a function of the ionization constant of the drug (Ka for both acids and bases) and the pH of the medium in which it is dissolved. Ionization constants are usually expressed in the form of their negative logarithm, pKa. Hence the pKa scale is analogous to the pH notation: the stronger an acid the lower its pKa and the stronger a base the higher its pKa. The relationship between pKa and the proportion of total drug in ionized form is represented by the Henderson—Hasselbalch equation:

$$\text{For weak acids pH--pKa} = \log \frac{\text{(Ionized drug)}}{\text{(Non-ionized drug)}}$$

$$\text{For weak bases pH--pKa} = \log \frac{\text{(Non-ionized drug)}}{\text{(Ionized drug)}}$$

Thus, when pKa = pH, the concentrations of ionized and non-ionized drug are equal.

Cell membranes are most permeable to substances that are lipid soluble and in the non-ionized, rather than the ionized, form. Thus, the rate of diffusion from the renal tubular lumen back into the circulation is decreased when a drug is maximally ionized. Because ionization of weak acids is increased in an alkaline environment, and that of basic drugs is increased in an acid solution, manipulation of the urinary pH enhances renal excretion. For acidic drugs there is a greater degree of ionization at pH 8 than 7.4 and for the basic drugs a greater degree at pH 6 than at 7.4. Thus, elimination of weak acids by the kidneys is increased in alkaline urine if the pKa (negative logarithm of the ionization constant) of the drug concerned lies in the range 3.0 to 7.5 for weak bases; elimination is increased in acid urine if the pKa of the drug lies in the range 7.5 to 10.5.

Forced diuresis will be effective if the following criteria apply:

1. A substantial proportion of the drug is excreted in the toxic and unchanged form, that is, it is not metabolized.

2. The drug is distributed mainly in the extracellular fluid.

3. The drug is minimally protein-bound.

The elimination of salicylates (pKa 3.5) and phenobarbitone (pKa 7.4) is increased by forced alkaline diuresis. Forced acid diuresis, which is very rarely employed, has a role only in the treatment of severe acute amphetamine, quinine, fenfluramine and phencyclidine poisoning.

As the procedure of forced diuresis is potentially harmful it should be considered only in moderately to severely poisoned patients. In assessing the need for forced diuresis it is important to take the clinical state into account as well as the plasma drug levels.

Technique

The state of hydration together with the renal, respiratory and cardiac function of the patient must be assessed and, if necessary, improved prior to commencing forced diuresis. Blood should be drawn for a base-line estimation of electrolytes, urea, blood sugar, drug level(s), arterial blood gases and pH. The urine pH should also be measured. A central venous pressure line is extremely useful in management and, in the first hour, 1500 ml fluid should be given intravenously as follows:

1. Forced alkaline diuresis: 500 ml 5 per cent dextrose
500 ml 1.2 or 1.4 per cent sodium bicarbonate
500 ml 5 per cent dextrose

2. Forced acid diuresis: 1000 ml 5 per cent dextrose
500 ml 0.9 per cent sodium chloride
10 g arginine or lysine hydrochloride i.v. over 30 minutes

From the outset potassium should be added to each 500 ml bag or bottle in a dose of 1 g potassium chloride [13.5 mmol (mEq)], adjusting this amount in relation to the plasma potassium levels. Bolus injections of frusemide (20 mg i.v.) may be needed to initiate and maintain an adequate urine flow.

The above sequence of infusions should be continued at such a rate that a urine flow of at least 500 ml per hour is achieved; a much higher urine flow rate is unnecessary and may be harmful. If less than 200 ml urine is produced in the first hour the diuresis should be discontinued and the patient reassessed to ensure that renal impairment is not present; dehydration is more likely in a younger patient.

The urine pH should be measured regularly (every 15 to 30 minutes) and for alkaline diuresis the urine pH should be maintained in the range 7.5 to 8.5 by adjusting the quantity of bicarbonate given. As much as 200 mmol (mEq) bicarbonate may be required in the first two hours of diuresis to achieve adequate alkalinization. This is important as little excretion of salicylate, for example, will occur unless the pH is in the correct range, no matter how profuse the diuresis. Care should also be taken to check the plasma pH at least two-hourly to ensure that it does not rise above 7.6. The plasma and urinary electrolytes are measured at the same time. For forced acid diuresis the urine pH should be maintained between 5.5 and 6.5 by giving oral ammonium chloride (4 g two-hourly).

The exact composition and amount of the fluid given intravenously must be adjusted in accordance with the patient's clinical and biochemical state. Volume requirements depend on changes in the central venous pressure and in the urine volume. Fluid intake and output should be recorded accurately. The indications and procedure for forced diuresis are shown in Figure 8.1, and the efficacy of forced alkaline diuresis is illustrated in Figures 8.2 and 8.3.

Contraindications and Complications

Forced diuresis should never be undertaken lightly as it is potentially hazardous in the elderly, in patients with cardiac and renal disease and in those who are 'shocked'. Well recognized complications include pulmonary oedema, water intoxication, cerebral oedema and electrolyte and acid–base disturbances. Unfortunately no record exists of the incidence of serious misadventures, though observation indicates it to be high. With care these complications can be minimized but this requires the co-operation of experienced medical, nursing and laboratory staff and, above all, the resources of an intensive care unit.

Dialysis

Peritoneal Dialysis

Although widely available, peritoneal dialysis is less effective than haemodialysis for the removal of

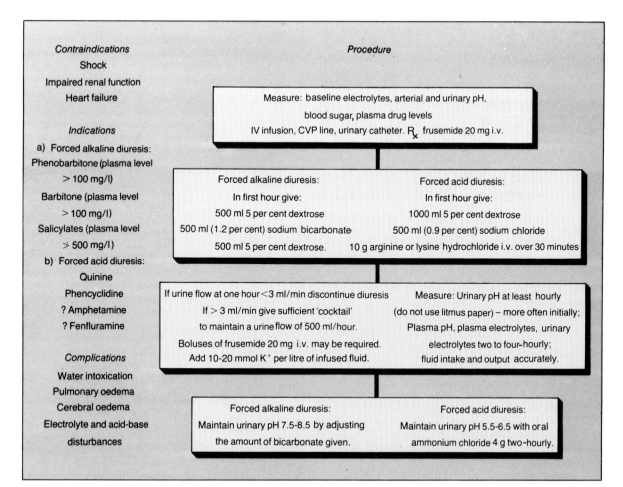

Figure 8.1. *Forced diuresis.*

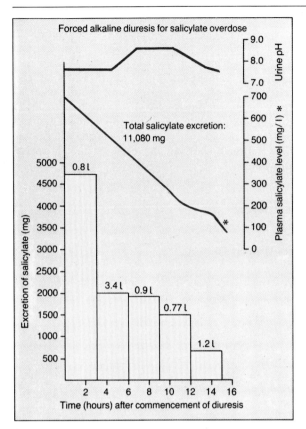

Figure 8.2. *Forced alkaline diuresis for salicylate overdose.*

poisons and, since the delivery of toxins to the peritoneum is dependent on blood flow rate, the efficiency of this technique is further reduced in the presence of hypotension. Peritoneal dialysis, therefore, has a very limited application, perhaps only in patients poisoned with lithium salts and ethylene glycol, though in the case of lithium, haemodialysis is more effective.

Haemodialysis

Haemodialysis was first used in 1913 for the removal of salicylic acid in experimental poisoning but was not applied clinically until 1950 when it was used for the treatment of aspirin poisoning. It was widely employed during the following two decades and, as a result, there are many reports of its apparent value in the treatment of acute poisoning (Winchester et al. 1977). Many of these accounts, however, are

little more than anecdotal, or even self-adulatory on the part of the authors. They often suffer from a dearth of analytical observations to support the published conclusions. Prescott (1974) has examined data purporting to demonstrate the efficacy of haemodialysis and has shown that this method of treatment has often been carried out in patients who have had less than therapeutic plasma concentrations of a drug, or that amounts equivalent to little more than one tablet have been removed.

Rationale for Dialysis

Schreiner (1958) stated that any substance should have the following characteristics before haemodialysis is employed:

1. It should diffuse easily through a dialysis membrane.

2. A significant proportion of the substance should be present in plasma water or capable of rapid equilibration with it.

3. The pharmacological effect should be directly related to the blood concentration.

4. Dialysis must add significantly to other body mechanisms of elimination.

These criteria have been further defined by Gibson and Nelson (1977) and the following properties of a substance should be known: molecular weight and volume, water solubility, protein binding, inherent plasma clearance and dialyser clearance. Even if a substance is known to be dialysable the criteria outlined below for haemoperfusion should be applied to decide whether or not to proceed with dialysis.

Haemodialysis is the treatment of choice in severe poisoning due to lithium and methyl and ethyl alcohol. Although this technique also effectively removes phenobarbitone, barbitone and salicylates, patients poisoned with these agents may be treated more simply by forced alkaline diuresis. Only rarely, therefore, is haemodialysis indicated for overdoses of these drugs unless the patient's condition is aggravated by concurrent renal impairment. Short-acting barbiturates and non-barbiturate hypnotics, which account for the majority of drug deaths in Great Britain, are not amenable to haemodialysis because of their high lipid solubility. An alternative means of removing poisons from the circulating blood and tissues has therefore been investigated.

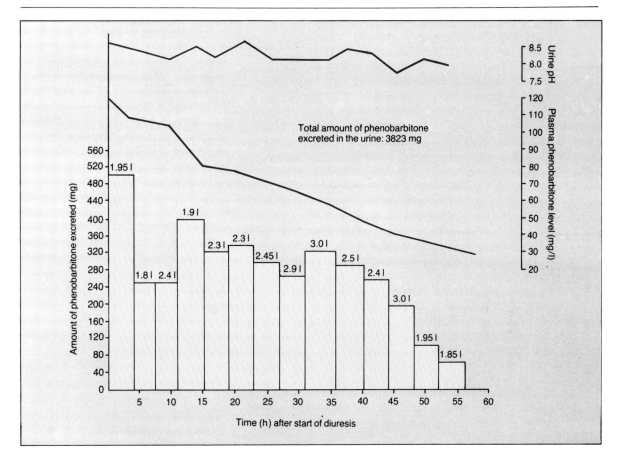

Figure 8.3. *Forced alkaline diuresis for phenobarbitone overdose.*

Haemoperfusion

Principle and Development

Haemoperfusion involves the passage of blood through devices containing adsorbent particles, e.g. activated charcoal, anion resins and uncharged resins such as Amberlite XAD-2 and XAD-4, to which drugs are adsorbed by surface forces.

In 1965, Yatzidis and his colleagues in Greece perfused the blood of two patients poisoned by barbiturates through an uncoated charcoal system. Although good drug removal was achieved a number of complications ensued including charcoal embolism, marked thrombocytopenia, fibrinogen loss and pyrogen reactions. Attempts were subsequently made

to eliminate these adverse effects by coating the carbon with a biocompatible polymer. Chang (1973) utilized cellulose nitrate and albumin as a coating and successfully perfused three patients. Vale et al. (1975) perfused 20 patients using a polyhydroxyethylmethacrylate coated carbon device, and this system has now been made available commercially in the form of the 'Haemacol' system (Table 8.1, **Plate 52**). Other devices marketed more recently include one containing cellulose acetate coated carbon ('Adsorba 300 C'), another utilizing uncoated carbon affixed to a polyester film, wound into a spiral coil and encased in a polycarbonate housing (Becton and Dickinson 'Hemo-detoxification' system), and charcoal columns manufactured in Italy and Japan (see Table 8.1, **Plate 52**).

In the early 1960s several workers investigated the

Table 8.1. Commercially available haemoperfusion devices. Each column costs £100—150.

Name of device	Manufacturer	Adsorbent	Coating
Adsorba 300c	Gambro	300g charcoal	Cellulose acetate
Haemacol	Smith & Nephew	300g charcoal	Polyhydroxyethylmethacrylate
Haemacol	Smith & Nephew	100g charcoal	Polyhydroxyethylmethacrylate
Hemo-detoxification system	B & D	87g charcoal	None
Euroadsorb	Biotec (Italy)	300g charcoal	Acrylic hydrogel
DHD—1	Kuraray (Japan)	160g charcoal	Polyhydroxyethylmethacrylate
ROO 4—haemoperfusion cartridge	Extracorporeal	650g XAD—4 resin	None

use of anion-exchange resins in an attempt to reduce or eliminate the haematological and other adverse effects which were common with uncoated charcoal devices. Complications persisted, however, but more recently Rosenbaum (1976) perfected a resin system using Amberlite XAD-4 and a cartridge containing 650 g XAD-4 has now been released for clinical use (Table 8.1) (Plate 52).

Contraindications to Haemoperfusion

Haemoperfusion is contraindicated or inappropriate if:

1. An antidote is available.

2. The toxic substance is a rapidly acting metabolic poison.

3. The substance is irreversibly acting, e.g. an organophosphorus insecticide.

4. The drug ingested is relatively non-toxic, e.g. a benzodiazepine.

5. The drug has a very large volume of distribution.

Indications for Haemoperfusion

The indications for haemoperfusion are based on general, clinical and biochemical considerations.

General Considerations

The main general considerations are as follows:

1. The toxic substance should be readily adsorbed onto charcoal or resin (Table 8.2).

2. A significant proportion of the substance should be present in plasma water or capable of rapid equilibration with it.

3. The pharmacological effect should be directly related to the blood concentration.

4. Haemoperfusion must add significantly to other body mechanisms of elimination.

Table 8.2. Drugs significantly adsorbed by charcoal.

All barbiturates
Ethchlorvynol
Glutethimide
Meprobamate
Methaqualone
Trichloroethanol derivatives
Ethyl alcohol
Salicylates
Theophylline

Clinical Considerations

Although the overall mortality of poisoned patients is low, that of patients in Grade IV coma ranges from 5 to 40 per cent. Based on this consideration the following criteria for haemoperfusion were agreed by a multi-centre group in Great Britain in 1974. A patient should meet three of the following criteria:

1. Be severely poisoned – as shown by, for example, Grade IV coma, hypotension, hypothermia, hypoventilation.

2. Show evidence of progressive clinical deterioration despite good supportive management.

3. Show no evidence of clinical improvement despite full resuscitative measures.

4. Have developed complications such as pneumonia, septicaemia, shock lung.

5. Have a high plasma drug level.

Biochemical Considerations (Table 8.3)

Haemoperfusion Technique

An arteriovenous shunt or a double lumen venous catheter is inserted into the patient's vascular tree. The haemoperfusion column and lines are primed with heparinized saline in accordance with the manufacturer's instructions and connected to the shunt or catheter. On commencement of perfusion a bolus of heparin is injected into the arterial line and heparinization is continued by administering an infusion of heparinized saline. The haemoperfusion circuit is shown diagrammatically in Figure 8.4 and in clinical use in Figure 8.5.

Table 8.3. Biochemical criteria for haemoperfusion.

The patient should have plasma drug levels not less than:

Phenobarbitone and barbitone	100 mg/l
Other barbiturates	50 mg/l
Glutethimide	40 mg/l
Methaqualone	40 mg/l
Salicylates	800 mg/l
Ethchlorvynol	150 mg/l
Meprobamate	100 mg/l
Trichloroethanol derivatives	50 mg/l
Theophylline	60 mg/l

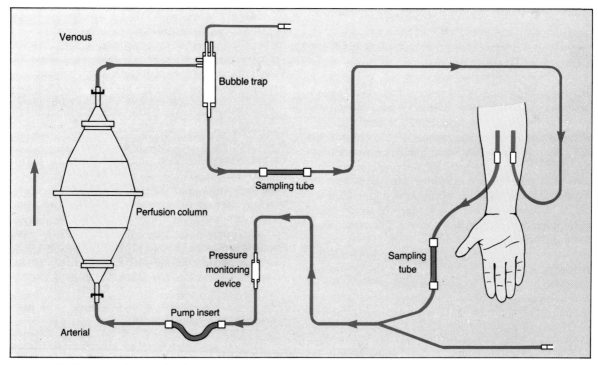

Figure 8.4. *Haemoperfusion circuit.*

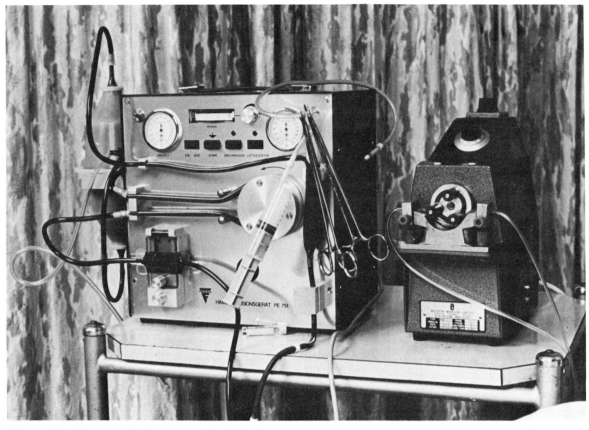

Figure 8.5. *Haemoperfusion system in clinical use.*

Efficacy of Haemoperfusion

Between 1973 and 1980 more than 60 severely poisoned patients were haemoperfused at Guy's Hospital following the ingestion of hypnotic drugs, theophylline, aspirin and paraquat. Clearance data are shown in Table 8.4. Haemoperfusion will reduce the time taken by a severely poisoned patient to recover consciousness following the ingestion of hypnotic drugs such as barbiturates, glutethimide, methaqualone, ethchlorvynol, meprobamate and trichloroethanol derivatives. As a result, complications such as pneumonia and shock lung develop less frequently and not only the morbidity but also the mortality can be expected to fall in this group of patients.

In all cases the plasma drug clearances achieved by haemoperfusion (Table 8.4) were superior to those obtained through haemodialysis, particularly for short- and medium-acting barbiturates and non-barbiturate hypnotics. When used for the treatment of poisoning due to long-acting barbiturates, haemo-

Table 8.4.   Efficacy of charcoal haemoperfusion

Drug	Clearance[1] (ml/min)	Amount removed (mg)
Amylobarbitone	80 (50–122)	2558 (567–7290)
Butobarbitone	72 (48–120)	1829 (375–4316)
Ethchlorvynol	124	3472
Glutethimide	125	1413
Meprobamate	153	2367
Methaqualone	100	976
Pentobarbitone	57 (50–63)	2823 (1590–4057)
Phenobarbitone	77 (44–120)	5256 (1302–7710)
Quinalbarbitone	68 (45–101)	1227 (312–2416)
Paraquat	125 (70–250)	96 (8–280)
Theophylline	97	920

[1] Blood flow 200–300 ml/min

perfusion is more efficient than forced diuresis and equally as efficient but less expensive and less complex than haemodialysis. In addition this technique may have an important diagnostic role to play in patients who are unconscious following a cardio-respiratory arrest and who have only moderately high plasma drug levels for which haemoperfusion would not normally be undertaken.

Complications of Haemoperfusion

The complications are summarized in Table 8.5. The haematological and biochemical effects are considered in greater detail below.

Haematological Effects

During perfusion there is a fall of approximately 30 per cent in the platelet count and a fall of up to 10 per cent in the leucocyte count, both of which are maximal within the first hour; thereafter the counts return to normal values. These reductions are similar to those seen during other extracorporeal procedures such as haemodialysis and cardiac-bypass surgery. Two mechanisms have been postulated to explain the thrombocytopenia:

1. The loss and possible destruction of platelets in the extracorporeal circuit. When blood comes into contact with the extracorporeal system ADP and serotonin are released and result in platelet aggregation. 'Sticky' platelets are removed in the first few minutes after perfusion has commenced and no further fall in the platelet count occurs if the lines and perfusion column are changed during the haemo-perfusion procedure. Moreover, it is known that platelet adhesiveness does fall during perfusion.
2. The reversible sequestration of platelets in the liver and possibly the spleen.

In addition to these two factors it is known that the degree of thrombocytopenia depends also on the rate of blood flow, the presence or absence, type and thickness of the carbon coating in the perfusion system and the type of adsorbent material used in the haemoperfusion column. The fall that occurs in platelet count may be reduced by the administration of sulphinpyrazone and prostacyclin. Aspirin does not appear to be protective in this respect.

Biochemical Effects

No biochemical changes of clinical significance occur, though sometimes there is a fall in the plasma glucose level on commencing haemoperfusion with the Becton and Dickinson system. Transient hypo-calcaemia has been reported in one patient but tetany did not occur. Small falls in plasma urate, urea, creatinine, bilirubin, phosphate and cholesterol levels have also been seen.

Conclusion

Whilst there is no substitute for supportive treatment there is, nonetheless, a small group of very severely poisoned patients in whom some active means of removing the drug or toxic chemical ingested is advantageous. Forced diuresis and peritoneal dialysis have limited clinical application and haemodialysis does not increase the elimination of short- and medium-acting barbiturates and the non-barbiturate hypnotics. Haemoperfusion, however, reduces both the morbidity and mortality in poisoning due to these drugs.

Table 8.5.   Complications of haemoperfusion.

Haemorrhage because of heparinization
Patient may disconnect shunt lines
Air embolism
Infection
Loss of peripheral artery
Thrombocytopenia, leucopenia
Loss of clotting factors
$Ca^{++}\downarrow$ Glucose$\downarrow$ Urea$\downarrow$ Creatinine$\downarrow$ Urate$\downarrow$

References

General

Prescott LF. Limitations of haemodialysis and forced diuresis. In: The Poisoned Patient: The Role of the Laboratory. Ciba Foundation symposium No. 26. North Holland: Excerpta Medica, 1974; 269–82.
Schreiner GE. The role of haemodialysis in acute poisoning. Arch Intern Med 1958; 102:896–913.
Winchester JF, Gelfand MC, Knepshield JH, Schreiner GE. Dialysis and haemoperfusion of poisons and drugs – update. Trans Am Soc Artif Intern Organs 1977; 23:762–842.

Pharmacokinetics and Drug Elimination

Gibson TP, Nelson HA. Drug kinetics and artificial kidneys. Clin Pharmacokinet 1977; 2:403–26.

Haemoperfusion

Chang TMS, Coffey JF, Barre P, Gonda A, Dirks JH, Levy M, Lister C. Microcapsule artificial kidney: treatment of patients with acute drug intoxication. Can Med Assoc J 1973; 108: 429–33.

Rosenbaum JL, Kramer MS, Raja R. Resin haemoperfusion for acute drug intoxication. Arch Intern Med 1976; 136: 263–6.

Vale JA, Thomas T, Widdop B, Goulding R. Use of charcoal haemoperfusion in poisoned patients: review of 20 cases. Pro Eur Soc Artif Organs 1975; 2:239–44.

Yatzidis H, Voudiclari S, Oreopoulos D, Tsaparas N, Triantaphyllidis D, Gavras C, et al. Treatment of severe barbiturate poisoning. Lancet 1965; ii:216–7.

Further Reading

General

Anonymous. When may eliminating poison save life? Drug. Therap Bull 1980; 18:41–42.

Pharmacokinetics and Drug Elimination

Pond S, Rosenberg J, Benowitz NL, Takki S. Pharmacokinetics of haemoperfusion for drug overdose. Clin Pharmacokinet 1979; 4:329–354.

Takki S, Gambertoglio JG, Honda DH, Tozer TN. Pharmacokinetic evaluation of haemodialysis in acute drug overdose. J Pharmacokinet Biopharm 1978; 6:427–42.

Tristone WJ, Winchester JF, Reavey PC. The use of pharmacokinetic principles in determining the effectiveness of removal of toxins from blood. Clin Pharmacokinet 1979; 4:23–37.

Haemoperfusion

Chang TMS Ed. Artificial Kidney, Artificial Liver and Artificial Cells. New York: Plenum Press. 1978.

De Groot G, Maes RAA, Van Heyst ANP. The use of haemoperfusion in the elimination of absorbed drug mixtures in acute intoxications. Neth J. Med 1977; 20:142–8.

Hampel G, Widdop B, Goulding R. Adsorptive capacities of haemoperfusion devices in clinical use. Artif Organs 1978; 2:363–6.

Hampel G, Crome P, Widdop B, Goulding R. Experience with fixed-bed charcoal haemoperfusion in the treatment of severe drug intoxication. Arch Toxicol 1980; 45:133–141.

Kenedi RM, Courtney JM, Gaylor JDS, Gilchrist T. Artificial Organs. London: Macmillan 1977.

Rosenbaum JL, Kramer MS, Raja MM. Haemoperfusion in the treatment of acute drug intoxication. Int J. Artif. Organs 1979; 2:316–8.

Torrente A de, Rumack BH, Blair DT, Anderson RJ. Fixed-bed uncoated charcoal haemoperfusion in the treatment of intoxications: Animal and patient studies. Nephron 1979; 24:71–7.

Winchester JF, Gelfand MC. Haemoperfusion in drug intoxication: clinical and laboratory aspects. Drug Metab Rev 1978; 8:69–104.

Chapter 9

Ramon Gardner

Psychiatric Aspects of Poisoning

Aspects of Poisoning

Self-poisoning by a deliberate overdose of drugs now accounts for about 15 per cent of all acute medical emergencies. Once such patients reach hospital few of them die. Most patients are given a stomach wash-out and, though some of them are then sent home and others discharge themselves from the accident department, most are admitted to general medical or even to surgical wards: few hospitals have a special poisons unit. After a psychiatric assessment, about one in five patients is recommended for treatment in a psychiatric ward, and as this is almost invariably on an informal basis, less than one per cent of all self-poisoned patients are detained under a section of the Mental Health Act. Most patients are discharged back into the community within 48 hours. Altogether about half of all the patients coming to hospital with self-poisoning are offered further psychiatric treatment and after-care.

Although they may have taken an overdose of drugs on impulse, perhaps after a family or marital quarrel, self-poisoned patients are a very high-risk group with respect to suicide. Within a year, 1 to 2 percent of such patients will have killed themselves compared to only 8 to 10 persons in 100,000 of the general population.

Risk Factors

Several lines of research have enabled us to recognize the sort of people who are most likely to commit suicide. Official mortality figures indicate that they are often men aged 40 or more in professional or managerial occupations, who are single, widowed, separated or divorced. In the UK the overall suicide rate has declined, but an increasing proportion of elderly women as well as men from unskilled occupations are killing themselves. There is also a rising suicide rate among young people and this is the fourth most common cause of death in the 15 to 34-year-old age group. Social factors are of great importance in contributing to suicide and research carried out by Sainsbury (1955) has shown that the socially isolated are most vulnerable.

Psychiatric illness

Retrospective studies suggest that nearly all known suicides are suffering from psychiatric illness. Robins et al. (1959) in the United States and Barraclough et al. (1974) in the UK interviewed the relatives, friends and doctors of consecutive cases of suicide soon after the event and found that over 90 per cent of the dead persons had had a psychiatric disorder (Table 9.1). About two-thirds of the suicides had been depressed. The majority had sought medical help within the three months prior to their death and in some cases the depression had been missed. It is well

Table 9.1.   Psychiatric diagnosis in American (A) and British (B) suicide studies.

Diagnosis	A	B
No mental illness	3	7
Depression	60	70
Alcoholism	31	15
Schizophrenia	3	3
Other	37	5
Total no. of suicides	134	100

documented that patients with a diagnosis of manic—depressive psychosis are liable to commit suicide at the onset of a depressive illness or within six months of being treated in hospital. The depressed person who lives by himself, particularly if he has been subject to a recent life change such as bereavement, marital separation or retirement, is much more likely to end his life than a person with a comparable degree of depression who is living with somebody else.

Alcoholism

In both the American and the British studies alcoholics were the second largest group to have committed suicide. Those who had a physical complication derived from their excessive drinking or had experienced a recent stressful life event were most susceptible.

Other Factors

Other persons who are liable to take their own lives include some schizophrenics, a few persons who are developing dementia and yet retain insight into their mental deterioration, and some elderly persons who realize that they have a fatal physical condition. There is an increased risk of suicide in epilepsy, and suicide also occurs in childhood, though it is rare in children under the age of 10 (Toolan 1962; Shaffer 1974). Any study of completed suicides contains examples of unstable personalities who have lacked the capacity to cope with adversity and the stresses of life. Such individuals may have been subject to mood swings (cyclothymic personalities), have abused alcohol or drugs (or both) or been in conflict with the law.

Clearly the chances of making a successful suicide attempt increase with repetition and when violent methods or non-ingestants are used.

'Attempted' Suicide

Most persons who have taken a deliberate overdose of drugs lack the social characteristics of successful suicides and many of them are found to be psychologically distressed rather than psychiatrically ill. About two-thirds of all self-poisoned patients are under the age of 35 and they are mostly women. Since they tend to belong to social classes III, IV and V, financial hardship is more often associated with attempted than with completed suicide. Difficulties in personal relationships, as shown by adolescent problems or by domestic and marital conflict, are

common. In many instances there is an element of appeal — the so-called cry for help — and the act of self-poisoning may be seen as a form of communication intended to change another person's attitude or behaviour, or both.

Stengel (1958) pointed out that most people who attempt suicide are governed by conflicting emotions and want both to live and to die or, conversely, do not care whether they live or die. He drew attention to the risk-taking element in many suicidal attempts so that some people who are determined to take their own lives survive through chance, while others who expect to live are unlucky. Recently the term 'attempted suicide' has fallen into disfavour because many persons who have taken an overdose of drugs deny afterwards that they had even thought of dying. For this reason Kessel (1965) prefers to describe their behaviour as self-poisoning or self-injury, while Kreitman et al. (1969) have coined the term 'parasuicide' meaning 'by the side of', 'irregular or perverted' suicide for all non-fatal acts of self-harm. However, many 'parasuicides' have in fact tried to kill themselves and it is essential to assess the suicidal risk in every such case.

Psychiatric Assessment

Nowadays, most patients who have taken an overdose of drugs are conscious when they reach hospital and few require intensive care. Yet the seriousness of the patient's physical condition bears little relationship to the suicidal risk or the need for psychiatric treatment. For example, a patient who has taken a couple of extra sleeping tablets may require psychiatric treatment in hospital, whereas another who has been resuscitated in the intensive care unit may be safely discharged home. In fact, more than half of all the patients who are either conscious or only drowsy on admission to hospital may be recommended for psychiatric treatment (Table 9.2).

Some patients may claim to have taken an overdose by mistake, but accidental overdosage is uncommon amongst adults and deliberate self-poisoning should always be carefully excluded.

Psychiatric History

Generally much of the information that is needed for a psychiatric assessment can be obtained when the patient and an accompanying relative or friend are first seen (see Appendix 1 on page 76). After the poisons history, inquiry is made about:

Table 9.2.   Levels of consciousness of self-poisoned patients[1] consecutively admitted to Addenbrooke's Hospital, Cambridge, and type of treatment recommended for them (Gardner et al 1978)

Treatment	Conscious or drowsy	Unconscious but responsive	Unconscious and unresponsive
Inpatient	107	20	14
Outpatient	249	28	16
Social worker	72	11	2
General practitioner	131	29	11

[1] 39 patients were excluded because one of the variables was not recorded.

1. The events preceding the overdose (including the motives).

2. Previous attempts and current and past psychiatric treatment.

3. The social circumstances of the patient, whether living alone or with others.

4. The reactions of the family or friends of the patient to the suicidal attempt.

5. Whether anyone will take the patient home and look after him or her on discharge from hospital.

Evaluation of the patient's mental state may have to be postponed until the effects of drugs and any alcohol have worn off. Once patients have been admitted to hospital, information concerning them reaches the ward from various sources and the nursing staff and social worker can all contribute towards the assessment.

Interview of Informants

It is always advisable to interview an informant. This may help to decide whether the overdose was accidental or deliberate, and whether there were any symptoms of depression which preceded it. Sometimes a depressed mood may colour the way patients think, not only about the future but also about the past, so that they give an unrealistic account of their problems (retrospective falsification). Patients may conceal a history of excessive drinking, or of violence — for example, the 'battered wife' or the mother who has engaged in child abuse. Interviewing an informant

enables a more accurate assessment to be made of the patient's personality and may throw some light on how or how not to treat the patient. The informant may be biased, however, and an estimate should also be made of his or her reliability.

Assessment of the Seriousness of the Suicidal Intent

A clue as to the seriousness of the suicidal intent may be provided by the nature of the poison taken, for example, it may have been a non-ingestant. Occasionally a person such as a doctor, nurse or pharmacist may knowingly use a more lethal poison or method.

Sometimes two methods are used, e.g. carbon monoxide from a car exhaust and an overdose of drugs. At least one-third of all self-poisoned patients have drunk alcohol within a short time of taking their overdose. This may enhance their depressed mood or disinhibit them, or both, so increasing the likelihood of a suicidal attempt. Some patients have deliberately drunk alcohol after taking their tablets in order to make the mixture a more lethal one.

It is important to find out whether the overdose was taken on impulse, perhaps in full view of the family, or whether there were any precautions taken to avoid discovery, or any other preparatory acts. Warning statements are commonly made and not infrequently (and mistakenly) ignored by exasperated relatives. Generally people swallow tablets or medicines that are to hand, but they may go to some lengths to procure the means. They may visit several chemist shops to acquire sufficient tablets or arrange to see their doctor to obtain a presciption. A few persons put their affairs in order and leave a will, while others write a suicide note.

Examination of the Mental State

Depression

In practice, examination of the mental state of the patient consists of eliciting the symptoms and signs of depression, and of asking about the patient's suicidal thoughts and intentions and about his or her attitude towards the future. The patient may look depressed, tearful, agitated or withdrawn. There may be early morning waking; lifting of depressed mood during the day (diurnal variation of mood); undue pessimism about his or her problems and the capacity to cope with them; guilt, self-blame and feelings of unworthiness; impaired appetite and weight loss. These symptoms and signs indicate some degree of endogenicity which should respond to physical methods of treatment. They are more likely to be found in the middle-aged and the elderly and in those patients who either have a family history or a past psychiatric history (or both) of depression or manic–depressive illness.

Reactive Depression

However, most self-poisoned patients are younger and their depressive symptoms are more reactive in nature. They lack the characteristic mood and sleep disturbance of patients with a depressive illness and some of them may have an atypical clinical picture, such as going to bed early to blot out their psychological distress, sleeping late or eating excessively and putting on weight. Yet they too may be severely depressed and represent a suicidal risk.

Functional Psychosis

Only a few self-poisoned patients are found to have a functional psychosis such as schizophrenia or mania (Table 9.3). This can be diagnosed after recovery from the overdose because any delusions and hallucinations or pressure of talk and elated mood occur in a setting of clear consciousness, and the patient is orientated for date and place.

Table 9.3. Illness diagnosis for self-poisoned patients[1] consecutively admitted to Addenbrooke's Hospital, Cambridge (Gardner et al 1978)

Illness diagnosis	No.
No psychiatric illness	87
Situational disturbance	222
Depressive illness or reaction	348
Mania	1
Organic psychiatric disorder	4
Schizophrenia	17
Epilepsy	7
Other	25

---

[1] 18 patients were excluded because the illness diagnosis was not recorded.

In all, 166 patients of those shown in Tables 9.3 and 9.4 had no psychiatric disorder — that is, they were given a diagnosis of normal personality and no psychiatric illness or situational disturbance.

Organic Confusional States

Other patients may have an organic confusional state — that is clouding of consciousness, disorientation

and impairment of recent memory — which persists after the effects of the overdose have worn off. If the patient is elderly, the possibility of an early dementia should be excluded. In the younger age group, drug abuse is a possible cause. LSD-type drugs give rise to visual illusions and hallucinations and the clinical picture has to be differentiated from schizophrenia in which the hallucinations are commonly auditory in nature, and there is no clouding of consciousness.

Amphetamine psychosis occurs in a setting of clear consciousness — in contrast to the psychotic states induced by other drugs — and so may be indistinguishable from paranoid schizophrenia. But a history of drug misuse can usually be obtained and amphetamines may be detected in the urine by gas chromatography for up to 48 hours after the last dose.

Sometimes an organic confusional state may be due to the abrupt withdrawal of alcohol or hypnotic–sedative drugs. Classically this is preceded by a major epileptic fit occurring within 36 hours of the patient's admission to hospital. The full-blown picture of delirium tremens may then develop in which visual hallucinations, misinterpretations or delusions, fear and motor restlessness may be seen.

Diagnosis

Tables 9.3 and 9.4 show the diagnoses, of both illness and personality, which are typically found in any series of self-poisoned patients. Women are more often diagnosed as being depressed and men as having a personality disorder. Alcoholism and, to a lesser

---

Table 9.4. Personality diagnoses for self-poisoned patients[1] consecutively admitted to Addenbrooke's Hospital, Cambridge (Gardner et al 1978)

Personality diagnosis	No.
Normal personality	345
Personality disorder	261
Subnormality	8
Drug dependence	21
Alcoholism	31
Other	23

---

[1] 40 patients were excluded because the personality diagnosis was not recorded.

In all, 166 patients of those shown in Tables 9.3 and 9.4 had no psychiatric disorder — that is, they were given a diagnosis of normal personality and no psychiatric illness or situational disturbance.

extent, drug abuse, occur more frequently than is indicated in the tables because these list only the primary diagnoses. Approximately one in five self-poisoned patients is found to have no demonstrable psychiatric disorder but is considered to have a normal personality and to have been psychologically distressed (diagnosed as 'situational disturbance' or 'no psychiatric illness' in Tables 9.3 and 9.4). Making a psychiatric diagnosis or, alternatively, excluding the presence of a psychiatric disorder, is of importance as it helps to determine the treatment (Table 9.5).

Table 9.5. Diagnostic categories of self-poisoned patients[1] consecutively admitted to Addenbrooke's Hospital, Cambridge, and type of treatment recommended for them (Gardner et al 1978)

Diagnostic category	Psychiatric treatment	Social worker	General practitioner
No psychiatric illness	127	50	117
Depressive illness or reaction	269	31	41
Other	41	4	14

[1] 35 patients were excluded because one of the variables was not recorded.

No psychiatric assessment of these patients is complete without an understanding of the motives which have led them to self-poisoning and of the reasons why they are unable to cope. Indeed, one of the aims of subsequent treatment is to help them to tackle their problems in a less disorganized and more effective way ('crisis intervention').

After carrying out a psychiatric assessment it is worthwhile summarizing the findings in a brief diagnostic formulation and treatment plan (see Appendix 2 on page 76 for examples). This should include the following:

1. The reasons why the overdose was taken.

2. An estimate of the degree of suicidal intent (based on the circumstances of the overdose).

3. The psychiatric diagnosis, both illness and personality. (There may be no demonstrable psychiatric disorder).

4. An assessment of the suicidal risk made after the patient has recovered from the effects of the overdose.

5. The main problem areas which have to be taken into account in deciding the patient's treatment and 'disposal'.

6. The action which is to be taken.

Management of Self-Poisoned Patients

Is Hospital Admission Warranted?

It may be relatively easy to decide in the accident department whether to admit self-poisoned patients to hospital if their physical condition warrants it, if there is some doubt as to the nature or the amount of the poison(s) taken, or if a physical complication is anticipated. But the decision becomes more difficult when the physical risk to the patient is too small to justify hospital admission. There may be a shortage of acute medical beds and some patients are reluctant to come into hospital.

Whenever possible, any patients who are suicidal or who are suspected of being so should be admitted to hospital — irrespective of their physical condition. Admission is also indicated when patients cannot be assessed adequately, either because they are too drowsy or uncooperative or because they have come to the accident department unaccompanied. It is inadvisable to send such patients home straight away if they live alone. Another reason for admitting some patients is to ensure that suitable arrangements are made for their further care. There is little point in offering them a psychiatric outpatient appointment or in asking them to make one at a later date if they are under the influence of drugs and alcohol and too emotionally distraught to heed this advice.

Some patients whose physical condition is found to be satisfactory may be dealt with directly in the accident department. For example, it may be possible to transfer patients to a psychiatric unit if they are already being treated there or if they are found to be suicidal. Other patients may be discharged from the accident department if their overdose was taken on impulse, they are not suicidal and repetition seems unlikely. Provided that a responsible adult is willing to look after the patient, many of the more trivial cases and some of those who need psychiatric outpatient treatment or social work support can be safely sent home. Good communication between the accident department and the patient's general practitioner is desirable.

Admission to Medical and Psychiatric Wards

Self-poisoned patients are more easily kept under observation in a general medical ward than in a sideward. If they are withdrawn or uncommunicative, they should be asked whether they have any suicidal thoughts and intentions. Some patients regret having failed in their suicidal attempt, are preoccupied with their depressive thoughts and may be quite unable to envisage resuming their normal activities. A few patients may contemplate a more violent method of suicide, such as jumping out of a window, and may have to be transferred to a psychiatric unit under a section of the Mental Health Act. While the necessary arrangements are being made, someone should stay with the patient and a major tranquillizer such as elixir chlorpromazine 100 mg can be given if necessary.

Admission to a psychiatric ward is usually on an informal basis and this must always be discussed first with the patient and often with a relative as well. If admission is declined, and the invoking of a section of the Mental Health Act is not justified, antidepressant medication may be commenced and the patient kept on the medical ward until any suicidal intentions have receded. Alternatively the patient may be discharged immediately for outpatient treatment. In either case, arrangements should be made for a relative or friend to look after the patient, once discharged, to take care of any medication and to accompany him or her to the outpatient clinic. Relatives often underestimate the amount of support they will need to give patients and the period for which it will be required. They should make plans for at least two or three weeks ahead and these may involve taking time off work, coming to live with the patient, or the patient going to stay with the relative or friend. Such arrangements can then be reviewed in the outpatient clinic.

Discharge from Hospital

Most self-poisoned patients, despite being depressed or psychologically distressed, do not regret having survived. Since the medical ward seems an inappropriate place for resolution of their personal difficulties, some patients will insist on discharging themselves prematurely. They can be allowed to go if a responsible adult is willing to look after them. Of course, this person must be told about the suicidal attempt and the medical staff should not collude with a patient who asks them to withhold this information. Patients will usually agree to the responsible adult being told if the implications of such a request are fully discussed with them. When a relative or friend cannot be contacted from the hospital, the police will often relay a message. Rarely a patient has to be detained under a section of the Mental Health Act.

Patients are less likely to leave hospital hurriedly if the attitude of the medical staff is favourably disposed towards them and concern is shown for their psychosocial difficulties as well as for their physical condition. No special training is needed for nurses to be able to take an interest in the events that precipitated the overdose, in the patient's attitude towards these since coming into hospital, and in the way the patient intends to cope with his or her problems. Nurses should be prepared to listen and not to offer solutions to personal difficulties since there is often another side to the story. Many crises are in fact resolved by the patients themselves and the other persons concerned without any professional intervention, though this process may be facilitated by one of the medical staff or a social worker seeing a relative or the patient and relative(s) together. Some patients derive considerable benefit from being kept in hospital for a few extra days. They gain respite, have time to think about their problems and to adopt a more realistic attitude towards them. They are thus better able to cope when they leave.

Outpatient Treatment and After-care

Patients may be anxious about seeing a psychiatrist for the first time in the outpatient clinic and the medical staff should ask them about their anxieties. These usually centre around the belief that psychiatrists treat only mad people and simple explanation and reassurance will help to ensure outpatient attendance. Generally the more depressed patients are referred to psychiatrists and those with the more obvious social problems to social workers. However, there is some overlap between the respective roles of these professionals (and that of the specially trained nurse) since they may all undertake counselling and supportive psychotherapy. Choice of referral may in fact depend on who is available. When there is any doubt as to whether a patient is able or willing to keep an outpatient appointment, a social worker or specially trained nurse should visit and take on the patient's after-care. Similar arrangements can be made for those patients who might benefit from being seen with their families at home. Sometimes the patient's general practitioner is the obvious choice for continuing any treatment. Whenever possible, all arrangements for further care should be made before the patient leaves hospital and this includes telephoning the general practitioner's surgery for an appointment. In addition, some system is needed to ensure that patients who are discharged at weekends or on bank holidays can be given an outpatient appointment or a time to see a social worker.

Many self-poisoned patients remain depressed or psychologically distressed after leaving hospital and need to be seen within a few days of going home. Arranging an outpatient appointment two or three weeks ahead is often of little value, particularly for those patients who are young and impulsive and have a low frustration threshold. Some of them will fail to turn up at the outpatient clinic, while others will have repeated their act(s) of self-poisoning before they are due to be seen. Figure 9.1 shows a typical repetition curve for self-poisoned patients followed up for one year. The steepest part occurs soon after the initial overdose and it is during this period that patients most need help.

Conclusion

Deliberate self-poisoning by an overdose of drugs is one of the commonest acute medical emergencies. Doctors and nurses need to be trained not only to resuscitate such patients but also to evaluate suicidal risk and their patients' psychosocial difficulties.

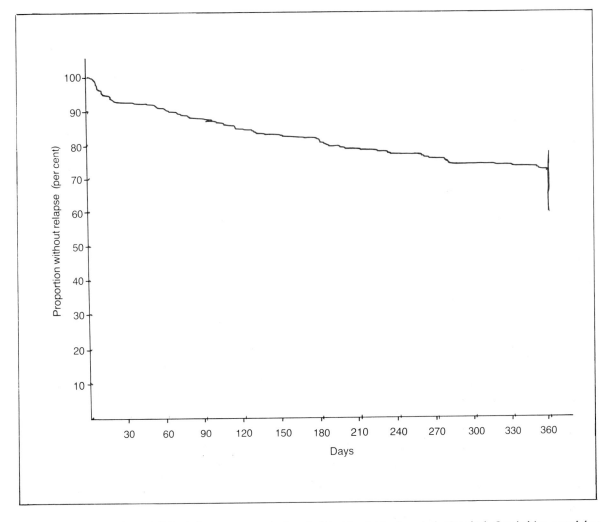

Figure 9.1. *Proportion of 276 patients consecutively admitted to Addenbrooke's Hospital, Cambridge, surviving one year without relapse (figures corrected for drop outs).*

Appendix 1 Psychiatric Assessment

HISTORY
Circumstances of the overdose
Precipitating events. Motives for taking overdose. Symptoms of depression preceding the attempt including listlessness and social withdrawal.
Precautions against discovery and preparatory acts — procuring means, affairs in order, warning statements, suicide note. Violent methods and more lethal drugs/poisons.

Past psychiatric history
Nature of any previous psychiatric disorder, suicidal attempt(s).
Details of current or past treatment — in- or out-patient/GP. Drugs. ECT or other treatment.

Present life situation
Housing, family, job (if unemployed, how long). Any stressful changes relating to these and other events. Is social worker/probation officer involved. Who can look after patient on discharge.

Family background
Father, mother, age, occupation. If dead, year and cause of death.
Number of siblings.
Family history of psychiatric illness — particularly depression, suicide, alcoholism.

Personal history
(Try and establish what sort of person the patient is, but be selective in your history taking)
Where born and brought up.
Age on leaving school and attainments there.
Further education.
Jobs — if many, the longest one held.
Sex and marriage. Date of marriage(s); if separated, divorced, widowed. Children.
Past medical history.

Previous personality (informant required)
(Try and decide, using your knowledge of human nature [and of society] whether the patient's enduring personality trait(s) deviate from the norm.) If delinquent, details of prison, borstal, probation; whether excessive drinking, drug abuse.

MENTAL STATE
Dejected appearance/agitated and restless, depressed. Ask whether depressed on waking and lifting of mood during the day (diurnal variation), impaired sleep — difficulty in getting off, frequent waking or early morning waking. Impaired appetite with weight loss. Pessimism about ability to resume (and cope with) normal activities.
Feelings of guilt, unworthiness, self blame.
Always ask about suicidal thoughts and intentions.

FORMULATION
The reason the overdose was taken.
Estimate the degree of suicidal intent.
Psychiatric diagnosis (illness and personality) — there may be no psychiatric disorder.
Assessment of suicidal risk (after recovery from overdose).
Problem areas having bearing on patient's treatment and 'disposal'.
Action to be taken.

Appendix 2 Examples of Formulations

1. *History and mental state* — A 17-year-old shop assistant admitted last night, drowsy but conscious after taking an overdose of diazepam (belonging to her mother) following a row with her boyfriend. She had a stomach washout and this morning is alert, does not appear depressed and realises that her action was an impulsive one. She wishes to go home. Her mother describes her as a somewhat jealous and possessive girl who became upset when her boyfriend refused to take her to the cinema and wanted to go out to a disco in a foursome.

Formulation — An acute situational disturbance in an apparently normal adolescent. The mother agrees to collect her this afternoon and the general practitioner is being notified of her discharge.

2. *History and mental state* — A 45-year-old single dustman admitted yesterday morning unconscious after an overdose of amitriptyline, having been found face downwards in a bath containing water, by a neighbour who had chanced to call. This morning there are no physical signs in his chest and an x-ray is normal. He has marked symptoms of depression with early morning waking (3.00 a.m.), diurnal variation of mood, ideas that life is not worth living and that there is no hope for the future. He regrets regaining consciousness. His appetite has been impaired and he has lost weight. His premorbid personality is described by his sister as sociable and outgoing. She states that his brother's death three months ago from a heart attack upset him. There is a family history of depression, his father having had treatment in a mental hospital.

Formulation — A middle-aged single man with a good premorbid personality who has made a serious suicidal attempt and is lucky to survive. He has a depressive illness which requires treatment with antidepressant medication and perhaps ECT. As he lives alone, he should be admitted to a psychiatric hospital. He has agreed to this, his sister has been told and the general practitioner will be informed.

3. *History and mental state* — A 29-year-old married woman with five children, admitted after an aspirin overdose for which she required a forced diuresis. She has been depressed and lacking in energy particularly since her husband lost his job three months ago. She took the overdose because she was at the end of her tether but now has no suicidal thoughts or intentions. There are underlying social problems relating to financial worries and coping with her four pre-school children. Her husband is to start a new job next week.

Formulation — A married woman with a depressive neurosis precipitated by a number of social and financial problems. She is no longer suicidal and wants to go home. The social worker is arranging some social support for the family and has already contacted the mother who will stay with the patient when she is discharged. In view of the duration of her depressive symptoms and some uncertainty as to how long she was suicidal before taking the overdose, she needs to be reassessed and is to be seen in the psychiatric outpatient clinic in five days time. Her mother has been asked to accompany her.

Acknowledgements

The data in Tables 9.2 to 9.5 and Figure 9.1 were obtained as part of a research project (No. 79/80) financed by the East Anglian Regional Health Authority. I am grateful to Dr R. Hanka and Miss S.J. Roberts for statistical advice, and to Mrs P. Mills for typing the manuscript.

References

Barraclough B, Bunch J, Nelson B, Sainsbury P. A hundred cases of suicide: clinical aspects. Br J Psychiatry 1974; 125: 355–373.

Gardner R, Hanka R, Evison B, Mountford PM, O'Brien VC, Roberts SJ. Consultation–liaison scheme for self-poisoned patients in a general hospital. Br Med J 1978; 2:1392–4.

Kessel N. Self-poisoning. Br Med J 1965; 2:1265–70.

Kreitman N, Philip AE, Greer S, Bagley CR. Parasuicide. Br J Psychiatry 1969; 115:746–7.

Robins E, Murphy GE, Wilkinson RH Jr, Grassner S, Kayes J. Some clinical considerations in the prevention of suicide based on a study of 134 successful suicides. Am J Public Health 1959; 49:888–99.

Sainsbury P. Suicide in London. London: Chapman and Hall, 1955.

Shaffer D. Suicide in childhood and early adolescence. J Child Psychol Psychiatry 1974; 15:275–91.

Stengel E, Cook NG. Attempted Suicide. London: Oxford University Press, 1958.

Toolan JM. Suicidal attempts in children and adolescents. Am J Psychiatry 1962; 118:719–24.

Further Reading

Gardner R, Hanka R, O'Brien VC, Page AJF, Rees R. Psychological and social evaluation in cases of deliberate self-poisoning admitted to a general hospital. Br Med J 1977; 2:1567–70.

Sainsbury P. Suicide: opinions and facts. Proc R Soc Med 1973; 66:579–587.

Stengel E. Suicide and Attempted Suicide. Harmondsworth: Penguin Books Ltd, 1973.

Chapter 10

R. Gardner, T. J. Meredith and J. A. Vale

Prevention of Poisoning

Prevention of Poisoning in Adults (R. Gardner)

In England and Wales the suicide rate declined by some 36 per cent between 1963 and 1974. Various reasons have been put forward to explain this. Domestic gas has been detoxified, and there has been an increasing tendency for men – who are more likely to kill themselves than women – to use poisons instead of more lethal methods. Prescribing habits have changed so that persons who would formerly have died after an overdose of barbiturates now survive after an overdose of benzodiazepines. Family doctors have been treating more of their patients with antidepressant drugs. In many parts of the UK distressed people are able to telephone a local branch of the Samaritans. Perhaps all of these factors have contributed towards the prevention of suicide.

Whether the trend towards community psychiatry has also helped to lower the suicide rate is a question that needs to be answered. To date research has provided some rather conflicting evidence. One study in Chichester, England concluded that the introduction of a community psychiatric service had succeeded in reducing the number of suicides in that area, whereas another study in Denmark found that a similar scheme had made no difference. Why the suicide rate should have fallen only in the UK is of great interest. It is possible that the National Health Service or the unique policy towards the assessment of self-poisoned patients, or both, have helped to lower the suicide rate, but these measures have certainly not prevented the growing 'epidemic' of deliberate self-poisoning.

Policies on the Hospital Treatment of Acute Poisoning

Policies on self-poisoning in the UK (Editorial, *British Medical Journal* 1979) have developed largely in response to the passing of the Suicide Act 1961. When attempted suicide ceased to be an indictable offence the then Ministry of Health advised all hospitals to see that suicidal patients received psychiatric attention. Later, the Department of Health (The Hill Report 1968) recommended that, in all cases of deliberate self-poisoning, patients should be referred to designated poisoning treatment centres in district general hospitals and be seen by psychiatrists. This plan has turned out to be impracticable and has been increasingly questioned. There is no convincing evidence that self-poisoned patients are more effectively treated in a special unit than in a general medical ward, and the assumption that only psychiatrists are competent to assess suicide risk and to decide the need for psychiatric or social work referral has proved to be unfounded.

Assessment of the Patient

In a prospective clinical trial carried out at Addenbrooke's Hospital, Cambridge, it was found that if junior doctors and nurses were suitably taught, medical teams could, in most instances, match psychiatrists at making diagnoses and identifying which patients needed further care. However, consultant physicians still needed a psychiatric opinion for roughly one in five of their patients (Gardner et al. 1977; Gardner 1978). As a result the physicians at Addenbrooke's have taken over the initial psychiatric assessment of all their self-poisoned patients as part of the routine clinical work. At Oxford, nurses with psychiatric experience and supervised by a consultant psychiatrist have proved equally reliable (Hawton et al. 1979). What seems to matter is the effectiveness of the training and of the arrangements for ensuring adequate psychiatric treatment and after care, and not the fact that a psychiatrist should see every patient.

If, as seems likely, the Department of Health amends its recommendation, physicians will be free to decide for each of their self-poisoned patients whether specialist psychiatric advice is necessary. Making a psychiatric diagnosis or, alternatively, excluding psychiatric disorder, is an important part of such an assessment. As doctors perform this task better than specially trained nurses or social workers they would be well advised to retain the responsibility for it.

Consultation – Liaison in the General Hospital

Once patients have been assessed it is important to ensure that they actually receive the treatment recommended for them. This is more likely to happen if self-poisoned patients are not placed throughout the general hospital but, whenever possible, are admitted into one of the medical wards. The sister-in-charge can then act as a source of reference for those wards which have less experience in handling this clinical problem. A social worker should give at least part of her time to the care of these patients on a regular basis. Psychiatrists can teach the junior staff how to carry out the initial psychiatric assessment, as well as providing prompt consultations when they are needed. They should also ensure arrangements for transferring patients to psychiatric wards and for seeing them in the psychiatric outpatient clinic shortly after their discharge from hospital.

Now that as many as one in seven of all acute medical admissions is for self-poisoning, liaison schemes of the kind developed at Addenbrooke's Hospital would enable doctors to be trained to evaluate suicidal risk and patients' psychosocial difficulties during their preregistration house jobs. Such training is important. Most known suicides have consulted a doctor before killing themselves, and most self-poisoned patients have taken prescribed drugs.

Psychiatric Treatment

Good communication between the medical and psychiatric ward is essential when transferring a suicidal patient. The most severely suicidal and depressed are best treated with a major tranquillizer such as chlorpromazine in addition to a tricyclic antidepressant or electroconvulsive therapy (ECT), or both. The retarded depressed patient is most likely to make a suicidal attempt when he or she has the energy to carry it out. Commonly this happens just after starting ECT or when an antidepressant drug begins to take effect.

Nowadays most patients are sent home for weekends and are discharged from psychiatric wards long before they have recovered from their psychiatric illness, and it is then that they are most at risk from a further suicidal attempt.

Careful follow up is probably necessary for at least six months after a patient's depression has been treated in hospital.

It is always advisable to see such a patient on each occasion to reassess the mental state, and not merely to give a repeat prescription. Since many depressed patients lack insight into their condition it is also important to interview a relative or friend and, when necessary, to ask one of them to take care of the patient's medication.

Prevention of Further Depressive Episodes

Some patients, who are recurrently depressed, can be maintained prophylactically on a tricyclic antidepressant. Others, particularly those who have a history of mania, may respond to lithium. The advantages of this drug are that it may protect the patient against both manic and depressive episodes, and patients generally find lithium more acceptable than the major tranquillizers which tend to make them feel drowsy or drugged.

Prevention of Further Self-Poisoning Incidents

In the year after their first overdose of drugs approximately 30 per cent of all self-poisoned patients will do it again. Paradoxically the more seriously ill patients respond relatively better to therapy since their risk of repetition is no greater than for those considered free of psychiatric illness. It can be seen from Figure 9.1. in the previous chapter that most patients who repeat their act of self-poisoning will have done so within three months of the initial attempt, and that any psychiatric treatment and after care must be started within days of patients leaving hospital if it is to prevent another attempt.

Since the first suicide prevention centre was set up in Vienna after the second world war, it has been assumed that the personnel who are going to follow up self-poisoned patients must see them first in hospital. But the clinical trial at Addenbrooke's Hospital suggests that such an arrangement is unnecessary in most cases. It was found that patients who were selected by the medical teams were as likely to attend the psychiatric outpatient clinic as those who had been assessed on the wards by psychiatrists.

What seems to matter is that patients should be properly informed about the arrangements for their further care and that they should be seen in the outpatient clinic within days of leaving hospital. In most cases no medication is required and patients are given supportive psychotherapy, counselling and perhaps family therapy – usually for only a few weeks after they have left hospital. Some patients require treatment with antidepressant drugs and may have to be followed up for a longer period.

Improvement of After Care

Recent studies have looked at different ways of improving after care using intensive social work, counselling by nurses and domiciliary visits. None of these methods reduced the repetition rate, but intensive social work did improve the social functioning of some of the more 'high-risk' patients (Chowdhury et al. 1973). Further research is needed to find the optimum care for the more vulnerable groups of patients such as those who are sent home from accident departments, who discharge themselves prematurely from medical wards or who fail to keep their psychiatric outpatient appointments.

Primary Prevention of Poisoning

Role of the Medical Profession

However well our overstretched hospitals cope with the 'epidemic' of deliberate self-poisoning, hopes of controlling it must rest largely on primary preventive measures. Too many drugs are too easily available. Simple precautions such as limiting the number of tablets that can be sold in a single container, a more

sparing use of repeat prescriptions and asking patients to bring back unwanted drugs, would diminish this availability. The reasons why so many psychotropic drugs are prescribed are complex, and their widespread use has to be seen in perspective. Alcohol is still more commonly used and misused than are the tranquillizers. Numerous persons are treated successfully with such drugs without ever taking an overdose and, when they do so, only a minority take another overdose. Nevertheless, the fact that one in five of all self-poisoned patients is found to have no demonstrable psychiatric disorder would suggest that there is scope for doctors to prescribe with greater care.

Retrospective studies (see Chapter 9) have shown that doctors often fail to detect that patients are suicidal because they have not enquired about suicidal thoughts and intentions and have omitted to interview an informant. Better medical training might also contribute towards the prevention of poisoning (Gardner et al 1978; Editorial, *British Medical Journal* 1979).

However, it would be idle to pretend that the problem of self-poisoning can be solved by the medical profession alone. Proportionately more self-poisoned patients than persons in the general population have come from 'broken' homes and not a few have unstable personalities. Prevention is likely to be applied too late to modify their self-destructive behaviour.

Voluntary Agencies and Self-Help

Trethowan (1975) has asked why an increasing number of people should be presenting themselves for medical help with difficulties which are primarily personal, interpersonal or environmental in origin. They seem to expect the doctor to find a solution for their psychosocial difficulties so that he or she all too readily resorts to prescribing a tranquillizer. Advertisements in newspapers and on television also tend to claim that for every disease there is a specific remedy – usually a drug – thus reinforcing patients' expectations of being given a prescription. The public has to be educated to seek appropriate help from other agencies and, in this respect, the media have played a more positive educational role. The growing interest in self-help groups and in voluntary work with young people, the elderly and the Samaritans, would suggest that the public is learning its lesson. Non-medically-qualified professionals and volunteers must in their turn learn to recognize those of their clients whom they cannot help by sympathetic listening and who need to be referred for psychiatric treatment.

References

Chowdhury N, Hicks RC, Kreitman N. Evaluation of an after care service for parasuicide (attempted suicide) patients. Social Psychiatry 1973; 8:67–81.

Editorial. Policies on self-poisoning. Br Med J 1979; 2: 1091–2.

Gardner R, Hanka R, O'Brien V, Page AJF, Rees R. Psychological and social evaluation in cases of deliberate self-poisoning. Br Med J 1977; 2:1567–70.

Gardner R, Hanka R, Evison B, Mountford PM, O'Brien VC, Roberts SJ. Consultation–liaison scheme for self-poisoned patients in a general hospital. Br Med J 1978; 2:1392–4.

Hawton K, Gath D, Smith E. Management of attempted suicide in Oxford. Br Med J 1979; 2:1040–42.

The Hill Report. Central and Scottish Health Services Councils, Hospital Treatment of Acute Poisoning. London: HMSO, 1968.

Trethowan WH. Pills for personal problems. Br Med J 1975; 3:749–51.

Prevention of Poisoning in Children
(T. J. Meredith and J. A. Vale)

Accidental poisoning is uncommon in children over five years of age. However, there is increasing evidence that children only nine or ten years old may indulge in deliberate self-poisoning. It has also become apparent that the deliberate administration of drugs to children by adults is a not infrequent form of child abuse. However, the preventive measures described in this chapter apply only to *accidental* poisoning in young children.

Many methods have been tried to prevent accidental poisoning in children.

Educational Campaigns

Campaigns to educate adults about the dangers of poisoning are often employed, e.g. 'Keep all medicines out of reach of children', but unfortunately they are of little proven value. Few families have lockable medicine cabinets, and those who do have them often do not use them properly. Even after a poisoning incident in the family many parents still do not take appropriate preventive measures. Furthermore, there is evidence that most families are under stress at the time of poisoning incidents and they are unlikely to remember either health education campaigns or to put poisons in safe places.

Child-Resistant Containers (CRCs)

The only measure that has been shown to definitely reduce the incidence of childhood poisoning is the use of child-resistant containers (CRCs). Scherz (1970), in an American study, reduced the number of poisoning episodes in a local community to less than 15 per cent of its former level by the use of such containers. The general introduction of these containers in the USA (Poison Prevention Packaging Act of 1976) led to a marked fall in the number of poisoned children. Since 1976 all solid analgesic preparations for children sold in Britain are required to be in opaque reclosable CRCs or dark unit packaging (strip or blister packs). The tablets must be white and the packs must not contain more than 25 doses. The effectiveness of this measure was assessed in a study of Newcastle and South Glamorgan hospital admissions of children under five in the period 1974 to 1976. The incidence of salicylate poisoning fell from 129 cases in 1975 to 48 cases in 1976; the number of hospital admissions also fell significantly.

Types of CRC Available

Three different reclosable CRCs are now used in Britain: 'Pop-lok' (Metal Box Ltd), 'Snap-safe' (Cope Allman Plastics Ltd) and 'Clic-loc' (UG Closures and Plastics Ltd) (Figure 10.1).

Pop-lok is a snap-fitting cap with an integral flush-fitting tab. A dot is moulded onto the hinge end of the cap and, when pressed, works against a fulcrum to lift the free end of the tab out of its slot. The tab can then be gripped and used to pull off the cap. This cap is not suitable for liquids.

Snap-safe is a snap-fitting cap that can be pushed off only when the arrow on the cap is aligned with an arrow on the bottle. It is not watertight.

Clic-loc is a screw cap comprising an inner and outer shell that cannot be unscrewed unless a downward force is applied while it is turned. It can be used on standard tablet or medicine bottles with a screw neck and is therefore a suitable closure for liquid as well as dry preparations.

BSI Test Protocol

The British Standards Institute has laid down a test protocol (BSI 5321) for reclosable CRCs, requiring that at least 85 per cent of a test panel of children aged less than five cannot open the containers and that at least 80 per cent still cannot open them after a single visual demonstration. Also, at least 90 per cent of a panel of adults must be able to open and properly reclose the containers using only written

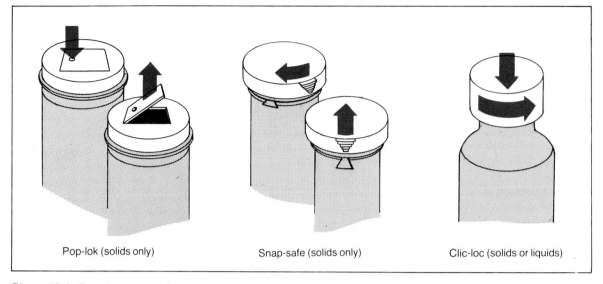

Figure 10.1. *Opening reclosable child-resistant containers.*

instructions. Pharmacists can give patients a visual demonstration which is more easily understood and which makes the containers no less childproof. Unfortunately many analgesic drugs are sold in shops and supermarkets where such help is not available.

Problems of Usage

Some elderly, arthritic and handicapped patients have difficulty opening CRCs and for this reason legislation in the UK and in the USA allows such patients to have their medications dispensed in normal containers. Fears have also been expressed that other patients will find child-resistant closures too much trouble to use and will either leave the tops off or transfer the contents to other containers. A survey in England found that nearly 90 per cent of patients found reclosable CRCs acceptable and that they could open and close them correctly (Anonymous 1977). However, a survey in America (Myers 1977) showed that 80 per cent of patients had initial difficulty in opening the containers. Of these, 87 per cent had not received instructions for use while 13 per cent had received instructions from people other than doctors, nurses and pharmacists. Of these, 47 per cent in some way diminished the child resistance of the container. Of those patients who received instructions from doctors, nurses or pharmacists, no one experienced difficulty in opening the containers and no one used the containers incorrectly.

Conclusion

There appears to be little doubt that the incidence of childhood poisoning has fallen since the introduction of child-resistant containers. It seems likely that the scheme will be extended in the UK to all dispensed and over-the-counter medicines implicated in childhood poisoning accidents. However, it is important that health care workers encourage their acceptance by patients.

References

Anonymous. Most people favour child-resistant closures — survey. J Pharm 1977; 216:297.

Myers CE. Patient experiences with a child-resistant prescription container. Am J Hosp Pharm 1977; 34:255–8.

Scherz RG. Prevention of childhood poisoning. A community project. Pediatr Clin North Am 1970; 17:713–27.

Further Reading

Craft AW, Jackson RH, Sibert JR. Child-resistant containers and child poisoning. Br Med J 1976; 2:301.

Craft AW, Sibert JR. Accidental poisoning in children. Br J Hosp Med 1977; 17:469–78.

Craft AW, Sibert JR. Preventive effect of CRCs. Pharm J 1979; 223:593.

Editorial. Childhood poisoning: prevention and first-aid managements. Br Med J 1975; 4:483–4.

Flanagan RJ, Huggett A, Jeffery DB, Raper SM. Child abuse. New Engl J Med 1980; 302:756.

Garrettson LK. The child-resistant container: a success and a model for accident prevention. Am J Public Health 1977; 67:135−6.

Holden JA. Factors related to accidental poisoning in pre-school children. J Environ Health 1979; 41:274−8.

McLean W. Child poisoning in England and Wales: some statistics on admissions to hospital, 1964-1976. Health Trends 1980; 12:9−12.

Rogers D, Tripp J, Bentovim A, Robinson A, Berry D, Goulding R. Non-accidental poisoning: an extended syndrome of child abuse. Br Med J 1976; 1:793−6.

Sherman FT. Child-resistant containers. Lancet 1980; i:97−8.

Sibert R. Stress in families of children who have ingested poisons. Br Med J 1975; 3:87−9.

Chapter 11

T. J. Meredith and J. A. Vale

Poisoning due to Hypnotics, Sedatives, Tranquillizers and Anticonvulsants

The mortality from barbiturate poisoning in the UK has fallen in recent years. This is partly due to a change in prescribing habits as alternative hypnotic, sedative and anticonvulsant drugs have become available. Many of these drugs are considerably safer than barbiturates when taken in overdose but they are nonetheless responsible for several hundred deaths each year (see Chapter 1).

The ingestion of an overdose of any of the barbiturate, hypnotic, sedative or anticonvulsant agents is usually associated with a depressed level of consciousness and some degree of respiratory and cardiovascular depression. The severity of these clinical features depends not only on the quantity ingested but also on the particular drug involved. There may be additional clinical features which either aid the diagnosis or are relevant to management. This chapter describes briefly the effects of overdose of individual drugs of the above groups but the principles of supportive care, management of shock and the treatment of respiratory complications are described in Chapters 4, 6 and 7 respectively. Furthermore, the use of specific elimination techniques, which may be appropriate to the management of certain severely poisoned patients, is described in Chapter 8.

Barbiturates

Whilst barbiturates are now prescribed infrequently in the UK, a large number remain available on prescription. These include amylobarbitone, barbitone, butobarbitone, cyclobarbitone, heptabarbitone, hexobarbitone, pentobarbitone, phenobarbitone and quinalbarbitone. Several of these drugs are combined in proprietary formulations, for example, amylobarbitone and quinalbarbitone. By convention, the barbiturates are divided into groups depending upon whether they have a long, medium, short or ultrashort duration of action. There is little merit in this classification so far as the treatment of overdose is concerned, although patients who ingest the short- to medium-acting barbiturates are often more severely poisoned than those who ingest the longer-acting preparations (barbitone and phenobarbitone).

Clinical Features

The typical features of a barbiturate overdose are impairment of the level of consciousness, respiratory depression, hypotension and hypothermia. In common with virtually all forms of hypnotic overdose, the severity of poisoning is increased if alcohol is also ingested. Hypotension is due not only to peripheral venous pooling but also to direct myocardial depression and, in very severely poisoned patients, there is also an element of medullary depression.

The overall mortality due to barbiturate poisoning is three to six per cent, but the mortality of patients admitted in Grade IV coma may be as much as 32 per cent (Arieff and Friedman 1973). The majority of these deaths are due to respiratory complications (see Chapter 7).

Bowel-sounds are often absent in barbiturate poisoning and when they do return, during the course of recovery, a relapse may occur as further drug is absorbed from the gut. Renal failure was once a common accompaniment to barbiturate overdose and a not infrequent cause of death. Modern management of hypotension and shock has now made this an uncommon complication. There are no specific neurological features of barbiturate overdose and the behaviour of the pupils, tendon reflexes and plantar responses is variable. Although fixed dilated pupils may be found in severe barbiturate poisoning, the possibility that cerebral anoxia may have occurred before arrival at hospital should be borne in mind.

Hypothermia and poor perfusion of skeletal muscle probably account for the finding of markedly elevated plasma concentrations of creatine phosphokinase during recovery from severe hypnotic overdoses. For the same reason, it is common to observe a peak of temperature during recovery as a reaction to tissue necrosis. Bullous lesions of the skin are said to occur in six per cent of cases of barbiturate poisoning although they may also be found in other forms of overdose. The bullae are most often found between the fingers, knees and the ankles.

Treatment

Gastric aspiration and lavage, where appropriate, and intensive supportive therapy should be administered. Forced alkaline diuresis (page 59) is effective only in cases of barbitone and phenobarbitone poisoning and it has no place in other forms of barbiturate intoxication. It is important, therefore, to use specific analytical techniques to detect and measure barbiturates in the blood (see Chapter 3). Haemoperfusion should be considered in patients with severe barbiturate poisoning. The indications for this treatment are described in Chapter 8.

References

Arieff AI, Friedman EA. Coma following non-narcotic drug overdosage: management of 208 adult patients. Am J Med Sci 1973; 266:405−26.

Further Reading

Ibe K, Barckow D, Loddenkemper R, Schmalisch N, Schopf U, Strey W. Complications pulmonaires secondaires aux intoxications aigues par les somniferes. Le Poumon et le Coeur 1970; 26:967−74.
Goodman JM, Bischel MD, Wagers PW, Barbour BH. Barbiturate intoxication. Morbidity and mortality. West J Med 1976; 124:179−86.
Jay SJ, Johanson Jr WG, Pierce AK. Respiratory complications of overdose with sedative drugs. Am Rev Respir Dis 1975; 112:591−8.
Matthew H. Barbiturates. Clin Toxicol 1975; 8:495−513.
Wright N, Clarkson AR, Brown SS, Fuster V. Effects of poisoning on serum enzyme activities, coagulation and fibrinolysis. Br Med J 1971; 3:347−50.

Non-Barbiturate Hypnotics

Chlormethiazole

Chlormethiazole has only recently been reported as a cause of severe poisoning. Coma, respiratory depression, reduced muscle tone, hypotension and hypothermia may all occur. Excessive salivation has been a prominent feature in some reported cases and the characteristic odour of chlormethiazole is often detected on the breath and in the gastric lavage fluid. Prognosis is poor in alcoholics and those with impaired liver function.

Treatment is supportive with pharyngeal suction and assisted ventilation as necessary.

Further Reading

Flanagan RJ, Lee TD, Rutherford DM. Analysis of chlormethiazole, ethchlorvynol and trichloroethanol in biological fluids by gas−liquid chromatography as an aid to the diagnosis of acute poisoning. J Chromatogr 1978; 153:473−9.
Illingworth RN, Stewart MJ, Jarvie DR. Severe poisoning with chlormethiazole. Br Med J 1979; 2:902−3.
Robinson AE, McDowall RD. Toxicological investigations of six chlormethiazole-related deaths. Forensic Sci Int 1979; 14:49−55.

Ethchlorvynol

Ethchlorvynol has a pungent odour which is often detectable on the breath and in the gastric lavage fluid. The clinical features of poisoning resemble those of overdosage with other hypnotic drugs but coma is often prolonged with severe respiratory depression. Bradycardia, hypotension and hypothermia are common and pulmonary oedema has been reported.

Treatment is supportive but haemoperfusion is of value in very severely poisoned patients (see page 63).

Further Reading

Benowitz N, Abolin C, Tozer T, Rosenberg J, Rogers W, Pond S. et al. Resin hemoperfusion in ethchlorvynol overdose. Clin Pharmacol Ther 1980; 27:236−42.
Glauser FL, Smith WR, Caldwell A, Hoshiko M, Dolan GS, Baer H, et al. Ethchlorvynol (Placidyl)-induced pulmonary edema. Ann Intern Med 1976; 84:46−8.
Pochopien DJ. Rate of decrease in serum ethchlorvynol concentrations after extreme overdosage − a case study. Clin Chem 1975; 21:894−5.
Teehan BP, Maher JF, Carey JJH, Flynn PD, Schreiner GE. Acute ethchlorvynol (Placidyl) intoxication. Ann Intern Med 1970; 72:875−82.

Glutethimide

Glutethimide exhibits a complex pattern of biotransformation and at least one of the metabolites, 4-hydroxyglutethimide, has potent pharmacological activity. A prominent feature of glutethimide poisoning, which resembles barbiturate intoxication in many other respects, is a characteristic fluctuation in the level of consciousness. This may be due to the formation of 4-hydroxyglutethimide but alternative explanations include further absorption from the gut after recovery from an ileus, enterohepatic circulation of glutethimide and its metabolites and release of the drug from body fat. The pupils are often dilated and unreactive to light in glutethimide poisoning because of the anticholinergic activity of the drug. Papilloedema, cerebral oedema and episodes of sudden apnoea may occur.

Treatment is essentially supportive but intravenous dexamethasone or mannitol should be given for cerebral oedema. Haemoperfusion should be considered in seriously poisoned patients (see page 63).

Further Reading

Chazan JA, Garella S. Glutethimide intoxication. Arch Int Med 1971; 128:215–9.

Decker WJ, Thompson HL, Arneson LA. Glutethimide rebound. Lancet 1970; i:778–79.

Editorial. Glutethimide: an unsafe alternative to barbiturate hypnotics. Br Med J 1976; 1:1424

Greenblatt DJ, Allen MD, Harmatz JS, Noel BJ, Shader RI. Correlates of outcome following acute glutethimide overdose. J Forensic Sci 1979; 24:76–86.

Hansen AR, Kennedy KA, Ambre JJ, Fischer LJ. Glutethimide poisoning. A metabolite contributes to morbidity and mortality. New Engl J Med 1975; 292:250–2.

Henderson LW, Metz M, Wilkinson JH. Serum enzyme elevation in glutethimide intoxication. Br Med J 1970; 3:751.

Methaqualone

Methaqualone is used as a hypnotic and sedative drug alone and in combination with diphenhydramine in proprietary preparations, e.g. Mandrax in the UK. Pyramidal signs are a prominent feature of overdosage. Depression of the level of consciousness may be accompanied by hypertonia, increased tendon reflexes and extensor plantar responses. Papilloedema and convulsions also occur, tachycardia is common and acute pulmonary oedema has been reported.

Treatment is supportive but haemoperfusion may be effective in severely poisoned patients (see page 63).

Further Reading

Bailey DN, Jatlow PI. Methaqualone overdose: analytical methodology and the significance of serum drug concentrations. Clin Chem 1973; 19:615–20.

Majelyne W, De Clerck F, Demeter J, Heyndrickx A. Treatment evaluation of a severe methaqualone intoxication in man. In: Human Toxicology. Heyndrickx A. Ed. Ghent: European Press, 1978: 175–82.

Trichloroethanol

Chloral hydrate, dichloralphenazone and triclofos are converted by liver alcohol dehydrogenase to the active metabolite, trichloroethanol, which in turn is further metabolized to the inactive compounds, trichloroacetic acid and trichloroethanol glucuronide.

The clinical features of acute overdosage with chloral hydrate and its derivatives are similar to those of barbiturate poisoning, although the patients may initially complain of a retrosternal burning sensation accompanied by vomiting. Cardiac arrhythmias have been described following chloral hydrate overdose but if they do occur it is important to exclude respiratory depression and hypoxia as the underlying cause.

Treatment should consist of gastric aspiration and lavage, where appropriate, together with intensive supportive therapy. Haemoperfusion should be considered in severely poisoned patients (see page 63).

Further Reading

Bowyer K, Glasser SP. Chloral hydrate overdose and cardiac arrhythmias. Chest 1980; 77:232–5.

Brown AM, Cade JF. Cardiac arrhythmias after chloral hydrate overdose. Med J Aust 1980; 1:28–9.

Wiseman HM, Hampel G. Cardiac arrhythmias due to chloral hydrate poisoning. Br Med J 1978; 2:960.

Other Sedatives and Tranquillizers

Antihistamines

Although antihistamines are used as sedatives, they are also commonly employed in the treatment of anaphylaxis, allergy and motion sickness. In addition, many antihistamines possess anticholinergic activity and some act as local anaesthetics. Although an ethylamine moiety is common to all antihistamines, their chemical structure may differ widely. The majority of antihistamines are derived either from an alkylamine, ethanolamine, ethylene diamine or a piperazine or phenothiazine. It is not surprising that several hundred preparations of antihistamines are available but those most commonly encountered are antazoline, brompheniramine, buclizine, carbinoxamine, chlorpheniramine, cinnarizine, clemastine, cyclizine, cyproheptadine, diphenhydramine, diphenylpyraline, embramine, meclozine, mepyramine, methapyrilene, orphenadrine, pheniramine, pyrrobutamine, tripelennamine and triprolidine.

Clinical Features

The anticholinergic properties of antihistamines are most prominent in cases of mild poisoning with dryness of the mouth, headache, nausea, tachycardia and urinary retention. The central effects of antihistamines become important in serious overdosage and they may both stimulate and depress the nervous system. In small children, the dominant effect is excitation and the clinical features include hallucinations, excitement, ataxia, incoordination, athetosis and convulsions. Fixed dilated pupils, a flushed face and hyperthermia are common and produce a clinical picture similar to that of atropine poisoning. Subsequently, coma and cardiorespiratory depression may develop and death can occur within 2 to 18 hours. Fever and flushing are uncommon in the adult, and the phase of excitement leading to convulsions is usually preceded by a period of drowsiness and coma.

Treatment

Treatment should consist of gastric aspiration and lavage and supportive measures. Diazepam may be required for treatment of convulsions.

Further Reading

Ainsworth CA, Biggs JD. A fatality involving methapyrilene. Clin Toxicol 1977; 11:281–6.

Backer RC, Pisano RV, Sopher IM. Diphenhydramine suicide – case report. J Anal Toxicol 1977; 1:227–8.

Barone DA, Raniolo J. Facial dyskinesia from overdose of an antihistamine. New Engl J Med 1980; 303:107.

Bayley M, Walsh FM, Valaske MJ. Report of a fatal, acute tripelennamine intoxication. J Forensic Sci 1975; 20:539–43.

Bozza-Marrubini M, Frigerio A, Ghezzi R, Parelli L, Restelli L, Salenati A. Two cases of severe orphenadrine poisoning with atypical features. Acta Pharmacol Toxicol 1977; 41:Suppl. II:137–52.

Fatteh A, Dudley JB. Fatal poisoning involving methapyrilene. J Am Med Assoc 1972; 219:756–7.

Gill DG, Sowerby HA. Orphenadrine poisoning in childhood. Practitioner 1975; 214:542–4.

Heinonen J, Heikkila J, Mattila MJ, Takki S. Orphenadrine poisoning. Arch Toxicol 1968; 23:264–72.

Leak D, Carroll D. Promethazine poisoning: clinical and electroencephalographic observations. Br Med J 1967; 2:31–2.

Robinson AE, Holder AT, McDowall RD, Powell R, Sattar H. Forensic toxicology of some orphenadrine-related deaths. Forensic Sci 1977; 9:53–62.

Sangster B, Van Heijst ANP, Zimmerman, ANE, De Vries HW: Intoxication by orphenadrine HCI; mechanism and therapy. Acts Pharmacol Toxicol 1977; 41 Suppl. II:129–36.

Winek CL, Fochtman FW, Trogus WJ, Fusia EP, Shanor SP. Methapyrilene toxicity. Clin Toxicol 1977; 11:287–94.

Wurmli K. Vergiftungen mit antihistaminica. Pharm Acta Helv 1973; 48:200–22.

Benzodiazepines

The benzodiazepines are widely used as mild tranquillizers and sedatives and there are numerous compounds encountered in clinical practice including bromazepam, chlordiazepoxide, clonazepam, desmethyldiazepam, diazepam, flunitrazepam, flurazepam, lorazepam, medazepam, nitrazepam, prazepam and temezepam.

The effect of these drugs in overdose is mild but, in the face of the most recent mortality statistics for the UK (see Chapter 1), it is difficult to support the view that overdosage with these drugs is never without harm. Dizziness, ataxia and slurred speech are common. Coma, respiratory depression and hypotension are usually mild but may be more prominent when alcohol has been ingested in addition to the drugs.

Gastric aspiration and lavage together with supportive therapy are the only necessary measures to be taken.

Further Reading

Busto U, Kaplan HL, Sellers EM. Benzodiazepine associated emergencies in Toronto. Am J Psychiatry 1980; 137:224–7.

Greenblatt, DJ, Allen MD, Noel BJ, Shader RI. Acute overdosage with benzodiazepine derivatives. Clin Pharmacol Ther 1977; 21:497–514.

Greenblatt DJ, Woo E, Allen MD, Orsulak PJ, Shader RI. Rapid recovery from massive diazepam overdose. J Am Med Assoc 1978; 240:1872–4.

Welch TR, Rumack BH, Hammond K. Clonazepam overdose resulting in cyclic coma. Clin Toxicol 1977; 10:433–6.

Butyrophenones

The butyrophenones (benperidol, haloperidol and triperidol) are used as antipsychotic and neuroleptic agents. Overdosage may result in drowsiness and hypotension but extrapyramidal side-effects are more common including akathisia and tardive dyskinesia.

Treatment is supportive but benztropine (2 mg i.v. or i.m.) may be used to control the extrapyramidal features.

Further Reading

Doenecke AL, Heuermann RC. Treatment of haloperidol abuse with diphenhydramine. Am J Psychiatry 1980; 137: 487–9.
Scialli JVK, Thornton WE. Toxic reactions from a haloperidol overdose in two children. Thermal and cardiac manifestations. J Am Med Assoc 1978; 239:48–9.
Sinaniotis CA, Spyrides P, Vlachos P, Papadatos C. Acute haloperidol poisoning in children. J Pediatr 1978; 93:1038–9.

Meprobamate

Meprobamate and related carbamates are still used as sedative and tranquillizing agents. Coma, respiratory depression and hypotension are the usual features of overdosage. Hypotension may be marked and pulmonary oedema has been reported in a number of patients.

Gastric aspiration and lavage should be performed where appropriate. Treatment is otherwise supportive although haemoperfusion may be necessary in very severely poisoned patients (see page 63).

Further Reading

Allen MD, Greenblatt DJ, Noel BJ. Meprobamate overdosage: a continuing problem. Clin Toxicol 1977; 11:501–15.
Crome P, Higgenbottom T, Elliott JA. Severe meprobamate poisoning: successful treatment with haemoperfusion. Postgrad Med J 1977; 53:698–9.
Lhoste F, Lemaire F, Rapin M. Treatment of hypotension in meprobamate poisoning. New Engl J Med 1977; 296:1004.
Schwartz HS. Acute meprobamate poisoning with gastrotomy and removal of a drug-containing mass. New Engl J Med 1976, 295:1177–78.

Phenothiazines

The phenothiazines are used primarily as antiemetic and antipsychotic drugs and their members include chlorpromazine, perphenazine, prochlorperazine, promethazine, promazine, trifluoperazine, thioridazine and trimeprazine. The phenothiazines have complex pharmacological properties and block peripheral cholinergic and α-adrenergic receptors, re-uptake of amines and the effects of histamine and 5HT.

The clinical features of phenothiazine overdosage include impairment of the level of consciousness, extrapyramidal signs (rigidity, tremor, hyper-reflexia, dyskinesia), marked restlessness and convulsions. Hypotension is common but respiratory depression is seen only in cases of severe poisoning. Tachycardia, ECG changes (prolongation of QT interval and T wave abnormalities) and arrhythmias may also occur. Hypothermia may be present and can be profound.

Treatment is supportive and gastric aspiration and lavage should be performed where appropriate. Benztropine (2 mg i.v. or i.m.) may be necessary to control the extrapyramidal features and diazepam should be given for convulsions.

Further Reading

Allen MD, Greenblatt DJ, Noel BJ. Overdosage with antipsychotic drugs. Am J Psychiatry 1980; 137:234–6.
Angle CR, McIntire MS, Zetterman R. CNS symptoms in childhood poisoning. Clin Toxicol 1968; 1:19–29.
Davis JM, Bartlett E, Termini BA. Overdosage of psychotropic dugs: a review. Dis Nerv Sys 1968; 29:157–64.
McKown CH, Verhulst HL, Crotty JJ. Overdosage effects and danger from tranquilizing drugs. J Am Med Assoc 1963; 185:425–30.

Anticonvulsants

Carbamazepine

Carbamazepine is structurally related to the tricyclic antidepressants and shares their anticholinergic activity. Overdosage may result in drowsiness, a dry mouth, coma and convulsions. Relapse into coma has been described during the course of recovery.

Treatment should include gastric lavage, if appropriate, and supportive therapy. Diazepam may be required to treat convulsions.

Further Reading

De Zeeuw RA, Westenberg HGM, Van der Kleijn E, Grimbrere JSF. An unusual case of carbamazepine poisoning with a near-fatal relapse after two days. Clin Toxicol 1979; 14: 263–9.
Salcman M, Pippenger CE. Acute carbamazepine encephalopathy. J. Am Med Assoc 1975; 231:915.

Ethosuximide and Methsuximide

The ingestion of either agent may cause anorexia, nausea, vomiting, drowsiness, dizziness, ataxia and coma. Treatment is supportive and gastric lavage should be performed where appropriate.

Further Reading

Karch SB. Methsuximide overdose. J Am Med Assoc 1973; 223:1463–5.

Paraldehyde

Paraldehyde is now rarely used as either a hypnotic or anticonvulsant agent. When ingested by mouth it causes marked gastrointestinal irritation with nausea and vomiting and it imparts a characteristic odour to the breath. Coma, respiratory and circulatory failure may occur and hepatic and renal damage have been reported. Severe metabolic acidosis may be a feature of paraldehyde intoxication but, although this substance is metabolized to acetic acid, other anions are thought to be involved.

Treatment is supportive and gastric lavage should be performed if appropriate.

Further Reading

Emmett M, Narins RG. Clinical use of the anion gap. Medicine 1977; 56:38–54.

Phenytoin and Hydantoin Derivatives

Acute overdosage of phenytoin results in nausea, vomiting, headaches, tremor, loss of consciousness, cerebellar ataxia and nystagmus. Respiratory depression may also occur.

Treatment should include gastric aspiration and lavage where appropriate, together with supportive therapy. Haemoperfusion should be considered in very severely poisoned patients.

Further Reading

Bruce AM, Smith H. The investigation of phenobarbitone, phenytoin and primidone in the death of epileptics. Med Sci Law 1977; 17:195–9.

Laubscher FA. Fatal diphenylhydantoin poisoning. J Am Med Assoc 1966; 198:1120–1.

Tenckhoff A, Sherrard DJ, Hickman RO, Ladda RL. Acute diphenylhydantoin intoxication. Am J Dis Child 1968; 116:422–5.

Primidone

Primidone is metabolized to phenobarbitone and phenylethyl malonamide, both of which are active anticonvulsants. The clinical features and management of primidone poisoning are the same as for barbiturate poisoning. Crystalluria has been noted.

Further Reading

Cate JC, Tenser R. Acute primidone overdosage with massive crystalluria. Clin Toxicol 1975; 8:385–9.

Sodium Valproate

Ingestion of sodium valproate in overdose may cause impairment of the level of consciousness and respiratory depression. Gastric lavage is of limited value because of rapid absorption of the drug. Treatment is supportive.

Further Reading

Tift JP. Valproic acid. New Engl J Med 1980; 303:394.

Sulthiame

Sulthiame is a sulphonamide derivative and possesses weak carbonic anhydrase inhibitory activity. Overdosage may result in headache, vomiting, ataxia, vertigo and hyperventilation. Hyper-reflexia, clouding of consciousness and catatonia may develop and renal tubular obstruction due to heavy crystalluria may occur.

Treatment is supportive but the urine should be kept alkaline to avoid crystalluria and renal impairment.

References

Rockley GJ. Attempted suicide with sulthiame. Br Med J 1965; 2:632.

Chapter 12

Peter Crome

Antidepressant Drug Poisoning

Over the last decade there has been a considerable increase in the mortality from antidepressant poisoning. In 1977, the last year for which statistics are available, 441 of the 3969 patients who died from acute poisoning in England and Wales had taken an antidepressant drug either alone or in combination with other agents. Two main reasons appear to account for this increase. First, antidepressant drugs are given to patients who are depressed and who are therefore more likely to poison themselves. Second, the number of prescriptions for antidepressant drugs has risen markedly over the same period; in 1977 nine-and-a-half million prescriptions for antidepressants were issued by general practitioners in England and Wales.

Tricyclic antidepressants are believed to act in mental depression by blockade of re-uptake of noradrenaline and/or 5-hydroxytryptamine into intracerebral neurones. This leads to increased concentrations of these monoamines in certain key areas of the brain. In addition, tricyclic antidepressants block the parasympathetic nervous system, the peripheral re-uptake of noradrenaline and also have a complex action on the heart. These diverse pharmacological properties account for the side-effects that complicate the therapeutic use of tricyclic antidepressants and cause their toxicity when taken in overdose.

The 13 tricyclic antidepressants currently available in the UK are all chemically related to either amitriptyline or imipramine (Table 12.1). They are the most common type of antidepressant prescribed and account for the majority of overdoses and deaths due to this group of drugs. In addition to their use in the treatment of depression, they are prescribed for anxiety, obsessional and phobic states and for childhood enuresis.

Table 12.1. Tricyclic antidepressants available in the UK.

Amitriptyline	*Imipramine*
Butriptyline	Clomipramine
Dothiepin	Desipramine
Doxepin	Dibenzepin
Maprotiline[1]	Opipramol
Nortriptyline	Trimipramine
Protriptyline	

[1] This drug, which has a four-ringed structure, is pharmacologically related to the tricyclic group and is included here.

Tricyclic Antidepressants

Clinical Features

These can be subdivided into those affecting the parasympathetic, the central and peripheral nervous systems, the cardiovascular and the respiratory systems (Table 12.2). In patients who are only mildly poisoned, drowsiness, sinus tachycardia, dry mouth, dilated pupils, increased tendon reflexes and extensor plantar responses are the most common clinical features. The morbidity and mortality in those who are severely poisoned are due largely to a cardiorespiratory depressant action, which produces hypoxia and either respiratory or metabolic acidosis. Grade IV coma and convulsions may also complicate the clinical picture.

Table 12.2. Clinical features of tricyclic antidepressant poisoning.

Effects on the parasympathetic nervous system	Effects on the central nervous system	Effects on the cardiovascular system	Effects on the respiratory system
Dry mouth	Agitation/delirium	Bradycardia	Respiratory depression
Blurred vision	Twitching	Sinus tachycardia	Aspiration pneumonia
Dilated pupils	Convulsions	Ventricular tachycardia	Intrapulmonary shunts
Constipation	Hallucinations	Ventricular fibrillation	Shock lung
Retention of urine	Pyramidal and extra-pyramidal signs	Conduction disturbances	Apnoea
Pyrexia	Coma	Asystole	
		Hypotension	

Symptoms usually appear within 30 to 60 minutes after ingestion of an overdose, except when a slow-release preparation has been taken, and usually reach maximum intensity in 4 to 12 hours. It is uncommon for coma to last for more than 24 hours, and even severely poisoned patients have usually recovered completely within 48 hours. Delirium may be a troublesome complication during the recovery phase.

Although there have been claims to the contrary, particularly by pharmaceutical companies, there appears to be little difference in the toxicity of the various tricyclic antidepressant drugs when taken in overdose. As a general rule, mild to moderate poisoning may be expected if less than 10 mg/kg body weight of the drug has been ingested. Severe poisoning is likely if 15 to 20 mg/kg body weight has been taken, though death in adults is rare when less than 1 g has been ingested.

Cardiovascular Complications

In therapeutic dosage tricyclic antidepressants may cause tachycardia, palpitations and postural hypotension. In addition, an increased incidence of sudden death and heart failure has been reported in patients with pre-existent cardiac disease. In the past these complications have been attributed to the anticholinergic activity of tricyclic antidepressants with potentiation of circulating noradrenaline and consequent cardiac arrhythmias. However, it has recently been established that tricyclic antidepressants have a dose-related quinidine-like action on the heart which results in decreased myocardial contractility and increased conduction time.

In overdose, the cardiac complications are likely to be due to a combination of these actions, but the quinidine-like activity probably accounts for the bizarre electrocardiographic changes that may be seen in severe poisoning (Figure 12.1, a and b). In very severely poisoned patients the increased heart rate returns to normal or there may be a bradycardia accompanied by varying degrees of heart block. Blood pressure and cardiac output also fall progressively. At the same time, the QRS complex becomes wider and P waves diminish in amplitude. This may make differentiation between sinus rhythm with prolonged intraventricular conduction and ventricular and supraventricular rhythms difficult, if not impossible. In common with hypnotic drugs taken in overdose there may be either a relative or absolute hypovolaemia which contributes to the hypotension seen.

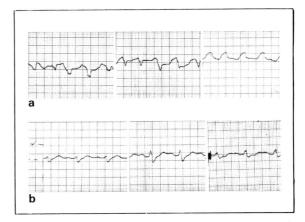

Figure 12.1. *Electrocardiogram (Leads I, II and III) of a patient with severe amitriptyline poisoning (a) on admission and (b) nine hours later. The first ECG shows the characteristic, bizarre, wide QRS complex seen in severe poisoning. The second ECG shows more obvious sinus rhythm with a bundle-branch block pattern.*

Respiratory Complications

Patients with tricyclic antidepressant poisoning are as likely as those with barbiturate poisoning to become hypoxic. This may be due either to depression of ventilation or to local pulmonary changes following aspiration of stomach contents. Patients poisoned by tricyclic antidepressants are particularly likely to develop cardiac complications if hypoxic.

Laboratory Investigations

There is often no difficulty in diagnosing tricyclic antidepressant poisoning, even when the patient is unconscious and unable to give a history, because the cardiac and neurological changes are usually characteristic. In some cases, however, diagnosis may not be easy if the patient presents atypically, for example in status epilepticus. In such cases laboratory confirmation of poisoning may be helpful.

Plasma drug concentrations above 1000 μg/l are associated with Grade IV coma (often prolonged), convulsions, cardiac complications and respiratory depression requiring mechanical ventilation. Nevertheless, patients have recovered with plasma concentrations over 5000 μg/l (therapeutic plasma levels are usually less than 250 μg/l).

Treatment

The majority of patients poisoned with tricyclic antidepressant drugs require no more than supportive care. A few require admission to an intensive care unit for cardiorespiratory support and to monitor and treat cardiac arrhythmias. The management of patients who are severely poisoned is summarized in Table 12.3.

Prevention of Further Absorption of the Drug

Gastric aspiration and lavage should be performed in all adults with tricyclic antidepressant poisoning when more than 250 mg of the drug has been taken. In children, emesis should be induced with syrup of ipecacuanha (Ipecacuanha Paediatric Emetic Draught BPC 10 to 15 ml, repeated once if necessary). Tricyclic antidepressants delay gastric emptying and large quantities of tablets may therefore remain in the stomach for some considerable time. For this reason,

Table 12.3. Treatment of severe tricyclic antidepressant poisoning.

Prevention of further absorption of drug
  Gastric aspiration and lavage (up to 12 hours)
  Activated charcoal 10 to 20 g by mouth

Cardiorespiratory support
  Correct hypovolaemia and hypoxia
  Correct acidosis with sodium bicarbonate
  Rx dopamine or dobutamine if above measures fail

Treat arrhythmias
  ? Drugs
  DC shock
  Pacemaker

Treat convulsions
  Diazepam or chlormethiazole intravenously

Physostigmine 2 to 4 mg intravenously

gastric lavage may be useful up to 12 hours after ingestion of an overdose. As in the case of all drugs taken in overdose, care should be taken to prevent aspiration of stomach contents, particularly in unconscious or uncooperative patients. Before gastric lavage is attempted a cuffed endotracheal tube should be inserted in all patients in whom a gag reflex is absent.

Absorption of drug from the GI tract may be further reduced by the oral administration of activated charcoal. This substance has been shown to reduce the absorption of large therapeutic doses of tricyclic antidepressants, but its efficacy in overdose has not been fully evaluated in man. It can be given as a drink, provided the patient is still conscious, or left in the stomach after gastric lavage. The optimum charcoal:drug ratio is 10:1, and a dose of 10-20 g should be sufficient to adsorb most of the drug left in the gut even after a severe tricyclic overdose. Activated charcoal may be given conveniently as two sachets of Medicoal dispersed in 200 to 300 ml of water. Other drugs should not be given by mouth as these may also be absorbed onto the charcoal.

Cardiorespiratory Support

When taken in overdose tricyclic antidepressant drugs decrease myocardial contractility and increase conduction times. If there is evidence of poor tissue perfusion (cold extremities, poor urine output and hypotension) after correction of any hypovolaemia, acidosis and hypoxia, then a positive inotropic drug, e.g. dopamine or dobutamine should be used. Physostigmine salicylate has been shown to have a positive inotropic activity in animal experiments but its effects in man are short-lived and unpredictable.

A variety of arrhythmias may occur in those who are severely poisoned. These include sinus bradycardia, supraventricular and ventricular tachycardias, ventricular fibrillation and sinus rhythm with grossly prolonged atrioventricular and intraventricular conduction times (Figure 12.1 a and b). Although there is a natural inclination to use an anti-arrhythmic drug to treat a tachycardia it should be remembered that disopyramide, lignocaine and β-adrenergic blocking drugs have been shown to potentiate tricyclic-induced cardiotoxicity both in animals and man. Moreover, the tachycardias which occur in this type of poisoning do not appear to have the same prognostic significance as similar arrhythmias occurring after a myocardial infarction and thus, in the majority of cases, anti-arrhythmic drugs are not required.

Transvenous cardiac pacing and direct current shock may be required for profound bradycardia or ventricular fibrillation respectively, although they are not always successful. A few patients have survived after their cardiac output has been maintained by external cardiac massage for several hours.

Sodium lactate (500 ml of a molar solution infused over 30 minutes) has been used to reverse the cardiotoxic effects of tricyclic antidepressant poisoning. It is claimed that this treatment is of particular value in shortening the width of the QRS complex. Whether this in turn has any beneficial effect on either blood pressure or cardiac output is not reported.

Sodium bicarbonate (10 mmol intravenously) has also been shown to reverse some cardiac arrhythmias in children. In animal experiments it was found that both sodium bicarbonate and artificial hyperventilation suppressed amitriptyline-induced arrhythmias. It is therefore probable that the beneficial action of bicarbonate is due solely to correction of the acidosis which is often present in severely poisoned patients.

Treatment of Convulsions

Fits, especially if repeated, may not only cause cerebral anoxia but may also precipitate cardiac arrest. For this reason prompt treatment is necessary. Diazepam and chlormethiazole intravenously are probably the agents of choice, but it needs to be emphasized that these drugs may further depress respiration. If the convulsions remain uncontrolled despite these measures, physostigmine (see below) may be tried cautiously. If drug therapy proves ineffective, and especially if the patient also has evidence of impaired cardiac function, mechanical ventilation and muscle paralysis should be instituted without delay. Ventilated patients should continue to receive anticonvulsants and their progress should, if possible, be observed using a cerebral function monitor.

The Use of Physostigmine

Coma may be reversed in tricyclic antidepressant poisoning by the intravenous injection of physostigmine salicylate, a cholinesterase inhibitor which crosses the blood—brain barrier. Unfortunately it has a short duration of action (usually less than 45 minutes) at the end of which time the patient may lapse back into coma. If too large a dose is injected marked cholinergic effects such as bradycardia and involuntary defaecation may ensue. The analeptic action of physostigmine is by no means specific to the anticholinergic group of drugs, and improvement in the level of consciousness in patients poisoned with barbiturates, benzodiazepines and glutethimide has also been reported. Like other analeptics it may precipitate convulsions. For these reasons physostigmine should not be used routinely. Its use should be restricted to patients in prolonged coma with complications such as pneumonia, or to exclude brain death in patients who have had an apnoeic episode. A suitable dose for an adult is 2 to 4 mg intravenously given over five minutes.

Delirium, choreoathetosis and tremor may all be reversed by physostigmine but because of its short duration of action these may all recur.

Active Elimination Techniques

As only a relatively small proportion of the body load of tricyclic antidepressants is circulating in the vascular compartment, forced diuresis and haemodialysis are able to remove only small amounts of the drug from the body. More recently, haemoperfusion with XAD-4 resin has been claimed to be effective in reversing coma and cardiotoxicity. However, although plasma clearance is high, only small amounts of drug are removed by this technique. None of these procedures can be recommended.

Monoamine Oxidase Inhibitors (MAOI)

These drugs are now used infrequently in the treatment of depression. They inhibit monoamine oxidase enzyme activity so that pressor substances naturally present in food, such as tyramine, are absorbed unchanged instead of being broken down in the gut and liver. This forms the basis of the so-called 'cheese reaction', when a patient taking monoamine oxidase inhibitors therapeutically may develop headache, coma, convulsions and severe hypertension following the ingestion of cheese. Other food substances such as broad beans and yeast extracts may produce similar reactions.

Clinical Features

Symptoms may be delayed for some hours after acute overdosage with MAOI. Symptoms are due principally to increased sympathetic activity and include excitement, pyrexia, increased tendon reflexes, convulsions, coma, sinus tachycardia and either hypo- or hypertension.

Treatment

Treatment of MAOI overdosage is essentially supportive. Hypotension should, in the first instance, be treated by fluid replacement to restore a normal circulating blood volume; a central venous pressure line may be needed to gauge fluid replacement. Elevation of the foot of the bed may also be useful. If possible, sympathomimetic drugs should be avoided in the treatment of hypotension due to MAOI overdosage for fear of potentiation of their pressor effect. Hypertension should be treated by the administration of an α-blocker such as phentolamine or phenoxybenzamine. Sedatives such as diazepam or chlormethiazole may be required for patients with severe excitement.

Lithium

Lithium carbonate is used in the treatment of manic depression both as a conventional formulation (Camcolit) and as sustained release formulations (Phasal and Priadel). The therapeutic range is small and toxicity may be either iatrogenic or the result of deliberate overdosage. Symptoms of overdosage include thirst, polyuria, diarrhoea and vomiting and in more serious cases, there may be impaired consciousness, hypertonicity and convulsions.

Laboratory Investigations

Measurement of the plasma lithium concentration is essential in cases of suspected toxicity. Levels above 1.5 mmol/l confirm toxicity. It is important to note that the sustained release formulations may delay and/or prolong both the symptoms and the timing of the peak plasma levels.

Treatment

In addition to supportive therapy the use of anticonvulsants, e.g. diazepam (10 mg i.v.), and active elimination therapy may be needed. The decision to use the latter is based on the severity of symptoms and the plasma lithium level (usually greater than 2 mmol/l). Forced alkaline diuresis is effective but peritoneal dialysis or haemodialysis may be needed if renal function is inadequate or if there is severe electrolyte imbalance.

Miscellaneous Drugs

The lack of predictable efficacy and the frequency of adverse side-effects of existing drugs have led to the development of a number of novel compounds for the treatment of depression. These drugs differ one from another not only pharmacologically but also toxicologically. It is likely that more drugs in this group will become available over the next few years.

Flupenthixol

This drug is a phenothiazine which in larger doses is used to treat schizophrenia. Overdose may cause loss of consciousness, dyskinesia, extrapyramidal signs and hypotension. In practice, however, symptoms are mild. Treatment is essentially supportive; benztropine and related drugs will reverse dyskinetic reactions.

Iprindole

This drug has a three-ringed structure but is not related to the other tricyclic drugs. It has little cardiotoxicity and has only mild anticholinergic properties. It is not prescribed widely and information on its effects in overdose is limited.

L-Tryptophan

This amino acid is a precursor of 5-hydroxytryptamine and it has been shown to increase the efficacy of monoamine oxidase inhibitors. Drowsiness may complicate its therapeutic use but cases of overdose have not been reported.

Mianserin

Mianserin has a four-ringed structure and it is believed to act in depression by increasing noradrenaline turnover. Drowsiness is a common side-effect of overdose but convulsions, cardiotoxicity and respiratory depression have not been reported, except when other drugs have been taken in addition. Treatment is symptomatic.

Nomifensine

This drug blocks the reuptake of both noradrenaline and dopamine into intracerebral neurones. Drowsiness, tremor and sinus tachycardia are the most common features of overdose but anticholinergic effects, convulsions and more serious cardiotoxicity have not been reported. Treatment is again symptomatic.

Pyridoxine

This vitamin is promoted for use in depression associated with the oral contraceptive pill. It is non-toxic.

Tofenacin

Tofenacin is a metabolite of the anti-Parkinsonian drug orphenadrine. Overdose resembles that caused by tricyclic antidepressants and should be treated similarly.

Viloxazine

This antidepressant not infrequently causes nausea and vomiting in therapeutic doses. More serious effects have not been reported when viloxazine has been taken in overdose.

Summary

The treatment of tricyclic antidepressant poisoning is essentially that of intensive supportive therapy. The stomach should be emptied by gastric aspiration and lavage and activated charcoal administered. Fluid depletion, acidosis, hypoxia and convulsions should be promptly treated along conventional lines. Drug treatment should be avoided, if at all possible, in the management of cardiovascular toxicity, but if supportive therapy alone fails, then drugs with positive inotropic actions should be tried first.

The treatment of poisoning due to monoamine oxidase inhibitors (MAOI) and lithium is essentially supportive, although severe hypertension due to MAOI may necessitate the use of an α-blocking agent. Also, active elimination therapy is sometimes required for lithium poisoning.

Further Reading

Bickel MH. Poisoning by tricyclic antidepressant drugs. Int J Clin Pharmacol Biopharm 1975; 11:145–76.

Biggs JT, Spiker DG, Petit JM, Ziegler VE. Tricyclic antidepressant overdose: incidence of symptoms. J Am Med Assoc 1977; 238:135–8.

Brown TCK. Tricyclic antidepressant overdosage: experimental studies on the management of circulatory complications. Clin Toxicol 1976; 9:255–72.

Brown TCK. Sodium bicarbonate treatment for tricyclic antidepressant arrhythmias in children. Med J Aust 1976; 2:380–2.

Brown TCK, Barker GA, Dunlop ME, Loughnan PM. The use of sodium bicarbonate in the treatment of tricyclic antidepressant-induced arrhythmias. Anaesthesia and Intensive Care 1973; 1:203–10.

Burrows GD, Vohra J, Sloman JG, Scoggins BA, Davies B. Cardiac effects of different tricyclic antidepressant drugs. Br J Psychiatry 1976; 129:335–41.

Crome P, Braithwaite RA. Relationship between clinical features of tricyclic antidepressant poisoning and plasma concentrations in children. Arch Dis Child 1978; 53:902–5.

Crome P, Newman B. The problem of tricyclic antidepressant poisoning. Postgrad Med J 1979; 55:528–32.

Crome P, Newman B. Fatal tricyclic antidepressant poisoning. J R Soc Med 1979; 72:649–53.

Dumovic P, Burrows GD, Vohra J, Davies B, Scoggins BA. The effect of tricyclic antidepressant drugs on the heart. Arch Toxicol 1976; 35:255–62.

Editorial. Sodium bicarbonate and tricyclic antidepressant poisoning. Lancet 1976, ii:838.

Goel KM, Shanks RA. Amitriptyline and imipramine poisoning in children. Br Med J 1974; 1:261–3.

Hansen HE, Amdisen A. Lithium intoxiciation. Q J Med 1978; 47:123–44.

Jefferson JW. A review of the cardiovascular effects and toxocity of tricyclic antidepressants. Psychosom Med 1975; 37:160–79.

Newton RW. Physostigmine salicylate in the treatment of tricyclic antidepressant overdosage. J Am Med Assoc 1975; 231:941–3.

Rumack BH. Physostigmine: rational use. J Am Coll Emerg Phys 1976; 5:541–2.

Starkey IR, Lawson AAH. Poisoning with tricyclic and related antidepressants – a ten year review. Q J Med 1980; 49:33–49.

Sutherland GR, Park J, Proudfoot AT. Ventilation and acid–base · changes in deep coma due to barbiturate or tricyclic antidepressant poisoning. Clin Toxicol 1977; 11:403–12.

Thorstrand C. Cardiovascular effects of poisoning with tricyclic antidepressants. Acta Med Scand 1974; 195:505–14.

Thorstrand C. Cardiovascular effects of poisoning with tricyclic antidepressants with special reference to the ECG. Acta Med Scand 1976; 199:337–44.

Chapter 13

T. J. Meredith and J. A. Vale

Salicylate Poisoning

Despite the introduction of alternative agents in recent years, aspirin remains one of the most commonly used analgesics and is found in most households in this country. It is not surprising, therefore, that aspirin poisoning is a common cause for admission to hospital. Although accidental consumption of aspirin by young children has been reduced as a result of new legal requirements for packaging, iatrogenic overdose in children is not uncommon. Moreover, aspirin is still commonly taken by many adults who choose deliberately to poison themselves.

Epidemiology

In the nine-year period, 1968 to 1977, there were 34 deaths attributed to aspirin poisoning in England and Wales in children under 14 years of age. Admission rates to hospital for poisoning in children remained constant over the same period until 1976, when a fall of five per cent was seen in those aged 0 to 4 years. It is possible that this reflects the introduction of new legislation in January 1976, which requires that all retail sales of solid aspirin are in opaque child-resistant containers or dark-tinted or opaque unit packaging. Furthermore, the tablets must be white and the packs must contain no more than 25 doses. In two areas of the country, Newcastle-upon-Tyne and South Glamorgan, marked falls in the number of hospital admissions for childhood salicylate poisoning have been observed since the introduction of child-resistant containers. So far as adults are concerned, approximately 200 deaths due to salicylate poisoning occur each year in England and Wales. In 1978 there were 215 deaths officially recorded as being due to the ingestion of aspirin alone.

Although ingestion of aspirin tablets (acetylsalicylic acid 300 mg) is the most frequent cause of salicylate poisoning, salicylic acid (a keratolytic agent) and methylsalicylate (oil of wintergreen) occasionally cause toxicity. This is most often the result of absorption through the skin. Methylsalicylate, if ingested by mouth, is particularly toxic due to rapid absorption and the fact that one teaspoonful is equivalent to 12 standard 300 mg tablets of aspirin.

Pharmacology and Pharmacokinetics

In therapeutic doses, aspirin is an effective analgesic, antipyretic and anti-inflammatory agent. All three properties are related to the ability of aspirin to inhibit the synthesis of prostaglandins.

Aspirin is rapidly absorbed from the stomach and small intestine although, in very large doses, absorption may occur more slowly. This is partly because the tablets adhere together to form a large bolus which dissolves slowly, and partly because gastric emptying is delayed. For these reasons, blood levels of aspirin may continue to rise for up to 24 hours after ingestion of an overdose.

The frequency with which therapeutic overdosage with aspirin occurs is often due to failure to understand the pharmacokinetics of elimination of the drug from the body. The most important biotransformation pathways, the formation of salicyluric acid and salicyl phenolic glucuronide (Figure 13.1), are saturable, a fact which has the following clinically important consequences.

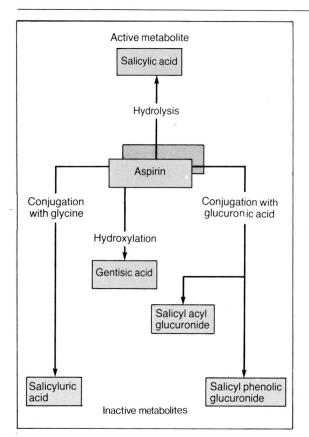

Figure 13.1. *The metabolism of aspirin.*

1. The time needed to eliminate a given fraction of a dose increases with increasing dose.

2. The steady-state blood level of a salicylate, particularly that of the pharmacologically active non protein-bound fraction, increases more than proportionately with increasing dose.

3. As the metabolic pathways of elimination become saturated, renal excretion of salicylic acid becomes increasingly important and this pathway is extremely sensitive to changes in urinary pH above pH 6. The ingestion of antacids, for example, increases elimination of the drug significantly and, in cases of salicylate intoxication, the use of forced alkaline diuresis exploits this particular aspect of salicylate excretion.

The therapeutic blood level of aspirin lies in excess of 150 mg/l, but symptoms of toxicity become apparent when the blood level exceeds 300 mg/l. In children the majority of fatalities from aspirin poisoning are the result of therapeutic overdose. For this reason a rational approach to long-term therapy should be employed, not only in children but also in

adults; 60 mg/kg/day in divided doses is a reasonable starting dose, but the blood salicylate level should be checked after five to seven days and the dose adjusted accordingly.

Pathophysiology of Salicylate Toxicity (Figure 13.2)

Fluid and Electrolyte Loss and Acid–Base Disturbances

In overdose salicylates directly stimulate the respiratory centre to produce both increased depth and rate of respiration, thereby causing a respiratory alkalosis to develop. In an attempt by the body to compensate, bicarbonate, accompanied by sodium, potassium and water, is excreted in the urine. Dehydration and hypokalaemia result but, more importantly, the loss of bicarbonate diminishes the buffering capacity of the body and allows an acidosis to develop more easily. Very high concentrations of salicylates in the tissues actually depress the respiratory centre and may further contribute to the development of a metabolic acidosis.

Metabolic acidosis in patients with salicylate poisoning is due not only to the presence of salicylic acid itself but also to interference with carbohydrate, lipid, protein and amino acid metabolism. Salicylates inhibit Kreb's cycle dehydrogenases, specifically α-keto glutaric dehydrogenase and succinic acid dehydrogenase. This inhibition produces an increase in circulating lactic and pyruvic acids. Salicylates affect lipid metabolism in several ways but essentially they stimulate fat metabolism and cause increased production of ketone bodies. Starvation and dehydration also contribute to the development of ketosis. Protein metabolism is accelerated, protein synthesis diminished and aminotransferases, responsible for the interconversion of amino acids, are inhibited. The result is increased circulating blood levels of amino acids together with aminoaciduria; this latter feature is further enhanced by inhibition of active tubular reabsorption of amino acids. The aminoaciduria increases the solute load on the kidneys and thereby increases water loss from the body.

Uncoupling of Oxidative Phosphorylation

Another primary effect of salicylates is to uncouple oxidative phosphorylation. The result is failure to

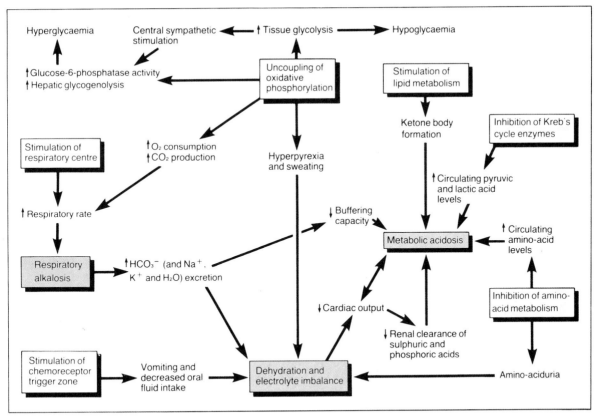

Figure 13.2. *The pathophysiology of salicylate toxicity.*

produce high-energy phosphates, so that ATP-dependent reactions are inhibited. Oxygen utilization and carbon dioxide production are increased. Energy normally used for the conversion of inorganic phosphate to ATP is dissipated as heat. Hyperpyrexia and sweating result and further dehydration occurs.

Central Emetic Effect

Fluid loss is enhanced by a central effect of salicylates which causes nausea and vomiting and, as a result, a diminished oral fluid intake. If dehydration is sufficiently severe, the low cardiac output and oliguria result in reduced clearance of sulphuric and phosphoric acids from the body; this aggravates the metabolic acidosis already present which, if severe, can itself diminish cardiac output.

Glucose Metabolism

Glucose metabolism also suffers as a result of uncoupled oxidative phosphorylation because of increased tissue glycolysis and peripheral demand for glucose. This is seen principally in skeletal muscle and may cause hypoglycaemia. The brain appears to be particularly sensitive to this effect and CNS glucose depletion may occur in the presence of a normal blood sugar level.

Increased metabolism and peripheral demand for glucose cause activation of hypothalamic sympathetic centres with adrenocortical stimulation and release of adrenaline. Increased glucose-6-phosphatase activity and hepatic glycogenolysis contribute to the hyperglycaemia sometimes seen following the ingestion of large amounts of salicylate. Increased circulating adrenocorticosteroid levels further contribute to the electrolyte and fluid imbalance.

Clinical Features of Salicylate Poisoning (Table 13.1)

The dose of salicylate ingested and the age of the patient are the most important factors which determine the severity of an overdose. Prior therapeutic

Table 13.1.   Clinical features of salicylate poisoning.

Nausea, vomiting and epigastric discomfort

Hyperpyrexia and sweating

Irritability, tremor, tinnitus and deafness

Tachypnea, hyperpnea and pulmonary oedema

Dehydration, hypokalaemia and hyper- or hyponatraemia

Respiratory alkalosis followed by metabolic acidosis (except in children)

Hyper- or hypoglycemia and hypoprothrombinaemia

administration of aspirin increases the toxicity of an acutely ingested overdose.

Children quickly develop a metabolic acidosis following the ingestion of aspirin in overdose and respiratory alkalosis is rare under the age of four years. The frequency with which the latter disturbance occurs increases with age until the usual adult picture of a respiratory alkalosis followed by a metabolic acidosis is seen by the age of 12 years. The reason for this changing pattern of response to salicylate has not been established. The development of an acidosis is followed by increasing central nervous system (CNS) toxicity and is associated with a poor prognosis.

Early Symptoms and Signs

In the early stages of moderate to severe salicylate poisoning, hyperpyrexia and sweating, vomiting and epigastric pain, and tinnitus and deafness may all occur. The latter disturbances are due to a direct effect of salicylate on the central nervous system. Early loss of consciousness does not occur following the ingestion of a salicylate overdose unless a hypnotic or sedative drug has been taken in addition. Drowsiness, stupor and even coma may occur in the late stages of very severe salicylate intoxication but are then almost invariably associated with the presence of a severe acidosis.

Respiratory Alkalosis

Adults, and children over the age of 12 years, generally exhibit a respiratory alkalosis in the early stages of salicylate poisoning. Dehydration occurs quickly and is due to the combination of sweating, vomiting,

overbreathing and an osmotic diuresis due to the presence of excess bicarbonate, sodium and potassium in the urine. Hypokalaemia may also be prominent and is due principally to the effects of the respiratory alkalosis, although vomiting, increased circulating adrenocorticosteroids and aminoaciduria (which is accompanied by loss of cations, especially potassium) also contribute. Although an alkaline urine is usually found in the early stages of salicylate poisoning, it is possible to find an acid urine if potassium loss from the body has been extreme.

Metabolic Acidosis

The loss of buffering capacity from the body and the various metabolic changes already discussed eventually lead to the development of a metabolic acidosis. This phase is seen much earlier in young children and accounts for the seriousness of salicylate overdose in this group of patients. To some extent the presence of an alkalosis affords protection against serious salicylate toxicity. At an alkaline pH salicylate becomes ionized and therefore penetrates cell membranes poorly. The development of a metabolic acidosis allows salicylate molecules to penetrate tissues more easily and leads, in particular, to CNS toxicity. Metabolic acidosis may occur early on in adults if a respiratory depressant drug has also been ingested, because the protective respiratory alkalotic phase is diminished or even abolished.

CNS Toxicity

The features of CNS toxicity seen in salicylate poisoning include general irritability and tremor, often soon after ingestion of the overdose. Subsequently hallucinations and delirium may occur and drowsiness and stupor sometimes develop. Deeper stages of coma are rare in salicylate poisoning. Central respiratory and cardiovascular depression may occur with very high tissue salicylate concentrations. It should be remembered that hypoglycaemia may be a feature of salicylate intoxication and CNS glucose depletion can occur in the presence of a normal blood sugar. Hypoglycaemia is less common in children than in adults, but when it does occur, it is more severe. Hyperglycaemia may also occur and persist for several days.

Pulmonary Oedema

One intriguing feature of salicylate poisoning is the occurrence of pulmonary oedema. Although this is most often due to fluid overload consequent upon overvigorous treatment, it can also occur in the presence of hypovolaemia. The pulmonary oedema fluid has the same protein and electrolyte composition as plasma, suggesting increased pulmonary vascular permeability. Although a neurogenic mechanism for the development of pulmonary oedema has not been completely excluded this is now thought to be unlikely. Platelets play an important role in the maintenance of vascular integrity, and it is possible that an effect of aspirin on prostaglandin synthesis and platelet function is responsible for the increased microvascular leak of proteins and fluid.

Hypoprothrombinaemia

Although aspirin overdose is associated with inhibition of platelet aggregation and hypoprothrombinaemia, it is unusual for significant bleeding problems to be seen. Aspirin-induced hypoprothrombinaemia is due mainly to decreased hepatic synthesis of factor VII, an action similar to that of warfarin. This effect is believed to be due to competition of aspirin with vitamin K and is reversed by the intravenous administration of vitamin K. Gastric erosions and gastrointestinal bleeding appear to be uncommon following salicylate overdose.

Oliguria

Oliguria is sometimes seen in patients following the ingestion of salicylates in overdose. The most common cause is dehydration but, very rarely, acute renal failure or inappropriate secretion of antidiuretic hormone may occur. These three conditions may readily be differentiated by measurement of the concentrations of sodium and urea together with osmolality in plasma and urine.

Laboratory Investigations

Most investigations necessary for the management of salicylate overdose have already been mentioned. The urinary pH is usually alkaline in the early stages and subsequently becomes acid. Measurement of arterial blood gases, pH and standard bicarbonate may show a respiratory alkalosis followed by the development of a metabolic acidosis. It is more usual, however, to find a mixed acid—base disturbance. Hypokalaemia is usual, but the plasma sodium concentration may be either high or low depending upon the principal source of fluid loss and the type of

replacement therapy given. The blood sugar may be high or low and the prothrombin time prolonged.

Assesssment of the Severity of a Salicylate Overdose

The dose of aspirin ingested and the age of the patient are important determinants of the severity of intoxication. In an adult, moderate to severe toxicity will result from the ingestion of about 50 standard 300 mg aspirin tablets.

Blood salicylate levels are the best guide to the severity of salicylate poisoning but they are less reliable when aspirin is already being taken therapeutically. The blood salicylate level should be determined six hours after ingestion of an overdose, and this should be repeated several hours later to make sure that the level is not continuing to rise because of slow absorption. Generally speaking, blood salicylate levels of less than 500 mg/l six hours after ingestion of an overdose are associated with only mild toxicity; levels between 500 and 750 mg/l are associated with moderate toxicity; levels in excess of 750 mg/l at six hours may be associated with severe toxicity.

The clinical features and the presence and type of acid—base disturbance are important guides to the prognosis and to the need for specific treatment. The presence of a metabolic acidosis is ominous even if the blood salicylate is not markedly elevated. Blood salicylate levels are difficult to interpret in the presence of an acidosis because salicylate is taken up into the tissues and blood levels fall, even though the salicylate is not being eliminated from the body.

Treatment (Table 13.2)

Gastric Aspiration and Lavage

Gastric aspiration and lavage is of value up to 24 hours after the ingestion of a large salicylate overdose because the drug tends to form a large insoluble mass in the stomach. Young children who have ingested aspirin tablets accidentally should be given syrup of ipecacuanha (Ipecacuanha Paediatric Emetic Draught BPC, 10 to 15 ml) rather than being subjected to gastric lavage.

Table 13.2.   Treatment of salicylate poisoning.

Gastric aspiration and lavage or, in a child, Ipecacuanha Paediatric Emetic Draught BPC. 10–15 ml

Correction of dehydration either orally or parenterally

Correction of hypokalaemia

Correction of severe metabolic acidosis with *cautious* administration of intravenous bicarbonate

Tepid sponging for hyperpyrexia

Intravenous vitamin K for hypoprothrombinaemia

Forced alkaline diuresis if blood salicylate level > 500 mg/l and marked clinical features or acidosis present

Consider haemoperfusion or haemodialysis if blood salicylate level > 900 mg/l

---

Activated Charcoal

Activated charcoal adsorbs aspirin in the stomach and small intestine, but the necessary charcoal:drug ratio is unfavourable. The ideal charcoal:drug ratio for maximum adsorption of most drugs is 10:1, and this means that 100 g of charcoal is needed to adsorb every 10 g of aspirin.

Fluid and Electrolyte Replacement

Fluid and electrolyte replacement is of paramount importance. Special attention should be paid to potassium supplementation because some degree of hypokalaemia is almost invariably present. The particular regime for the replacement of sodium and water depends upon the principal source of loss, i.e. vomiting, hyperventilation or osmotic diuresis. The fluid regime should include at least some dextrose to prevent the development of hypoglycaemia. If hyperpyrexia is severe, tepid sponging is the easiest and the most appropriate treatment.

Intravenous Vitamin K

Hypoprothrombinaemia may readily be corrected by the use of intravenous vitamin K.

Correction of Acid–Base Disturbances

The presence of a respiratory alkalosis requires no specific treatment, but a severe metabolic acidosis may require at least partial correction with bicarbonate. However, patients with severe metabolic acidosis usually receive a forced alkaline diuresis and this serves to correct the acidosis as well as to enhance excretion of the drug. Bicarbonate should be administered cautiously because hypokalaemia is aggravated and the sodium and water load may precipitate pulmonary oedema. Sedatives and respiratory depressant drugs should be avoided because they hasten the development of metabolic acidosis and CNS toxicity. Tetany is occasionally seen in salicylate poisoning because of alkalosis, which may be either primarily respiratory in origin or due to the administration of bicarbonate as part of a forced alkaline diuresis regime. Very rarely, tetany is due to loss of calcium or magnesium in the urine. Tetany may be corrected with the use of calcium gluconate (10 ml of a 10 per cent solution, intravenously), together with cessation of intravenous bicarbonate if appropriate.

Treatment of Pulmonary Oedema

This complication is seen occasionally in salicylate poisoning. Fluid overload should be excluded so far as possible but, if increased pulmonary vascular permeability is suspected, measurement of the pulmonary artery wedge pressure (using a flow-directed pulmonary artery line) may be needed, both for confirmation of the diagnosis and to monitor subsequent fluid administration. Hypovolaemia should be corrected and the colloid osmotic pressure returned to normal with the use of colloid infusions. Assisted ventilation may prove necessary to correct the ventilation–perfusion imbalance, and this also allows the use of positive end expiratory ventilation (PEEP) which appears to be beneficial in this form of pulmonary oedema.

Forced Alkaline Diuresis (see Chapter 8)

Mild cases of salicylate poisoning may be managed with either oral or parenteral fluid and electrolyte replacement. However, more severely poisoned patients who exhibit marked symptoms or signs of salicylism and whose blood salicylate levels are in excess of 500 mg/l (and particularly if acidosis is present) should receive specific elimination therapy in the form of a forced alkaline diuresis. Although the volume of the diuresis achieved is important it need not be more than 500 ml/hour, and the pH of the urine is of far greater significance (Figure 8.2, page 62). The urinary pH should be in excess of 7.5 and should ideally lie between 8.0 and 8.5. Occasionally it proves difficult to achieve this degree of urinary alkalinization without causing the blood pH to rise above 7.6. In this case it is important to establish that any potassium deficit has been fully corrected and the administration of potassium, either orally or intravenously, will often allow the development of satisfactory urinary alkalinization.

Haemoperfusion and Haemodialysis

Very rarely, severely poisoned patients (blood salicylate level > 900 mg/l) prove refractory to forced alkaline diuresis despite full potassium supplementation. Haemoperfusion or haemodialysis may then prove necessary, both forms of treatment removing salicylate from the bloodstream extremely effectively. It should be remembered, though, that even if forced alkaline diuresis is 'ineffective', any correction of acidosis affords some protection against penetration of salicylate into tissues.

Summary

Salicylate poisoning remains an important cause of morbidity and mortality in adults. The introduction of child-resistant containers, however, has resulted in a decline in the number of hospital admissions for salicylate poisoning among children. Unhappily most fatalities from salicylate intoxication in young children are the result of therapeutic overdosage. The amount of salicylate taken, and the blood salicylate level measured six hours after ingestion, provide a good guide to the likely toxicity. Although correction of fluid and electrolyte balance is all that is required in mild cases of poisoning, forced alkaline diuresis, or even haemoperfusion or haemodialysis, may be necessary in severely poisoned patients.

Further Reading

General

Done AK. Aspirin overdosage: incidence, diagnosis and management. Pediatrics 1978; 69: Suppl. 890–7.
Miller RR, Jick H. Acute toxicity of aspirin in hospitalized medical patients. Am J Med Sci 1977; 274:271–9.

Epidemiology

Sibert JR, Craft AW, Jackson RH. Child-resistant packaging and accidental child poisoning. Lancet 1977; ii:289–90.

Pharmacokinetics

Levy G. Clinical pharmacokinetics of aspirin. Pediatrics 1978; 69:Suppl. 867–72.
Levy G, Giacomini KM. Rational aspirin dosage regimens. Clin Pharmacol Ther 1978; 23:247–52.

Pathophysiology

Pearson HA. Comparative effects of aspirin and acetaminophen on hemostasis. Pediatrics 1978; 69:Suppl. 926–9.
Smith MJH. The metabolic basis of the major symptoms in acute salicylate intoxication. Clin Toxicol 1968; 1:387–407.
Temple AR. Pathophysiology of aspirin overdosage toxicity, with implications for management. Pediatrics 1978; 69: Suppl. 873–6.

Pulmonary Oedema

Bowers RE, Brigham KL, Owen PJ. Salicylate pulmonary oedema: the mechanism in sheep and review of the clinical literature. Am Rev Resp Dis 1977; 115:261–8.
Hormaechea E, Carlson RW, Rogove H, Uphold J, Henning RJ, Weil MH. Hypovolaemia, pulmonary edema and protein changes in severe salicylate poisoning. Am J Med 1979; 66: 1046–50.

CNS Toxicity

Hill JB. Salicylate intoxication. New Engl J Med 1973; 288: 1110–3.
Thurston JH, Pollock PG, Warren SK, Jones EM. Reduced brain glucose with normal plasma glucose in salicylate poisoning. J Clin Invest 1970; 49:2139–45.

Treatment

Done AK, Temple AR. Treatment of salicylate poisoning. Modern Treatment 1971; 8:528–51
Lawson AAH, Proudfoot AT, Brain SS, MacDonald RH, Fraser AG, Cameron JC, Matthew H. Forced diuresis in the treatment of acute salicylate poisoning in adults. Q J Med 1969; New Series 38:31–48.

Chapter 14

T. J. Meredith and J. A. Vale

Paracetamol Poisoning

Paracetamol (acetaminophen) is a non-steroidal analgesic and antipyretic agent. It was first marketed for use as a drug in the UK in 1956 and since then it has become popular with the medical profession and the general public as a safe alternative to aspirin.

The first two cases of fulminant hepatic failure due to paracetamol poisoning occurred in 1966. Since then the incidence of paracetamol poisoning has increased progressively and this condition is now responsible for more cases of hepatic failure in the UK than any other cause. In 1978 there were 492 deaths associated with paracetamol poisoning in England and Wales (Figure 14.1). Of these, 196 deaths were recorded as being due to paracetamol alone and 296 occurred when paracetamol was taken in combination with other drugs. Of the latter, 229 were said to be associated with ingestion of the respiratory-depressant drug, dextropropoxyphene, which may be prescribed in fixed combination with paracetamol as 'Distalgesic'. The acute toxicity of this combination presents differently from that due to paracetamol alone (see page 109).

Adults account for the majority of serious and fatal cases of paracetamol poisoning and, although adolescents are occasionally involved, it is extremely rare for young children to ingest sufficient paracetamol to cause more than minimal liver damage.

Metabolism of Paracetamol

The major metabolites of paracetamol are the glucuronide and sulphate derivatives. Smaller proportions of the drug are excreted in the urine either as free paracetamol or as one of the products of microsomal oxidation. A proportion of the metabolite formed by microsomal oxidation is conjugated with glutathione (Figure 14.2) and is excreted subsequently as the cysteine or mercapturate conjugates.

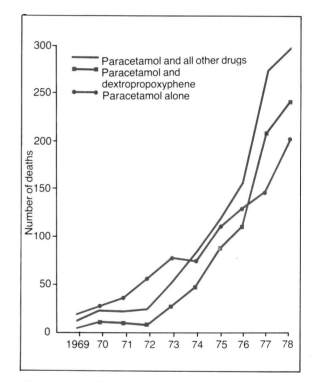

Figure 14.1. *The mortality in England and Wales from paracetamol alone and in combination with other drugs in the period 1969–1978 (from statistics published by the Office of Population Censuses and Surveys).*

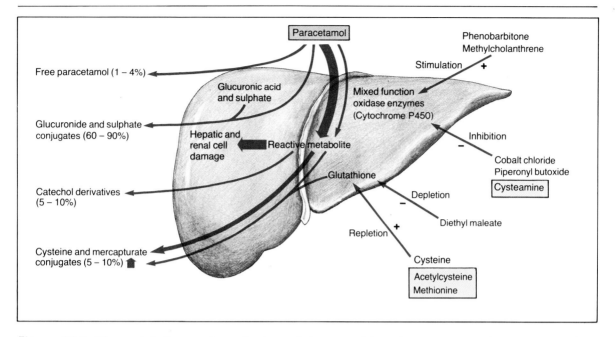

Figure 14.2 *The metabolism and mechanism of hepatotoxicity of paracetamol. The principal urinary metabolites of paracetamol are shown on the left, and the changes that occur in overdose are indicated by the use of broad arrows. The sites of action of the protective agents cysteamine, acetylcysteine and methionine are shown on the right.*

Mechanism of Hepatotoxicity

It has been shown experimentally in mice and rats, that the severity of liver necrosis is not directly related to the concentration of unchanged paracetamol present at any given time. Pretreatment of the animals with either phenobarbitone or 3-methylcholanthrene (Figure 14.2) stimulates the disappearance of paracetamol from the tissues, although both markedly potentiate the hepatic necrosis. [Phenobarbitone and 3-methylcholanthrene both stimulate the mixed function oxidase (cytochrome P_{450}) enzyme system.] Piperonyl butoxide and cobalt chloride inhibit the metabolism and disappearance of paracetamol from the tissues and protect the liver from necrosis. (Piperonyl butoxide combines with cytochrome P_{450} and inactivates the enzyme, whereas cobalt chloride blocks the synthesis of cytochrome P_{450}.) The above results suggest that the development of hepatic necrosis in paracetamol poisoning is mediated by a metabolic product of the drug.

The use of tritium-labelled paracetamol in mice has shown that a small proportion of the radioactivity becomes covalently bound to proteins in the liver, and that the amount of binding is related to the extent of the necrosis. A fall in hepatic glutathione levels is seen following the administration of large doses of paracetamol, and there appears to be a critical level below 30 per cent of the normal value) at which covalent binding and necrosis occurs. Pretreatment with diethyl maleate depletes the liver of glutathione and exacerbates paracetamol-induced necrosis, whereas the administration of glutathione precursors, such as cysteine, affords protection.

In summary, the current theory concerning the mechanism of paracetamol hepatotoxicity is that a small fraction of paracetamol is oxidized by the mixed function oxidase system to a reactive product which normally complexes with glutathione. This complex is further degraded and appears in the urine as either cysteine or mercapturate conjugates. When very large quantities of paracetamol are presented to the liver, the glutathione stores become depleted and, below a certain critical level, insufficient remains to 'mop up' the oxidized metabolite. The metabolite then becomes free to combine covalently with liver cell macromolecules and cause hepatic necrosis. Further evidence for this hypothesis is provided by the pattern of metabolites excreted in the urine of different animal species.

The evidence for a similar mechanism in humans

is not so clearly defined. However, an increased susceptibility to paracetamol-induced liver damage has been reported in a retrospective study of patients with a history of drug ingestion likely to cause liver enzyme induction. Moreover, prestimulation of microsomal enzymes with phenobarbitone in man leads to an increase in mercapturic acid excretion after therapeutic doses of paracetamol. Davis et al (1976) compared the urinary excretion of paracetamol and its conjugates in volunteers taking therapeutic doses of the drug and in patients admitted soon after an overdose of the drug. In the latter group there was a greatly increased production of the cysteine and mercapturic acid conjugates of paracetamol, which is now known to occur after the sulphate and glucuronide pathways have become saturated.

Renal Toxicity of Paracetamol

Acute tubular necrosis is occasionally seen in patients following the ingestion of an overdose of paracetamol. This usually occurs in the context of fulminant liver failure, but there is now experimental evidence that the toxic metabolite of paracetamol may be formed in situ by cytochrome P_{450} enzyme systems in the kidney parenchyma. The formation of this metabolite, and the early development of acute renal failure in man due to paracetamol poisoning, may be prevented by the use of those same agents that protect against hepatic toxicity (see below).

Clinical Features of Paracetamol Poisoning (Table 14.1)

Few symptoms or signs appear on the first day after ingestion of a paracetamol overdose, although pallor, anorexia, nausea and vomiting may occur. Despite the paucity of symptoms more than 75 per cent of patients attend hospital within eight hours of the overdose. No disturbance of consciousness occurs at this early stage unless a sedative drug has been taken in addition to the paracetamol. If liver damage develops, and is of sufficient severity, abdominal pain and hepatic tenderness appear on the second day. Liver function tests become abnormal 12 to 36 hours after ingestion of an overdose, with elevation of the serum aminotransferase and bilirubin concentrations and prolongation of the prothrombin time. Peak disturbance of liver function occurs four to six days

Table 14.1. Clinical features of paracetamol overdose.

1st day	Anorexia
	Nausea
	Vomiting
1st–2nd day	Abdominal pain
	↑ Bilirubin
	↑ Aspartate aminotransferase
	↑ Prothrombin time
2nd–7th day	Hepatic failure (jaundice, hepatic encephalopathy)
	Acute renal failure

after the overdose and frank liver failure, preceded by jaundice and hepatic encephalopathy, may ensue.

Necrosis of hepatocytes in the centrilobular areas of the liver is the principal histological change seen in less severe cases of paracetamol poisoning. In those patients who progress to fulminant hepatic failure, wide areas of confluent necrosis are seen, often with survival of only a few hepatocytes in the periportal areas.

Mild or moderate liver damage due to paracetamol overdose may be accompanied by transient glucose intolerance, while severe liver damage may be associated with hypoglycaemia. Disseminated intravascular coagulation sometimes occurs in severe paracetamol overdose as may metabolic acidosis and acute renal failure. Cardiac arrhythmias and electrocardiographic abnormalities have been reported in severely affected patients as have necrosis and fatty infiltration of the myocardium at autopsy. However, cardiac arrhythmias and histological abnormalities of the myocardium are found commonly in patients with fulminant hepatic failure from any cause, and it is unlikely that they occur specifically as a consequence of paracetamol overdose.

The overall mortality rate of patients admitted to hospital with paracetamol poisoning before effective treatment became available was two to three per cent. However, in a series of 60 severely poisoned patients admitted to the Liver Unit at King's College Hospital, the mortality was 20 per cent. Those patients who do not succumb to liver failure make a full recovery. Liver function tests return to normal within three to six months of the overdose although, very rarely, hepatic fibrosis may persist.

Prediction of Liver Damage

It is possible to extrapolate from animal data and calculate the dose of paracetamol in man that would deplete the liver of sufficient glutathione to cause accumulation of the toxic metabolite and subsequent hepatic damage. In normal individuals this would amount to 15 g of paracetamol and, in those whose enzymes are 'induced' by previous alcohol or drug consumption, the hepatotoxic dose of paracetamol would be about 10 g. These amounts correspond well with those found clinically to cause liver damage in adults.

Nevertheless, it is unwise to rely upon an estimate (particularly one made by the patient) of the dose of paracetamol ingested. A more reliable indicator of the likelihood of liver damage is the plasma level of paracetamol. Significant liver damage is likely to occur if the level at 4 hours exceeds 200 mg/l and at 12 hours exceeds 70 mg/l.

However, a few patients with high paracetamol levels in the early hours after overdose subsequently develop only minimal liver damage (Gazzard et al. 1977).

One would expect the half-life of unchanged paracetamol to be a more reliable predictor of liver damage. The half-life for elimination is usually of the order of two to three hours, but in overdose complicated by liver damage it will exceed four hours. This is due to saturation of sulphation and glucuronidation processes rather than liver damage per se. Unfortunately calculation of the half-life requires two plasma paracetamol estimations separated by a reasonable period of time, and by the time the second value is available it may be too late to offer effective treatment to the patient.

Despite the limitations detailed above the most efficient and reliable way to determine which patients need specific treatment is by measurement of a single plasma paracetamol level, provided that more than four hours have elapsed since ingestion of the overdose (Figure 14.3). This may be done within minutes with the necessary degree of accuracy with the aid of a blood paracetamol estimation kit.

Treatment of Paracetamol Poisoning

Gastric Aspiration and Lavage

Gastric aspiration and lavage has been shown to be of value for up to six hours after ingestion of a paracetamol overdose. However, because small children of less than five years old tend to swallow only small amounts of paracetamol, gastric lavage is unnecessary and syrup of ipecacuanha is all that is usually required in children.

Activated Charcoal

Activated charcoal has been advocated as an additional means of preventing absorption of paracetamol from the stomach. It has been shown, for example, that 10 g of charcoal administered *immediately* after ingestion of 1 g paracetamol will reduce absorption by about 70 per cent. Similar results have been achieved with cholestyramine. It seems unlikely, therefore, that either form of treatment would be of value more than a few hours after ingestion of an overdose of paracetamol. Furthermore, the ideal charcoal:paracetamol

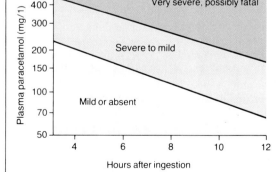

Figure 14.3. *Measurement of the plasma paracetamol levels gives an indication of the likely prognosis in a given case of paracetamol poisoning and the need, therefore, for the administration of either oral methionine or intravenous acetylcysteine.*

ratio is 10:1, and a patient who ingested 50 g of paracetamol would be required to swallow half a kilogram of charcoal.

General Treatment

General treatment may include parenteral fluid replacement for the first one to two days because of the nausea and vomiting that sometimes occur. Intravenous vitamin K (10 mg daily for three days) may be given to severely poisoned patients although it is unlikely to be very effective. Fresh frozen plasma or clotting factor concentrate may be used to maintain the prothrombin time within safe limits, although such treatment does not appear to influence either the morbidity or mortality. The further management of hepatic failure is beyond the scope of this book.

Forced Diuresis, Haemodialysis and Haemoperfusion

The use of forced diuresis has been suggested for paracetamol poisoning because excretion of the unchanged drug is related to urine flow. However, early forced diuresis does not prevent liver damage and may even be dangerous because paracetamol has an antidiuretic affect. Haemodialysis and haemoperfusion have both been used early in paracetamol poisoning but neither form of treatment has been shown to prevent the development of hepatic damage. It is possible, however, that haemoperfusion may prove to have a role in the treatment of those patients who present to hospital too late for the administration of protective agents (see below).

Protective Agents

Cysteamine

Treatments directed towards prevention of hepatic damage caused by the active metabolite of paracetamol have been more successful. Cysteamine, for example, will effectively protect against paracetamol-induced liver damage. This compound is rapidly oxidized to cystamine in vivo and these two substances remain in equilibrium in the body. Both cysteamine and cystamine strongly inhibit cytochrome P_{450} activity, and probably act by reducing formation of the active paracetamol metabolite (Figure 14.2).

The first report on the use of cysteamine in man came from Prescott and his associates (1974) who described its use in five patients with high paracetamol

levels. A total of 3.2 g of the base was given over 20 hours. All the patients survived and developed only minimal liver damage. It was emphasized that, to be of value, cysteamine should be given as soon as possible after ingestion, and certainly within 10 hours.

All subsequent reports of the use of cysteamine in paracetamol poisoning have shown it to be effective in the prevention of hepatic damage provided that it is administered within 10 hours of ingestion of the overdose.

Unfortunately the use of cysteamine is associated with a number of distressing side-effects. These include nausea, vomiting and abdominal pain. Of more significance, cardiac arrhythmias, including ventricular tachycardia, have been observed during the administration of cysteamine. The drug is not available as a pharmaceutical preparation and it has in many cases to be made up and filtered immediately prior to use.

Methionine

In contrast to cysteamine, methionine and acetylcysteine are remarkably free of side-effects. Methionine (Figure 14.2) speeds the synthesis of liver glutathione, and, in the experimental situation, effectively prevents liver damage. Although results from a controlled trial are not available, many hundreds of patients have been given methionine on the advice of the London Centre of the National Poisons Information Service. Detailed information is available on 96 patients who had high plasma paracetamol levels (falling above a line joining semi-logarithmic plots of 200 mg/l at 4 hours and 70 mg/l at 12 hours) on admission and who were treated with oral methionine within 10 hours of ingestion of the overdose. Only seven patients developed severe liver damage (aspartate aminotransferase >1000 i.u./l); one of these exhibited hepatic encephalopathy and one developed transient renal failure. There were no deaths from hepatic failure.

The use of oral methionine is not associated with any serious side-effects. Sometimes, however, there is difficulty with oral administration of the drug because of vomiting, although this occurs rarely and may be controlled with the use of an antiemetic drug. More commonly, difficulties are encountered because the patient is unconscious as a result of ingestion of another drug. This is often due to dextropropoxyphene and, in these circumstances, naloxone should be administered. Even if the patient remains unconscious, methonine may be given with the aid of a nasogastric tube provided that the tablets are crushed beforehand. The dose of methonine is shown in Table 14.2. Young children rarely require the administration of anything other than an emetic because of their tendency to ingest small quantities of paracetamol.

Older children may be given the adult dose of oral methonine.

N-Acetylcysteine

N-acetylcysteine (Figure 14.2) is rapidly hydrolyzed in vivo to cysteine which acts as a precursor to glutathione. Acetylcysteine has proved to be as effective a treatment as cysteamine and methionine in man. Acetylcysteine may be administered either by injection or orally and is available as 'Parvolex' (Duncan Flockhart) which is a 20 per cent solution suitable for intravenous use. 'Airbron' (Duncan Flockhart) and 'Mucomyst' (McNeil Laboratories) are 20 per cent solutions intended as mucolytic agents but they are sterile and, although not necessarily pyrogen free, can be used intravenously in an emergency. Acetylcysteine may also be used orally but requires dilution in a soft drink because of its unpleasant taste, and even then causes vomiting in many patients. The rather complicated dosage regimes for both parenteral and oral administration are shown in Table 14.2.

Comparative data for methionine and N-acetylcysteine are shown in Tables 14.3 and 14.4. There is no evidence that either agent is effective once more than 10 hours have elapsed from the time of ingestion of the overdose, and certainly neither compound should be administered if gross disturbance of hepatic function is present. Finally, in these days of economic constraint it is worth mentioning that, at the time of writing (October 1980), the recommended course of oral methionine attracts a charge of some 80p, whereas the corresponding course of N-acetylcysteine costs more than £30. The latter treatment seems reasonable, however, should a patient be either unconscious or suffering from intractable nausea and vomiting.

Dextropropoxyphene Poisoning

Dextropropoxyphene, a substance chemically similar to methadone, was first synthesized in 1953 and its analgesic properties were described two years later. It was said to resemble codeine in its potency and toxicity but to have fewer side-effects. It was marketed in the USA as the hydrochloride salt under the proprietary names of 'Darvon', 'Dolene', 'Progesic'' 'SK-65' and later as the napsylate salt in 'Darvon-N' and 'Darvocet-N'.

In the UK, dextropropoxyphene is a constituent of a number of preparations. These include 'Depronal SA', 'Doloxene', 'Doloxene Compound', 'Dolosan', 'Distalgesic', 'Napsalgesic' and 'Cosalgesic'' all of

---

Table 14.2.   Management of paracetamol poisoning.

The prevention of gastrointestinal absorption

Gastric lavage or, in children, Syrup of Ipecacuanha, 10—15 ml.

Protective agents

Methionine 2.5 g orally stat., then 2.5 g four-hourly for a further three doses. Total dose: 10 g methionine over 12 hours

or

N-Acetylcysteine 150 mg/kg i.v. over 15 minutes in 200 ml of 5 per cent dextrose, then 50 mg/kg in 500 ml of 5 per cent dextrose i.v. in the next four hours and 100 mg/kg in 1000 ml of 5 per cent dextrose i.v. over the ensuing 16 hours. Total dose: 300 mg/kg over 20 hours. Alternatively, the 20 per cent solution may be diluted to a 5 per cent solution in a soft drink for oral administration. A single loading dose of 140 mg/kg is given, followed by 17 doses of 70 mg/kg every four hours.

N.B. Protective agents should be administered only so long as no more than 10 hours have elapsed from the time of ingestion of the paracetamol overdose (see text).

Supportive measures

Five per cent dextrose solution to correct dehydration.
Correction of electrolyte imbalance.
Vitamin K 10 mg i.v. for three days if the prothrombin time is prolonged.

Treatment of hepatic failure

---

which are available only on prescription. The most commonly prescribed preparation in the UK is Distalgesic; each tablet contains 325 mg of paracetamol and 32.5 mg of dextropropoxyphene.

The number of deaths due to the ingestion of paracetamol and dextropropoxyphene in combination has risen markedly in recent years (Figure 14.1). The signs of overdosage with compound preparations of paracetamol and dextropropoxyphene are those of opiate poisoning (see Chapter 15) with early onset of 'pin-point' pupils, depressed respiration and loss of consciousness. The respiratory depression and hypoxia may further lead to cardiac arrhythmias and convulsions. Respiratory arrest is the usual mode of death and this occurs typically within a few hours of the overdose. In common with other forms of opiate poisoning, pulmonary oedema may also occur. Liver

Table 14.3.   Hepatic and renal damage in patients poisoned with paracetamol.

Treatment	No. of patients	No. (%) with severe liver damage (AST > 1000 i.u./l)	Mean maximum AST (i.u./l)	No. (%) with acute renal failure	Mortality
Oral methionine < 10 hours	96	7 (7)	294	1 (1)	0
Oral N-acetylcysteine < 10 hours (Rumack and Peterson 1978)	49	8 (16)	210	0	0
Intravenous N-acetylcysteine < 10 hours (Prescott et al. 1979)	62	1 (2)	113	0	0
Oral methionine 10–24 hours	36	17 (47)	1464	2 (6)	2 (6)
Oral N-acetylcysteine 10–24 hours (Rumack and Peterson 1978)	51	23 (45)	2207	0	0
Intravenous N-acetylcysteine 10–24 hours (Prescott et al. 1979)	38	20 (53)	3814	5 (13)	2 (5)
Supportive treatment only (Prescott et al. 1979)	57	33 (58)	> 2022	6 (11)	3 (5)

Table 14.4.   Hepatic and renal damage in 'high-risk' patients[1] poisoned with paracetamol.

Treatment	No. of patients	No. (%) with severe liver damage (AST > 1000 i.u./l)	Mean maximum AST (i.u./l)	No. (%) with acute renal failure[2]	Mortality
Oral methionine < 10 hours	43	6 (14)	464	1 (2)	0
Intravenous N-acetylcysteine < 10 hours (Prescott et al. 1979)	33	1 (3)	185	0	0
Oral methionine 10–24 hours	31	14 (45)	1532	2 (6)	2 (6)
Intravenous N-acetylcysteine 10–24 hours (Prescott et al. 1979)	27	18 (67)	4919	5 (19)	2 (7)
Supportive treatment only (Prescott et al. 1979)	28	25 (89)	> 3186	6 (21)	3 (11)

[1] Plasma paracetamol levels > 300 mg/l at 4 hours and > 75 mg/l at 12 hours
[2] Plasma creatinine > 300 μ mol/l

failure is an uncommon cause of death. Ingestion of more than 20 tablets of Distalgesic is dangerous, particularly if alcohol or other central depressants have been taken at the same time.

Early diagnosis of Distalgesic poisoning is important because respiratory arrest and death may be averted by the use of the opiate antagonist naloxone. There is no reason why such patients should die provided that they reach hospital and cerebral anoxic damage has not already occurred. The use of one of the protective agents, methionine or acetylcysteine, may also be necessary if the blood paracetamol concentration is high (Figure 14.3), but there is experimental evidence that dextropropoxyphene actually inhibits mixed function oxidase enzyme activity. It is possible, therefore, that formation of the toxic paracetamol metabolite is reduced by dextropropoxyphene.

Conclusion

Paracetamol, when used in therapeutic doses, is a safe and effective analgesic and antipyretic agent. It is, however, predictably hepatotoxic in man when ingested in single quantities of more that 10 to 15 g. The current 'antidotes' of choice are oral methionine and intravenous N-acetylcysteine, either of which should be administered within 10 hours of ingestion of a paracetamol overdose.

References

Mechanism of Hepatic and Renal Toxicity

Davis M, Simmons CJ, Harrison NG, Williams R. Paracetamol overdose in man: relationship between pattern of urinary metabolites and severity of liver damage. Q J Med 1976; New Series 45: 181–91.

Prediction of Outcome

Gazzard BG, Hughes RD, Widdop B, Goulding R, Davis M, Williams R. Early prediction of the outcome of paracetamol overdose based on an analysis of 163 patients. Postgrad Med J 1977; 53:243–7.

Treatment

Prescott LF, Newton RW, Swainson CP, Wright N, Forrest ARW, Matthew H. Successful treatment of severe paracetamol overdosage with cysteamine. Lancet 1974; i:588–92.
Prescott LF, Illingworth RN, Critchley JAJH, Stewart MJ, Adam RD, Proudfoot AT. Intravenous N-acetylcysteine: the treatment of choice for paracetamol poisoning. Br Med J 1979; 2:1097–100.
Rumack BH, Peterson RG. Acetaminophen overdose: incidence, diagnosis and management in 416 patients. Pediatrics 1978; 69:Suppl. 898–903.

Further Reading

General

Black M. Acetaminophen hepatotoxicity. Gastroenterology 1980; 78:382–92.
Meredith TJ, Goulding R. Paracetamol. Postgrad Med J 1980; 56:459–473.

Clinical Features

Meredith TJ, Newman B, Goulding R. Paracetamol poisoning in children. Br Med J 1978; 2:478–9.
Prescott LF, The nephrotoxicity and hepatoxicity of antipyretic analgesics. Br J Clin Pharmacol 1979; 7:453–62.

Epidemiology

Meredith TJ, Vale JA, Goulding R. The epidemiology of acetaminophen poisoning in England and Wales. Arch Int Med 1981; In press.

Mechanisms of Hepatic and Renal Toxicity

Jollow DJ, Mitchell JR, Potter WZ, Davis DC, Gillette JR, Brodie BB. Acetaminophen-induced hepatic necrosis. II Role of covalent binding in vivo. J Pharmacol Exp Therap 1973; 187:195–202.
McMurtry RJ, Snodgrass WR, Mitchell JR. Renal necrosis, glutathione and covalent binding after acetaminophen. Toxicol Appl Pharmacol 1978; 46:87–100.
Mitchell JR, Jollow DJ, Potter WZ, Davis DC, Gillette JR, Brodie BB. Acetaminophen-induced hepatic necrosis. I Role of drug metabolism. J. Pharmacol Exp Therap 1973; 187: 185–94.
Mitchell JR, Jollow DJ, Potter WZ, Gillette JR, Brodie BB. Acetaminophen-induced hepatic necrosis. IV Protective role of glutathione. J Pharmacol Exp Therap 1973; 187:211–7.
Potter WZ, Davis DC. Mitchell JR, Jollow DJ, Gillette JR, Brodie BB. Acetaminophen-induced hepatic necrosis. III Cytochrome P_{450}-mediated covalent binding in vitro. J Pharmacol Exp Therap 1973; 187:203–10.
Slattery JT, Levy G. Acetaminophen kinetics in acutely poisoned patients. Clin Pharmacol Therap 1979; 25:184–95.

Treatment

Meredith TJ, Volans GN. Paracetamol toxicity and its treatment. In: Recent Advances in Clinical Pharmacology 2. Edinburgh: Churchill Livingstone, 1980; 130–48.
Prescott LF, Park J, Ballantyne A, Adriaenssens P, Proudfoot AT. Treatment of paracetamol (acetaminophen) poisoning with N-acetylcysteine. Lancet 1977; ii:432–4.
Vale JA, Meredith TJ, Goulding R. The treatment of paracetamol (acetaminophen) poisoning: the use of oral methionine. Arch Int Med 1981; In press.
Winchester JF, Gelfand MC, Helliwell M, Vale JA, Goulding R, Schreiner GE. Extracorporeal treatment of salicylate or acetaminophen poisoning – is there a role? Arch Int Med 1981; In press.

Dextropropoxyphene Poisoning

Bogartz LJ, Miller WC. Pulmonary edema associated with propoxyphene intoxication. J Am Med Assoc 1971; 215: 259–62.
Carson DJL, Carson ED. Fatal dextropropoxyphene poisoning in Northern Ireland. Review of 30 cases. Lancet 1977; i: 894–7.
Editorial. Treatment of dextropropoxyphene poisoning. Lancet 1977; ii:542.

Moore RA, Rumack BH, Conner CS, Peterson RG. Naloxone. Underdosage after narcotic poisoning. Am J Dis Child 1980; 134: 156−8.

Peterson GR, Hostetler RM, Lehman T, Covault HP. Acute inhibition of oxidative drug metabolism by propoxyphene (Darvon). Biochem Pharmacol 1979; 28:1783−9.

Sturner WQ, Garriott JC. Deaths involving propoxyphene. A study of 41 cases over a two-year period. J Am Med Assoc 1973; 223:1125−30.

Tennant FS. Complications of propoxyphene abuse. Arch Intern Med 1973; 132:191−4.

Whittington RM. Dextropropoxyphene (Distalgesic) over-dosage in the West Midlands. Br Med J 1977; 2:172−3.

Young RJ, Lawson AAH. Distalgesic poisoning − cause for concern. Br Med J 1980; 1:1045−7.

Chapter 15

T. J. Meredith and J. A. Vale

Poisoning due to Opiates and Morphine Derivatives

The deliberate self-administration of an opiate drug is a relatively common cause of poisoning in Great Britain, the USA and Europe. The group of opiate drugs is large and includes apomorphine, buprenorphine, codeine and dihydrocodeine (DF 118), dextromoramide, dextropropoxyphene (propoxyphene), diamorphine (diacetylmorphine, heroin), dipipanone, diphenoxylate, methadone, morphine, pentazocine and pethidine (meperidine).

Clinical Features

Acute opiate overdose most often occurs in addicts, in whom the presence of infected venepuncture marks and thrombosed veins over the arms and legs is characteristic. Veins in the lower rectum and vagina are sometimes used for covert administration of one of these drugs. Heroin may also be 'snorted' rather than parenterally administered and this leads to inflammation and oedema of the nasal mucosae.

Coma, respiratory depression (often accompanied by cyanosis) and pinpoint pupils are the cardinal signs of opiate overdose. The frequency and severity of additional clinical features depends upon the particular drug ingested and these are discussed later in this chapter. Skeletal muscles are usually flaccid but the ingestion of some opiate drugs in overdose may be associated with increased muscle tone and twitching. Convulsions may also occur, particularly in children.

Respiratory depression is the usual cause of death in opiate poisoning but it is striking that patients appear to tolerate the consequences of severe respiratory depression due to an opiate drug much better than when it is caused by a non-specific depressant such as a barbiturate. In the latter instance respiratory depression is accompanied by severe cardiovascular depression (see Chapter 11), whereas marked hypotension is found in less than 10 per cent of cases of opiate poisoning and, when it occurs, is usually due to peripheral vasodilatation. Opiate poisoning, particularly that due to dextropropoxyphene, diamorphine, methadone and morphine, may be complicated by non-cardiogenic pulmonary oedema.

Treatment of Opiate Overdose

Naloxone has revolutionized the treatment of opiate overdose. It is a pure narcotic antagonist and thus has no intrinsic agonist activity (see Chapter 5). Naloxone should be given immediately to reverse severe respiratory depression and coma due to opiate poisoning. The adult dose is 0.4 to 0.8 mg given either intravenously or intramuscularly; the dose in children is 0.005 to 0.01 mg/kg body weight. The onset of action of naloxone occurs within minutes and, if the diagnosis is correct, the patient should respond with an increase in respiratory rate, an improvement in the level of consciousness and dilatation of the pupils. If the patient fails to respond, a second and larger dose of naloxone may be given within 5 to 10 minutes. The duration of action of naloxone (one to four hours) is often less than that of the opiate drug taken in overdose and, for this reason, careful observation of the level of consciousness and either respiratory rate or tidal or minute volume is necessary and repeated doses of either intravenous or intramuscular naloxone may be required.

In opiate-dependent subjects, even small doses of naloxone will precipitate a moderate-to-severe withdrawal syndrome. This is very similar to that seen after the abrupt withdrawal of opiates except that the syndrome appears within minutes after the administration of naloxone and subsides in about two hours. The severity and duration of the syndrome are related to the dose of the antagonist and the degree of dependence.

Opiate drugs delay gastric emptying and increase antral tone. Gastric lavage is of value if the drug has been ingested (rather than administered parenterally) and if the patient is conscious. In view of the high risk of pulmonary complications in unconscious patients, it is wise to avoid the further risk of aspiration of stomach contents by delaying gastric lavage until the effects of the opiate drug have been reversed by naloxone (see below). If the patient is unconscious, or has a depressed cough reflex as the result of ingestion of another drug, then a cuffed endotracheal tube should be inserted to protect the airway (see Chapter 7).

Intensive supportive therapy, directed particularly towards the respiratory system, is important and, in cases of non-cardiogenic pulmonary oedema refractory to normal therapeutic measures, positive end expiratory pressure (PEEP) ventilation may be necessary.

Further Reading

Moore RA, Rumack BH, Conner CS, Peterson RG. Naloxone. Underdosage after narcotic poisoning. Am J Dis Child 1980; 134:156–8.

Apomorphine

Apomorphine is obtained by treating morphine with strong mineral acids. It has diminished analgesic properties and produces a combination of CNS excitation and depression. Apomorphine has been used to induce vomiting in poisoned patients but this action is often prolonged and can be accompanied by respiratory depression. Furthermore, excessive doses of apomorphine are associated with convulsions and cardiac toxicity. The toxic effects of apomorphine are counteracted by naloxone, although it is rarely taken in overdose.

Buprenorphine

Buprenorphine is a new narcotic antagonist analgesic similar to pentazocine. Little information is available concerning its effects in overdose. It may have greater maximum analgesic activity than pentazocine and it does have a longer duration of action. However, it is more sedative than pentazocine and is prone to cause vomiting. In contrast to other opiate derivatives the analgesic and respiratory-depressant effects of buprenorphine are only reversed partially, if at all, by naloxone. Doxapram may be used to stimulate respiration, but mechanical ventilation may be necessary for severe respiratory depression.

Further Reading

Banks CD. Overdosage of buprenorphine. NZ Med J 1979; 89:255–6.

Codeine and Dihydrocodeine (DF 118)

Codeine is used widely as an oral analgesic agent and as a cough suppressant. Approximately 10 per cent of an ingested dose of codeine is metabolized to morphine. In addition to the usual clinical features of opiate overdose, codeine may also cause convulsions. Pulmonary oedema has been reported following the intravenous self-administration of codeine.

Dihydrocodeine is structurally closely related to codeine and behaves in a pharmacologically similar manner. There is little information concerning its effects in overdose.

Further Reading

Huffman DH, Ferguson RL. Acute codeine overdose: correspondence between clinical course and codeine metabolism. Johns Hopkins Medical Journal 1975; 136:183–6.

Nakamura GR, Greisemer EC, Noguchi TT. Antemortem conversion of codeine to morphine in man. J Forensic Sci 1976; 21:518–24.

Pearson MA, Poklis A, Morrison RR. A fatality due to the ingestion of (methyl morphine) codeine. Clin Toxicol 1979; 15:267–71.

Sklar J, Timms RM. Codeine-induced pulmonary edema. Chest 1977; 72:230–1.

Winek CL, Collom WD, Wecht CH. Codeine fatality from cough syrup. Clin Toxicol 1970; 3:97–100.

Wright JA, Baselt RC, Hine CH. Blood codeine concentrations in fatalities associated with codeine. Clin Toxicol 1975; 8: 457–63.

Dextromoramide and Dipipanone

Dextromoramide and dipipanone are both high-potency, narcotic, analgesic agents, structurally related to methadone. They are rarely taken in over-dose and are not associated with any specific clinical features other than those that occur with any form of opiate poisoning.

Dextropropoxyphene (propoxyphene)

The analgesic activity of propoxyphene resides in the D-isomer of α-propoxyphene which is structurally related to methadone. The L-isomer is devoid of analgesic activity but it has been used as an antitussive agent. Respiratory depression, convulsions and pulmonary oedema occur in dextropropoxyphene over-dose, which is discussed in detail on page 109.

Further Reading

See pages 111–112.

Diamorphine (Diacetyl-morphine, Heroin)

Heroin is a semisynthetic derivative of morphine with potent analgesic activity. It is frequently abused and it is usually administered either by injection ('main-lining') or by inhalation ('snorting'). 'Street-grade' heroin is usually only 2 to 6 per cent pure and may contain codeine as an impurity.

In addition to the typical features of opiate poisoning, hypothermia may also occur due to vaso-dilation and loss of temperature regulation. Hypo-glycaemia has been reported in up to seven per cent of cases of heroin overdose, although this is thought to be multifactorial in origin (alcohol ingestion, liver disease, malnutrition and the narcotic agent itself).

As many as 50 per cent of heroin overdose patients develop pulmonary oedema. Duberstein and Kaufman (1971) reported on a series of 149 patients in which the overall mortality was 8.7 per cent. However, over 20 per cent of those with pulmonary oedema died, and all those who did die suffered from this compli-cation. In addition, up to 75 per cent of patients with pulmonary oedema subsequently developed bacterial pneumonia. The management of pulmonary oedema is discussed in Chapter 7.

References

Duberstein JL, Kaufman DM. A clinical study of an epidemic of heroin intoxication and heroin induced pulmonary edema. Am J Med 1971; 51:704–14.

Further Reading

Garriott JC, Sturner WQ. Morphine concentrations and survival periods in acute heroin fatalities. N Engl J Med 1973; 289:1276–8.
Levine SB, Grimes ET. Pulmonary edema and heroin over-dose in Vietnam. Arch Pathol Lab Med 1973; 95:330–2.
Steinberg AD, Karliner JS. The clinical spectrum of heroin pulmonary edema. Arch Intern Med 1968; 122:122–7.

Diphenoxylate

Diphenoxylate is a complex molecule linking the cyanide precursor of normethadone to norpethidine. It has both a slower onset and a greater duration of action than pethidine. Diphenoxylate is most com-monly used as an antidiarrhoeal agent in conjunc-tion with atropine. In the UK it is available in the form of 'Lomotil' tablets which contain 2.5 mg diphenoxylate hydrochloride and 0.025 mg atropine sulphate. Diphenoxylate and its salts are virtually insoluble in aqueous solution and this precludes the possibility of parenteral abuse. This is further dis-couraged by the presence of atropine in tablet formu-lations.

Unfortunately paediatric poisoning is not uncom-mon, particularly in children aged less than five years, and a number of fatalities have occurred.

The combination of diphenoxylate and atropine markedly reduces gastric emptying and intestinal motility. For this reason, the onset of symptoms following an overdose may be delayed for up to 12 hours and it is wise to continue observation for 48 hours. Relapses are common during the course of recovery.

Respiratory depression is the major complication of diphenoxylate poisoning and, typically, a gradual reduction in the respiratory rate is followed by total apnoea. Vomiting, abdominal pain, drowsiness and coma also occur. Even though Lomotil tablets incor-porate only a small amount of atropine this is often toxic to children who exhibit variable sensitivity to this drug. Tachycardia, anxiety, restlessness and flushing may be seen, but the pupils are more often constricted (due to diphenoxylate) than dilated. Hypotension, loss of tendon reflexes and convulsions have also been reported in Lomotil poisoning.

Gastric aspiration and lavage should be performed if an overdose has been ingested within the preceding 12 hours. Repeated doses of naloxone are necessary to reverse respiratory depression because of the long duration of action of diphenoxylate and the prolonged absorption of the drug due to intestinal stasis.

Further Reading

Curtis JA, Goel KM. Lomotil poisoning in children. Arch Dis Child 1979; 54:222–5.

Cutler EA, Barrett GA, Craven PW, Cramblett HG. Delayed cardiopulmonary arrest after Lomotil ingestion. Pediatrics 1980; 65:157–8.

Editorial. Lomotil intoxication in children. Br Med J 1973; 2:678–9.

Penfold D, Volans GN. Overdose from Lomotil. Br Med J 1977; 2:1401–2.

Rumack BH, Temple AR. Lomotil poisoning. Pediatrics 1974; 53:495–500.

Wasserman GS, Green VA, Wise GW. Lomotil ingestions in children. Am Fam Physician 1975; 11:93–7.

Methadone

Methadone is a completely synthetic narcotic analgesic whose chemical structure only remotely resembles that of morphine but whose properties are remarkably similar. It is often used in maintenance therapy for heroin addicts but it is also a potent oral analgesic agent. Methadone causes marked sedation and respiratory depression in non-tolerant subjects and pulmonary oedema is well recognized in methadone overdose.

Further Reading

Dole VP, Foldes FF, Trigg H, Robinson JW, Blatman S. Methadone poisoning. NY State J Med 1971; 71:541–3.

Fraser DW. Methadone overdose. J Am Med Assoc 1972; 217:1387–9.

Garriott JC, Sturner WQ, Mason MF. Toxicologic findings in six fatalities involving methadone. Clin Toxicol 1973; 6: 163–73.

Kjeldgaard JM, Hahn GW, Heckenlively JR, Genton E.

Methadone induced pulmonary edema. J Am Med Assoc 1971; 218:882–3.

Schaaf JT, Spivack ML, Rath GS, Snider GL. Pulmonary edema and adult respiratory distress syndrome following methadone abuse. Am Rev Respir Dis 1973; 107:1047–51.

Sey MJ, Rubenstein D, Smith DS. Accidental methadone intoxication in a child. Pediatrics 1971; 48:294–6.

Smialek JE, Nonforte JR, Aronow R, Spitz WU. Methadone deaths in children: a continuing problem. J Am Med Assoc 1977; 238: 2516–7.

Morphine

Morphine is the standard narcotic analgesic agent to which other analgesics are compared. The clinical features of acute morphine poisoning are similar to those due to heroin, although morphine overdose is much less commonly seen.

Further Reading

Felby S, Christensen H, Lund A. Morphine concentrations in blood and organs in cases of fatal poisoning. Forensic Sci 1974; 3:74–81.

Pentazocine

Pentazocine is a synthetic compound which has both agonist and partial antagonist activity. Pentazocine causes respiratory depression in overdose and it is unusual in that hypotension is uncommon but rather hypertension and tachycardia may occur. The respiratory depression is reversed by naloxone but not by the partial antagonist, nalorphine.

Pethidine (Meperidine)

Pethidine is a synthetic narcotic analgesic. In addition to the usual clinical features of opiate poisoning, pethidine toxicity causes muscular twitching, increased tendon reflexes and convulsions, all of which are thought to be due to formation of the metabolite, norpethidine. Death in man has resulted from ingestion of 1.2 g of the drug, though recovery has followed the ingestion of 2 g.

Chapter 16

J. A. Vale and T.J. Meredith

Poisoning due to Cardiovascular Drugs

Beta-Adrenergic Blocking Drug Poisoning

Beta-adrenergic blocking drugs are now used widely for the treatment of hypertension, angina pectoris, thyrotoxicosis and cardiac arrhythmias. These drugs antagonize the effects of endogenous catecholamines on the heart and other tissues by competitive inhibition at β-adrenergic receptors. In addition each β-adrenergic blocking drug differs qualitatively and quantitatively in its pharmacological actions. Membrane stabilizing activity is the least important of these actions, but some have intrinsic sympathomimetic activity while others are cardioselective.

In overdose these drugs have a marked negative intropic action and this probably explains the lack of response to pharmacological and electrical stimulation in some cases of overdose. Up to March 1980 43 cases of poisoning due to β-adrenergic drugs had been described in the literature, of which nine died. Over the same period 40 cases were referred to the London Centre of the National Poisons Information Service, of which eight died.

Clinical Features

Drowsiness, delirium, unconsciousness, fits and hallucinations.
Bradycardia, hypotension, low output cardiac failure.
Cardiorespiratory arrest (asystole or ventricular fibrillation).
Bronchospasm.
Hypoglycaemia.

Treatment

1. Gastric lavage if appropriate.
2. Supportive measures.
3. If marked bradycardia is present:
(a) Give atropine 0.6 to 3 mg (50 μg/kg in children) intravenously and repeat as necessary.
(b) Insert a cardiac pacemaker.
4. If hypotension is present:
(a) Give glucagon 50 to 150 μg/kg intravenously over one minute followed by an infusion of 1 to 5 mg/hour.
It is thought that glucagon activates myocardial adenyl cyclase by a different mechanism from the β-adrenergic catecholamines. This effect is not blocked by β-adrenergic blocking drugs (Parmley 1971).
(b) Give dobutamine infusion (2.5–20 μg/kg/min).
5. If bronchospasm is present:
Give salbutamol (albuterol) by nebulizer, or salbutamol or aminophylline by intravenous infusion.
6. Give intravenous glucose for hypoglycaemia.

Note: Cardiac massage was continued for two hours in one patient with a successful outcome.

References

Parmley WW. The role of glucagon in cardiac therapy. New Engl J Med 1971; 285:801–2.

Further Reading

Editorial. Self-poisoning with β-blockers. Br Med J 1978; 1: 1010–1011.

Editorial. Beta-blocker poisoning. Lancet 1980; i:803–4.

Frishman W, Jacob H, Eisenberg E, Ribner H. Clinical pharmacology of the new β-adrenergic blocking drugs. Part 8. Self-poisoning with β-adrenoceptor blocking agents: recognition and management. Am Heart J 1979; 98:798–811.

Illingworth RN. Glucagon for β-blocker poisoning. Practitioner 1979; 223:683–5.

Kosinski EJ, Malindzak GS, Winston-Salem NC. Glucagon and isoproterenol in reversing propranolol toxicity. Arch Intern Med 1973; 132:840–3.

Richards DA, Prichard BNC. Self-poisoning with β-blockers. Br Med J 1978; 1:1623–4.

Clonidine Poisoning

The chemical structure of clonidine is closely related to that of phentolamine and tolazoline. Clonidine exerts its hypotensive activity by reduction of sympathetic tone mediated by a central action on postsynaptic α-receptors in the medulla. Clonidine, therefore, decreases heart rate, cardiac output and total peripheral resistance. In the presence of high plasma clonidine concentrations peripheral α-agonistic activity predominates, which probably accounts for the vasoconstriction and hypertension reported following clonidine overdose.

Clonidine is used both for the treatment of hypertension and, in low dosage, in the prophylaxis of migraine and the suppression of menopausal flushing. Interestingly, in Great Britain 'Catapres' (clonidine hydrochloride 0.1 mg and 0.3 mg) is seldom taken in overdose but 'Dixarit' (clonidine hydrochloride 0.025 mg) is a frequent cause of poisoning, particularly in children. It has been suggested that this is because Dixarit is produced as an attractive, blue, sugar-coated sweet-tasting tablet whereas Catapres is a white uncoated tablet.

Clinical Features

A review of 170 cases by Stein and Volans (1978) of the Poisons Unit, Guy's Hospital, indicates that poisoning with this drug may be severe and life-threatening, particularly in children, though no deaths occurred in their series. In contrast to other reports, peripherally mediated α-sympathomimetic effects (such as hypertension and severe vasoconstriction) were unusual, while bradycardia, hypotension, coma and respiratory depression (due to the central effects of the drug) were common (Table 16.1).

Table 16.1   Clinical features of acute clonidine overdosage in 133 children aged under 10 years (mean age 2 years 8 months) and in 37 adults (mean age 29). Mean clonidine dosage: children 0.509 mg (range 0.025 to 3.000 mg), adults 2.096 mg (range 0.250 to 7.000 mg).[1]

Signs and symptoms	No. (%) of children	No. (%) of adults
Impaired consciousness	113 (85)	29 (78)
Pallor	36 (27)	6 (16)
Bradycardia[2]	32 (24)	18 (49)
Cardiac arrhythmias	6 (5)	
Cardiac arrest		1 (3)
Hypotension[3]	28 (21)	12 (32)
Depressed respiration	20 (15)	2 (5)
Apnoea	3 (2)	
Miosis	18 (14)	3 (8)
Unreactive pupils	7 (5)	
Hypotonia	14 (11)	2 (5)
Irritability	14 (11)	1 (3)
Hyporeflexia	5 (4)	1 (3)
Extensor plantar reflex	4 (3)	
Hypertension	3 (2)	4 (11)
Dry mouth	3 (2)	4 (11)
Mean duration of effects (hr)	16.2 (range 3.5–48.0)	15–96
Mean period of hospitalization (hr)	32.5 (range 1.0–72.0)	24–96

1   Stein and Volans, 1978 – Reproduced by kind permission of the authors and the Editor of the *British Medical Journal.*

2   Bradycardia defined as a pulse of < 80/min, age 1–4 years; < 75/min age 4–6 years; < 70/min, age 6–10 years; < 60/min, age > 10 years.

3   Hypotension defined as a systolic blood pressure of < 75 mm Hg, age 1–2 years; < 80 mm Hg, age 2–40 years; < 90 mm Hg, age > 40 years.

Treatment

1. Gastric lavage or emesis if appropriate.

2. Supportive measures.

3. Atropine 0.6 to 2 mg i.v. for bradycardia.

4. Alpha-adrenergic blocking drugs (tolazoline or phentolamine) have been advocated and used in severely poisoned patients, in the hope that both the peripheral and central actions of clonidine might be blocked.

Although forced diuresis has been advocated (Hunyor et al. 1975, Poyner et al. 1976), there is no evidence that it is effective (Wing et al. 1978). Moreover, this technique might potentiate the hypotensive effects of the drug.

References

Hunyor SN, Bradstock K, Somerville PJ, Lucas N. Clonidine overdose. Br Med J 1975; 4:23.

Poyner TE, Gennery BA, Vassey RH. Management in cases of clonidine overdosage. Practitioner 1976; 217:132–4.

Stein B, Volans GN. Dixarit overdose: the problem of attractive tablets. Br Med J 1978; 2:667–8.

Wing LMH, Davies DS, Reid JL, Dollery CT. Clonidine overdose. Br Med J 1975; 4:408–9.

Further Reading

Conner CS, Watanabe AS. Clonidine overdose: a review. Am J Hosp Pharm 1979; 36:906–11.

De Nayer-Van Der Wielen B, Guidée M. Intoxication par la clonidine et hypertension sévère. Louvain Med 1978; 97: 113–7.

Grabert B, Conner CS, Rumack BH, Peterson RG. Clonidine – recurrent apnea following overdose. Drug Intell Clin Pharm 1979; 13:778–80.

MacFaul R, Miller G. Clonidine poisoning in children. Lancet 1977; i:1266–7.

Mendoza JE, Medalie M. Clonidine poisoning with marked hypotension in a two-and-a-half-year-old child. Clin Pediatr 1979; 18:123; 7.

Mofenson HC, Greensher J, Weiss TE. Clonidine poisoning: is there a single antidote? Clin Toxicol 1979; 14:271–5.

Moore MA, Phillipi P. Clonidine overdose. Lancet 1976; ii: 694.

Neuvonen PJ, Vilska J, Keranen A. Severe poisoning in a child caused by a small dose of clonidine. Clin Toxicol 1979; 14: 369–74.

Pai GS, Lipsitz DJ. Clonidine poisoning. Pediatr 1976; 58: 749–50.

Digoxin and Digitoxin Poisoning

Important differences exist between the clinical features and treatment of patients who exhibit toxicity whilst taking either digoxin or digitoxin for therapeutic reasons and those who deliberately poison themselves by the ingestion of a single large dose of one of these drugs. Digitoxin poisoning is manifested by the same clinical signs that are seen with digoxin and the following discussion applies to both drugs.

Clinical Features

Nausea and vomiting.
Cardiac arrhythmias (supraventricular arrhythmias, with or without heart block, bradycardia, ventricular premature beats).
Hyperkalaemia (inhibition of the $Na^+ - K^+$ activated ATPase by digoxin).
High serum digoxin concentration.

Treatment

1. Gastric aspiration and lavage. (Activated charcoal adsorbs digoxin in the stomach and small intestine but, in order to be effective, it needs to be administered within one hour of the overdose.)

2. Intensive supportive therapy.

3. Treat arrhythmias:
(a) Atropine for digoxin-induced heart block and bradycardia.
(b) Phenytoin suppresses ventricular ectopic beats and improves conduction through the atrioventricular node.
(c) Propanolol and lignocaine suppress ventricular arrhythmias but are negatively inotropic and should be avoided if the cardiac output is low.

4. Pacemaker.

5. Correct hyperkalaemia with glucose and insulin infusion. Severe hyperkalaemia may be corrected by the use of sodium resonium ion-exchange resins or dialysis.

6. High urine output to eliminate digoxin.

7. Use of digoxin-specific Fab antibody fragments (Chapter 5, p 36).

Note: Haemodialysis and haemoperfusion are unlikely to remove significant quantities of digoxin from the body because of the large apparent volume of distribution of the drug (350 l).

Further Reading

Ahlmark G. Extreme digitalis intoxication. Acta Med Scand. 1976; 200:423–5.

Bremner WF, Third JLHC, Lawrie TDV. Massive digoxin ingestion. Report of a case and review of currently available therapies. Br Heart J 1977; 39:688–92.

Citrin DL, O'Malley K, Hillis WS. Cardiac standstill due to digoxin poisoning successfully treated with atrial pacing. Br Med J 1973; 2:526–7.

Dunea G. Digoxin ups and downs. J Am Med Assoc 1979; 242:2106.

Editorial. Treating poisoning with antibodies. Lancet 1980; 2:628.

Ekins BR, Watanabe AP. Acute digoxin poisonings: review of therapy. Am J Hosp Pharm 1978; 35:268–77.

Hess T, Stucki P, Barandun S, Scholtysik G, Riesen W. Treatment of a case of lanatoside C intoxication with digoxin-specific F(ab')₂ antibody fragments. Am Heart J 1979; 98: 767–71.

Holt DW, Trail TA, Brown CB. The treatment of digoxin overdose. Clin Nephrol 1975; 3:119–22.

Lely AH, Van Enter CHJ. Large-scale digitoxin intoxication. Br Med J 1970; 3:737–40.

Rotmensch HH, Graff E, Terdiman R, Aviram A, Ayzenberg O, Laniado S. Furosemide-induced forced diuresis in digoxin intoxication. Arch Intern Med 1978; 138:1495–7.

Smith TW, Haber E, Yeatman L, Butler VP. Reversal of advanced digoxin intoxication with Fab fragments of digoxin-specific antibodies. New Engl J Med 1976; 294: 797–800.

Smith TW, Willerson JT. Suicidal and accidental digoxin ingestion. Circulation 1971; 44:29–36.

Warren SE, Fanestil DD. Digoxin overdose. Limitations of haemoperfusion–haemodialysis treatment. J Am Med Assoc 1979; 242:2100–1.

5. Cardiodepressant drugs such as quinidine and procainamide should be avoided for the treatment of arrhythmias as they may well increase the mortality.

6. If asystole occurs, transvenous pacing should be tried, but the ventricular response is often poor.

7. Haemoperfusion may be of value in those who are severely poisoned (Hayler et al. 1979).

References

Hayler AM, Medd RK, Holt DW, O'Keefe BD. Experimental disopyramide poisoning: treatment by cardiovascular support and with charcoal haemoperfusion. J Pharm Exp Ther 1979; 211:491–5.

Further Reading

Anderson WH, Stafford DT, Bell JS. Disopyramide distribution at autopsy of an overdose case. J Forensic Sci 1980; 25:33–9.

Hayler AM, Holt DW, Volans GN. Fatal overdose with disopyramide. Lancet 1978; i:968–9.

Holt DW, Helliwell M, O'Keeffe BD, Hayler AM, Marshall CB, Cook G. Successful management of serious disopyramide poisoning. Postgrad Med J 1980; 56:256–60.

Hutchison A, Kilham H. Fatal overdosage of disopyramide in a child. Med J Aust 1978; 2:335–6.

O'Keeffe Bd, Hayler AM, Holt DW, Medd RK. Cardiac consequences and treatment of disopyramide intoxication: experimental evaluation in dogs. Cardiovasc Res 1979; 13:630–4.

Powell F, Smith P, Carey O. Fatal disopyramide overdosage. J Irish Med Assoc 1978; 71:552.

Tempe JD, Hasselmann M, Jaeger A, Haegy JM, Checoury A, Sauder Ph. Intoxication aigues par le disopyramide. J Med Strasbourg 1979; 10:21–7.

Wayne K, Manolas E, Sloman G. Fatal overdose with disopyramide. Med J. Aust, 1980; 1:231–2.

Disopyramide Poisoning

Disopyramide not only possesses membrane-stabilizing (i.e. local anaesthetic-like) activity but it also prolongs the action potential of normal cardiac cells. It thus has the properties of both Class I and Class III anti-arrhythmic agents. Anticholinergic effects are common even in therapeutic doses. Disopyramide is rapidly absorbed and peak plasma levels are attained within two hours. It has a relatively small volume of distribution and is not highly protein bound.

Clinical Features

Following a severe overdose of disopyramide a steady decline in cardiac output is seen, although the blood pressure is relatively well maintained until circulatory collapse occurs. Typically respiratory depression and serious arrhythmias do not occur until after circulatory collapse has supervened. The mortality is high in those who are severely poisoned.

Treatment

1. Gastric lavage if appropriate.

2. Monitor blood pressure regularly, preferably with an indwelling arterial cannula to provide immediate warning of cardiovascular collapse which may occur suddenly.

3. Isoprenaline infusion to maintain blood pressure.

4. Raise the serum potassium level 5 to 6.6 mmol/l; correct any acidosis.

Mexiletine Poisoning

Mexiletine depresses the maximum rate of depolarization of cardiac muscle with little or no modification of resting potentials or the duration of action potentials. It is rapidly absorbed following ingestion and peak plasma levels are achieved within two to four hours. Less than 15 per cent of the administered dose is recovered unchanged in the urine.

Clinical Features

Nausea, vomiting, unpleasant taste, hiccoughs.
Light-headedness, drowsiness, confusion, dizziness, diplopia, blurred vision, nystagmus, dysarthria, ataxia, tremor, paraesthesiae, convulsions.

Palpitations, hypotension, sinus bradycardia, atrial fibrillation.

Treatment

1. Emesis or gastric lavage, if appropriate.

2. Supportive measures.

3. Atropine 1 to 2 mg i.v. for bradycardia.

4. Isoprenaline infusion for severe hypotension.

5. Transvenous cardiac pacing — but ventricular response is usually poor.

Further Reading

Jequier P, Jones R, Mackintosh A. Fatal mexiletine overdose. Lancet 1976; i:429.

Quinidine and Quinine Poisoning

Quinine and quinidine are optical isomers and share many pharmacological properties, although the latter compound is more toxic. Both alkaloids depress skeletal and cardiac muscle function though quinidine does so to a greater degree.

Quinidine is rapidly and completely absorbed after ingestion and has a half-life of about five hours. It is rapidly bound to plasma albumin. Between 10 and 50 per cent of the unchanged drug appears in the urine within 24 hours.

Peak plasma concentrations of quinine are reached within one to three hours after oral administration. Seventy per cent is protein bound and less than five per cent of the administered dose is excreted unaltered in the urine. Renal excretion of quinine is twice as rapid when the urine is acid as when it is alkaline.

Clinical Features

Ringing in the ears, headache, nausea, vomiting, diarrhoea, abdominal pain.
Blurred vision, disturbed odour perception, photophobia, diplopia, night blindness, constricted visual fields, scotomata and, in severe cases, optic atrophy. (It is not known whether these changes are primarily neural or vascular in origin. The rapid response to stellate ganglion block supports the latter view). Collapse with impairment of consciousness, shallow rapid breathing, sinus tachycardia and hypotension. Cardiac arrhythmias may follow.
ECG changes include widening of the QRS complex and flattening of the T-waves.

Treatment

1. Gastric lavage, if appropriate.

2. Supportive measures.

3. In severe poisoning forced acid diuresis. (See Chapter 8)

4. Prophylactic stellate ganglion block in severe cases to prevent blindness.

Dialysis probably does not substantially increase the elimination of either quinine or quinidine.

Further Reading

Bankes JLK, Hayward JA, Jones MBS. Quinine amblyopia treated with stellate ganglion block. Br Med J 1972; 4:85–6.
Gerhardt RE, Knouss EF, Thyrum PT, Luchi RJ, Morris Jr. JJ. Quinidine excretion in aciduria and alkaluria. Ann Intern Med 1969; 71:927–33.
Reimold EW, Reynolds WJ, Fixler DE, McElroy L. Use of haemodialysis in the treatment of quinidine poisoning. Pediatrics 1973; 52:95–9.
Robertson DH, Kothanda Raman KR. Quinine poisoning — an unusual indication for stellate ganglion blockage. Anaesthesia 1979; 34:1041–42.
Shub C, Gau GT, Sidell PM, Brennan LA. The management of acute quinidine intoxication. Chest 1978; 73:173–8.
Valman HB, White DC. Stellate block for quinine blindness in a child. Br Med J 1977; 1:1065.
Winek CL, Davis ER, Collom WD, Shanor SP. Quinine fatality — a case report. Clin Toxicol 1974; 7:129–32.

Verapamil Poisoning

Verapamil has a specific inhibitory effect on the transmembranal passage of calcium ions in the myocardial cell, and thereby reduces the activity of calcium-dependent adenosine triphosphatase. In addition, verapamil diminishes peripheral resistance and so relieves the work load on the heart.

Clinical Features

In overdose, verapamil may cause dizziness, nausea, vomiting, atrioventricular conduction defects and hypotension, which can be severe. After a large overdose, the prognosis is poor in those with ischaemic heart disease and in those who are taking β-adrenergic blocking agents. Intravenous injection of verapamil may cause cardiac arrest (asystole, ventricular fibrillation and total atrioventricular block), particularly when a β-blocker has been given within the preceding 12 hours.

Treatment

1. Emesis or gastric lavage if appropriate.

2. Supportive measures.

3. Calcium gluconate 10 to 20 ml of a 10 per cent solution.

4. Dobutamine infusion to maintain cardiac output.

Further Reading

Da Silva OA, De Melo RA, Filho JPJ. Verapamil acute poisoning. Clin Toxicol 1979; 14:361–7.

de Fair U, Lundman T. Attempted suicide with verapamil. Eur J Cardiol 1977; 6:195–8.

Madera F, Wenger R. Zur frage von vergiftung mit Isoptin S. Intensivmed 1977; 14:373–7.

Perkins CM. Serious verapamil poisoning: treatment with intravenous calcium gluconate. Br Med J 1978; 2:1127.

Chapter 17

J. A. Vale and T. J. Meredith

Poisoning due to Bronchodilator Drugs

Beta₂ Adrenoceptor Stimulant Drug Poisoning

Beta$_2$ adrenoceptor stimulant drugs (salbutamol [albuterol], terbutaline) are widely used in the treatment of obstructive airways disease and, less commonly, in the management of premature labour. Poisoning with these drugs has followed either deliberate or accidental ingestion or confusion over the parenteral and oral doses (Brandsetter and Gotz 1980).

Clinical Features

Tremor, 'bursting feeling', agitation.
Palpitations, tachycardia, peripheral vasodilation.
Lactic acidosis, hyperglycaemia, hypokalaemia (Fahlen and Lapidus 1980).

Treatment

1. Emesis or gastric lavage, if appropriate.

2. Supportive measures.

3. A cardioselective β-adrenergic blocking drug should be given if rate-related chest pain or arrhythmias occur.

References

Brandsetter RD, Gotz V. Inadvertent overdose of parenteral terbutaline. Lancet 1980; i:485.
Fahlen M, Lapidus L. Lactic acidosis and beta-adrenergic agents. Br Med J 1980, 281:390.

Further Reading

Gluckman L. Ventolin psychosis. NZ Med J 1974; 80:411.
Gomolin I, Ingelfinger JA. Terbutaline overdose. New Engl J Med 1979; 300:143.
Kinney EL, Traultein JJ, Harbaugh CV, Lambert D, Zelis RF Ventricular tachycardia after terbutaline. J Am Med Assoc 1978; 240:2247.
Lawyer C, Pond A. Problems with terbutaline. New Engl J Med 1977; 296:821.
Ray I, Evans CJ. Paranoid psychosis with ventolin. Can Psychiatr Assoc J 1978; 23:427.

Theophylline Poisoning

Iatrogenic poisoning from theophylline, often by the intravenous route, is not uncommon, and it has been suggested therefore that it is important to monitor plasma drug levels during therapy (Hendeles and Weinberger 1979).

Self-poisoning with theophylline compounds appears to be increasing and it has an appreciable mortality (Helliwell and Berry 1979). Factors which may increase the susceptibility of patients to the toxic effects of theophylline include chronic obstructive pulmonary disease, liver dysfunction and heart failure. Hypotension, cardiac arrhythmias and convulsions indicate a poor prognosis, particularly in patients greater than 50 years of age.

Iatrogenic poisoning can generally be managed symptomatically while the drug is eliminated by endogenous metabolic pathways. In cases of severe poisoning, with marked cardiovascular and neurological effects, more rapid removal of the drug may be necessary to prevent potentially fatal complications.

Clinical Features

Nausea, vomiting, abdominal discomfort, diarrhoea, thirst, diuresis.
Palpitations, cardiac arrhythmias, hypotension.
Agitation, tremor, convulsions.

Treatment

1. Emesis or gastric lavage, if appropriate. Activated charcoal should be left in the stomach.

2. Symptomatic and supportive measures.

3. Treat convulsions with diazepam 5 to 10 mg intravenously.

4. Charcoal haemoperfusion (see Chapter 8) if patient is severely poisoned (plasma level >60 mg/l). Peritoneal and haemodialysis appear to be ineffective.

References

Helliwell M, Berry D. Theophylline poisoning in adults. Br Med J 1979; 2:1114.

Hendeles L, Weinberger M. Guidelines for avoiding theophylline overdose. New Engl J Med 1979; 300:1217.

Further Reading

Ehlers SM, Zaske DE, Sawchuk RJ. Massive theophylline overdose: rapid elimination by charcoal haemoperfusion. J Am Med Assoc 1978; 240:474–5.

Iberti TJ, Hammond RS. Massive oral theophylline poisoning. South Med J 1978; 71:965–6.

Jefferys DB, Raper SM, Helliwell M, Berry DJ, Crome P. Haemoperfusion for theophylline overdose. Br Med J 1980; 280:1167.

Levy G, Gibson TP, Whitman W, Procknal J. Haemodialysis clearance of theophylline. J Am Med Assoc 1977; 237: 1466–7.

Russo ME. Management of theophylline intoxication with charcoal column haemoperfusion. New Engl J Med 1979; 300:24–6.

Sintek C, Hendeles L, Weinberger M. Inhibition of theophylline absorption by activated charcoal. J Pediatr 1979; 94: 314–6.

Weinberger M, Hendeles L. Management and prevention of theophylline toxicity: is dialysis helpful. Dev Pharm Ther 1980; 1:26–30.

Zwillich CW, Sutton FD, Neff TA, Cohn WM, Matthay RA, Weinberger M. Theophylline induced seizures in adults. Ann Intern Med 1975; 82:784–7.

Chapter 18

J. A. Vale and T. J. Meredith

Poisoning due to Non-Catecholamine Sympathomimetic Drugs

In contrast to the catecholamines, most of the clinically useful non-catecholamines are effective when given orally and many act for long periods.

Amphetamine Poisoning

The amphetamines have many properties in common with other sympathomimetic amines, but they possess marked central stimulatory activity in doses that do not produce marked peripheral side-effects. Amphetamines have been used as appetite depressants, though this use is now unwarranted. They are now most often used in the treatment of narcolepsy and in hyperkinetic states in children who have minimal brain damage. In addition, amphetamines have been widely misused 'for kicks' because of their stimulant effects.

Amphetamines are readily absorbed both from the GI tract and from parenteral sites. Excretion is pH-dependent and is increased considerably if the urine is acid; about 50 per cent of an administered dose may be recovered in the urine as unchanged drug.

Clinical Features

Restlessness, tremor, irritability, insomnia.
Dryness of the mouth, nausea, vomiting, diarrhoea, abdominal pain.
Flushing, sweating, hyperpyrexia, cardiac arrhythmias, marked hypertension, tachypnoea, circulatory collapse.
Delirium, hallucinations, coma and convulsions.

Treatment

1. Gastric lavage, if indicated.

2. Supportive treatment.

3. Chlorpromazine 50 to 100 mg intravenously for sedation, or droperidol 5–15 mg intravenously (200–600 μg/kg body weight in children).

4. Forced acid diuresis may be valuable in those who are severely poisoned.

Dialysis and haemoperfusion probably have no part to play in treatment.

Further Reading

Adjutantis G, Coutselinis A, Dimopoulous G. Fatal intoxication with amphetamines. Med Sci Law 1975; 15:62–3.

Anonymous. Clinical aspects of amphetamine abuse. J Am Med Assoc 1978; 240:2317–9.

Beckett AH, Rowland M, Turner P. Influence of urinary pH on excretion of amphetamine. Lancet 1965; i:303.

Connell PH. Clinical manifestations and treatment of amphetamine type of dependence. J Am Med Assoc 1966; 196: 718–23.

Gary NE, Saidi P. Methamphetamine intoxication. Am J Med 1978; 64:537–40.

Jordan SC, Hampson F. Amphetamine poisoning associated with hyperpyrexia Br Med J 1960; 2:844

Patuck D. Acute dexamphetamine sulphate poisoning in a child. Br Med 1956; 1:670–1.

Van Hoof F, Hendrickx A, Timperman J. Report of a human fatality due to amphetamine. Arch Toxicol 1974; 32:307–12.

Pemoline Poisoning

Pemoline is a central nervous system stimulant drug which is structurally different from the amphetamines and methylphenidate though pharmacologically it has similar actions. It has been used in adults with 'psychogenic fatigue' and in children with hyper-activity and minimal brain dysfunction.

Clinical Features

As for amphetamine poisoning. In addition, frequent sucking movements of the tongue and choreiform movements have been described.

Treatment

As for amphetamine poisoning except that there is no evidence that forced diuresis is effective.

Further Reading

Alsop JA. Pemoline adverse reactions. Drug Intell Clin Pharm 1977; 11:367.
McNeil JR. Accidental ingestion of pemoline. Clin Pediatr 1979; 18:761–2.

Ephedrine Poisoning

Ephedrine differs from adrenaline (epinephrine) in several respects. It may be administered orally, it has a much longer duration of action and exerts more pronounced central effects, although it is of lower potency. The cardiovascular effects are similar to those of adrenaline but persist for much longer; bron-chial muscle relaxation is less prominent than with adrenaline. On the other hand, the effects on the nervous system are similar to those of amphetamine although they are much less marked.

Clinical Features

Nausea, vomiting.
Irritability, fever, tachycardia, sweating, praecordial pain, palpitations.
Dilated pupils, blurred vision, paranoid psychosis, delusions and hallucinations (auditory and visual).
Convulsions and coma.
Respiratory depression and hypertension.

Treatment

1. Emesis or gastric lavage, if appropriate.

2. Supportive treatment.

3. Practolol 5 to 20 mg i.v. or labetalol 50 to 200 mg i.v. for supraventricular tachycardia.

Further Reading

Adams RD, Robertson C, Jarvie DR, Stewart MJ, Proudfoot AT. Clinical and metabolic features of overdosage with Amesec. Scott Med J 1979; 24:246–9.
Herridge CF, A'Brook MF. Ephedrine psychosis. Br Med J 1968; 2:160.
Kane FJ, Florenzano R. Psychosis accompanying use of bron-chodilator compound. J Am Med Assoc 1971; 215:2116.
McCleave DJ, Phillips PJ, Vedig AE. Compartmental shift of potassium – a result of sympathomimetic overdose. Aust NZ J Med 1978; 8:180–3.
Roxanas MG, Spalding J. Ephedrine abuse psychosis. Med J Aut 1977; 2:639–40.
Meigham W Van, Stevens E, Cosemans J. Ephedrine – induced cardiopathy. Br Med J 1978; 1:816.

Fenfluramine Poisoning

Fenfluramine is an amphetamine derivative which is a popular anorectic agent in Western Europe. Fenflura-mine is rapidly and completely absorbed after the oral administration of therapeutic doses in man. Eighty per cent of a 60 mg dose is excreted within 48 hours and elimination is complete 72 hours after ingestion. Excretion is considerably higher when the urine is acid (Beckett and Brookes 1967).

In a recent review of 53 cases of fenfluramine poisoning (15 taken from the literature) by Von Muhlendahl and Krienke (1979), there was a 20 per cent mortality (10 patients). This occurred after fenfluramine was taken in overdoses ranging from 28.7 to 70 mg/kg body weight. In 9 out of 10 patients who died, cardiac arrest occurred one to four hours after ingestion. None of the surviving patients developed major symptoms later than four hours after ingestion.

Clinical Features

In acute overdosage the clinical features are similar to those of amphetamine:
Excitability and restlessness.
Sweating, hyperpyrexia, redness of the face.
Mydriasis, sluggish or absent pupillary reaction to light.
Nystagmus
Tachycardia and tachypnoea.
Hyper-reflexia, tremor, clonus, convulsions, coma.

Treatment

1. Gastric lavage, if appropriate. (Note: activated charcoal adsorbs fenfluramine.)

2. Supportive therapy.

3. Diazepam intravenously for convulsions, excitability and restlessness.

4. Chlorpromazine for marked hyperthermia.

5. Forced acid diuresis enhances renal elimination, though the amount recovered in one report was low (Riley et al. 1969)

References

Beckett AH, Brooks LG. The absorption and urinary excretion in man of fenfluramine and its main metabolite. J Pharm Pharmacol 1967; 19:Suppl. 42–49.

Riley I, Corson J, Haider I, Oswald I. Fenfluramine overdosage. Lancet 1969; ii: 1162–3.

Von Muhlendahl KE, Kreinke EG. Fenfluramine poisoning. Clin Toxicol 1979; 14:97–106.

Further Reading

Campbell DB, Moore BWR. Fenfluramine overdosage. Lancet 1969; ii:1307.

Darmady JM. Diazepam for fenfluramine intoxication. Arch Dis Child 1974; 49:328–30.

Fleisher MR, Campbell DB. Fenfluramine overdosage. Lancet 1969; ii:1306–7.

Gold RS, Gordon HE, Da Costa RWD, Porteous IB, Kimber KJ. Fenfluramine overdosage. Lancet 1969, ii:1306.

Richards AJ. Fenfluramine overdosage. Lancet 1969; ii:1367.

Simpson H, McKinlay I. Poisoning with slow-release fenfluramine. Br Med J 1975; 4:462–3.

Veltri JC, Temple AR. Fenfluramine poisoning. J Pediatr 1975; 87:119–21.

White AG, Beckett AH, Brookes LG. Fenfluramine overdosage. Br Med J 1967; 1:740.

Chapter 19

T. J. Meredith and J. A. Vale

Alcohol Poisoning

Methyl Alcohol Poisoning

Methyl alcohol (methanol) is widely used as a solvent and to denature solutions of ethanol. It is also found in paint, varnishes, duplicating fluid and antifreeze solutions, and it may prove to be an important alternative energy source. The ingestion of as little as 10 ml of methanol may cause permanent blindness and 30 ml is potentially fatal, although individual susceptibility varies widely. Toxicity may also occur through inhalation or percutaneous absorption of the alcohol.

Clinical Features

Methanol causes only mild and transient inebriation and drowsiness when ingested alone but, after a latent period of 8 to 36 hours, nausea, vomiting, abdominal pain, headaches, dizziness and coma supervene. Blurred vision and diminished visual acuity may also occur and the development of dilated pupils, unreactive to light, suggests that permanent blindness may ensue. A severe metabolic acidosis with an increased anion gap is found in serious cases of methanol poisoning and, in some instances, this may be accompanied by raised blood sugar and serum amylase concentrations. A blood methanol level of > 500 mg/l is indicative of serious methanol poisoning.

Pathophysiology

In man, methanol is metabolized by alcohol dehydrogenase and catalase enzyme systems, although the quantitative importance of the latter enzyme is not known. In monkeys, and in rats rendered folate-deficient, it has been demonstrated that formic acid is further metabolized to carbon dioxide by means of a folate-dependent one carbon pool pathway. It is not certain whether the visual effects of methanol toxicity are due either to formaldehyde or to formic acid, although it is possible that formaldehyde is formed locally in the retina. Furthermore, the metabolic acidosis of methanol poisoning has not been fully explained because formate accounts for only half of the increased anion gap. Recently, however, formate has been shown to inhibit cytochrome oxidase activity and other organic anions may therefore be involved in the development of the acidosis.

Treatment

The treatment of methanol poisoning should include gastric aspiration and lavage, provided that the alcohol has been ingested within the preceding four hours. Bicarbonate should be given intravenously to correct the metabolic acidosis.

Administration of Ethanol

Specific inhibition of the metabolism of methanol to formaldehyde and formic acid is achieved by the administration of ethanol (loading dose of 50 g orally followed by an intravenous infusion of 10 to 12 g/hour), in order to obtain circulating ethanol levels of 1000 to 2000 mg/l.

Haemodialysis

Haemodialysis is indicated if the blood methanol level exceeds 500 mg/l, if the metabolic acidosis cannot be corrected, if mental, visual or fundoscopic complications develop or if more than 30 ml of methanol has been ingested. The infusion of ethanol will need to be increased by at least 7 to 10 g/hr during haemodialysis because this substance too is readily dialysable. Peritoneal dialysis is less effective than haemodialysis.

4-Methyl Pyrazole

It is possible that, in the future, 4-methyl pyrazole may be used in the treatment of severe methanol poisoning. This substance inhibits alcohol dehydrogenase activity by forming a ternary complex with the enzyme and NAD. Methyl pyrazole has been used successfully to treat methanol poisoning in monkeys, and in man it has been used to inhibit the oxidation of ethanol for experimental purposes.

Folinic Acid

An alternative approach recently employed in the treatment of experimental methanol poisoning in monkeys has been the administration of synthetic folate analogue (leucovorin calcium, folinic acid) to enhance the metabolism of formate to carbon dioxide.

Further Reading

Anonymous. Use of folate analogue in treatment of methyl alcohol toxic reactions is studied. J Am Med Assoc 1979; 242:1961–2.

Bennett Jr IL, Cary FH, Mitchell Jr GL, Cooper MN. Acute methyl alcohol poisoning: a review based on experiences in an outbreak of 323 cases. Medicine 1953; 32:431–63.

Billings RE, Tephly TR. Studies on methanol toxicity and formate metabolism in isolated hepatocytes. Biochem Pharmacol 1979; 28:2985–91.

Blomstrand R, Ostling-Wintzell H, Lof A, McMartin K, Tolf BR, Hedstrom KG. Pyrazoles as inhibitors of alcohol oxidation and as important tools in alcohol research: an approach to therapy against methanol poisoning. Proc Natl Acad Sci USA 1979; 76:3499–503.

Gonda A, Gault H, Churchill D, Hollomby D. Hemodialysis for methanol intoxication. Am J Med 1978; 64: 749–58.

McCoy HG, Cipolle RJ, Ehlers SM, Sawchuk RJ, Zaske DE. Severe methanol poisoning. Application of a pharmacokinetic model for ethanol therapy and hemodialysis. Am J Med 1979; 67:804–7.

Naraqi S, Dethlefs RF, Slobodniuk RA, Sairere JS. An outbreak of acute methyl alcohol intoxication. Aust NZ J Med 1979; 9:65–8.

Schneck SA. Methyl alcohol. In: Handbook of Clinical Neurology Vol 36. Vinken PJ, Bryn GW Eds. Amsterdam: Elsevier, 1979; 351–60.

Ethyl Alcohol Poisoning

Ethyl alcohol (ethanol) is widely available in concentrations of up to 50 per cent in cosmetic preparations and beverages. It is also used as a solvent and as an antiseptic agent. Ethyl alcohol is rapidly absorbed through the gastric and intestinal mucosa and is distributed throughout the body water. Approximately 90 per cent of an ingested dose is oxidized to acetaldehyde, acetic acid and then carbon dioxide and water at a rate of about 10 to 20 ml/hr.

Ethyl alcohol acts as a central nervous depressant. In small doses it interferes with cortical processes but in large doses it may depress medullary function. It is important to remember that the effects of alcohol may be exacerbated by other central nervous depressants, for example, some hypnotic agents. The fatal dose of ethyl alcohol for an average adult lies between 300 and 500 ml if this amount is ingested in less than an hour (strong spirits, such as whisky and gin, contain 40 to 55 per cent ethanol).

Clinical Features

The clinical features of ethanol intoxication are well known and are related to blood alcohol levels as follows:

1. *Mild intoxication (500 to 1500 mg/l)*; emotional lability, slight impairment of visual acuity, muscular coordination and reaction time, slurred speech.

2. *Moderate intoxication (1500 to 3000 mg/l)*; visual impairment, sensory loss, muscular incoordination, slowed reaction time.

3. *Severe intoxication (3000 to 5000 mg/l)*; marked muscular incoordination, blurred or double vision, sometimes stupor and hypothermia and occasionally hypoglycaemia and convulsions.

4. *Coma (> 5000 mg/l)*; depressed reflexes, respiratory depression, hypotension, hypothermia. Death may occur from respiratory or circulatory failure or from aspiration pneumonia.

Hypoglycaemia

Severe hypoglycaemia may sometimes accompany alcohol intoxication. This effect is largely due to inhibition of gluconeogenesis and occurs more commonly in children who have accidentally drunk alcohol. Alcohol-induced hypoglycaemia typically occurs within 6 to 36 hours of ingestion of a moderate to large amount of alcohol by a previously mal-nourished individual, or one who has fasted for the previous 24 hours. The patient is often in coma and hypothermic; the usual features of hypoglycaemia, such as flushing, sweating and tachycardia, are frequently absent.

Treatment

The treatment of ethanol poisoning should include gastric aspiration and lavage, where appropriate, together with intensive supportive therapy. Naloxone (0.4 to 1.2 mg i.v.) has recently been shown to im-prove the level of consciousness in a proportion of patients with ethanol-induced coma, but the reason for this has not been fully established.

Hypoglycaemia

Hypoglycaemia should be treated with either oral or intravenous glucose. Glucagon is ineffective in the treatment of ethanol-induced hypoglycaemia.

Use of Fructose

The administration of fructose may sometimes be useful in the treatment of severe alcohol poisoning because the metabolism of this carbohydrate results in the conversion of $NADH_2$ to NAD, the supply of which may be rate-limiting for alcohol metabolism. Unfortunately the use of fructose may be accompanied by retrosternal and epigastric discom-fort as well as metabolic acidosis.

Haemodialysis and Haemoperfusion

Haemodialysis and haemoperfusion both remove alcohol from the blood effectively and the use of one of these techniques may occasionally be necessary in very severe cases of ethyl alcohol poisoning.

Further Reading

Brown SS, Forrest JAH, Roscoe P. A controlled trial of fructose in the treatment of acute alcoholic intoxication. Lancet 1972; ii:898—900.

Elliott RW, Hunter PR. Acute ethanol poisoning treated by haemodialysis. Postgrad Med J 1974; 50:515—7.

Jeffcoate WJ, Herbert M, Cullen MH, Hastings AG, Walder CP. Prevention of effects of alcohol intoxication by naloxone. Lancet 1979; ii:1157—9.

Mark V. Alcohol and changes in body constituents; glucose and hormones. Proc R Soc Med 1975; 68:377—80.

Ragen FA, Samuels MS, Hite SA. Ethanol ingestion in children. J Am Med Assoc 1979; 242:2787—8.

Wagner JG, Wilkinson PK, Sedman AJ, Kay DR, Weidler DJ. Elimination of alcohol from human blood. J Pharm Sci 1976; 65:152—4.

Isopropyl Alcohol Poisoning

Isopropyl alcohol (isopropanol) is used as a sterilizing agent and as rubbing alcohol. It is also found in after-shave lotion and window-cleaning solutions.

Clinical Features

The systemic effects and toxicity of isopropanol are similar to those of ethyl alcohol although the former is twice as potent, largely because of a slower rate of metabolism. Approximately 10 to 15 per cent of an ingested dose of isopropyl alcohol is metabolized to acetone and, for this reason, ketonuria is a common finding in isopropanol poisoning. Symptoms and signs persist for two to four times as long as those in cases of ethyl alcohol poisoning.

Treatment

Isopropyl alcohol is readily dialysable and haemo-dialysis is indicated in severely poisoned patients although, in most instances, gastric lavage and sup-portive therapy are the only necessary measures.

Further Reading

Adelson L. Fatal intoxication with isopropyl alcohol (rub-bing alcohol). Am J Clin Pathol 1962; 38:144—51.

Agarwal SK. Non-acidotic acetonemia: a syndrome due to isopropyl alcohol intoxication. J Med Soc NJ 1979; 76:914—6.

Freireich AW, Cinque TJ, Xanthaky G, Landau D. Haemo-dialysis for isopropanol poisoning. New Engl J Med 1967; 277:699—700.

Juncos L, Taguchi JT. Isopropyl alcohol intoxication. J Am Med Assoc 1968; 204:732—4.

King LH, Bradley KP, Shires DL. Haemodialysis for isopropyl alcohol poisoning. J Am Med Assoc 1979; 211:1855.

Chapter 20

J. A. Vale and T. J. Meredith

Ethylene Glycol Poisoning

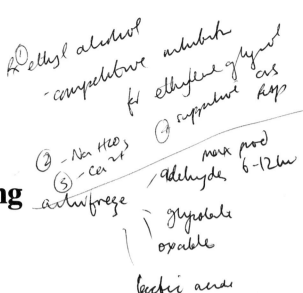

Ethylene glycol $(CH_2OH)_2$, is a colourless, odourless, water-soluble liquid that has a variety of commercial applications. It is, however, most commonly used as an antifreeze fluid to protect car radiators. Its sweet taste and ready availability have contributed to its popularity as a suicide agent and as a poor man's substitute for alcohol. Ethylene glycol came into widespread use in the 1920s and the first case of poisoning was described in 1930. The toxicity of the glycols was, however, not fully appreciated until 1937 when 76 people died following the use of an elixir of sulphanilamide which contained 72 per cent diethylene glycol. Even in 1969 seven children died in Cape Town as a result of the ingestion of a hypnotic containing this substance.

It is thought that the minimum lethal dose of ethylene glycol is about 100 ml for an adult, although recovery after treatment has been reported following the ingestion of 240 ml, 400 ml and 970 ml. Deaths from ethylene glycol are uncommon in England and Wales; only 31 cases have been reported in 34 years (1954 to 1978), though 15 of these occurred in one year (1977).

Why is Ethylene Glycol Toxic?

Ethylene glycol itself appears to be non-toxic. Until metabolized it has no effect on respiration, the citric acid cycle or other biochemical pathways. Metabolism takes place in the liver and kidneys and proceeds as shown in Figure 20.1. The toxicity of ethylene glycol may be explained on the basis of accumulation of the following four metabolic products:

1. Aldehydes, which inhibit oxidative phosphorylation, cellular respiration and glucose metabolism, protein synthesis, DNA replication and ribosomal RNA synthesis, central nervous system respiration, serotonin metabolism, and alter central nervous system amine levels. The cerebral symptoms that occur 6 to 12 hours after the ingestion of ethylene glycol coincide with the maximum production of aldehydes.

2. Glycolate, which, at least in monkeys and in the rat, is largely responsible for the marked acidosis that occurs.

3. Oxalate, which may produce renal damage and acidosis. It is thought, however, that only about one per cent of ethylene glycol is converted to this compound. The production of oxalate is also important in that it may chelate calcium ions to form relatively insoluble calcium oxalate crystals; hypocalcaemia may result. As well as renal intratubular obstruction, impairment of cerebral function also follows deposition of calcium oxalate.

4. Lactic acid, which is produced as a result of large amounts of nicotinamide adenine dinucleotide being formed during the breakdown of ethylene glycol. In addition, some of the condensation products of glyoxylate metabolism inhibit the citric acid cycle, thereby increasing lactic acid production (Figure 20.1).

Ethylene Glycol Poisoning

Clinical Features

The clinical features of ethylene glycol poisoning may be divided into three groups depending on the

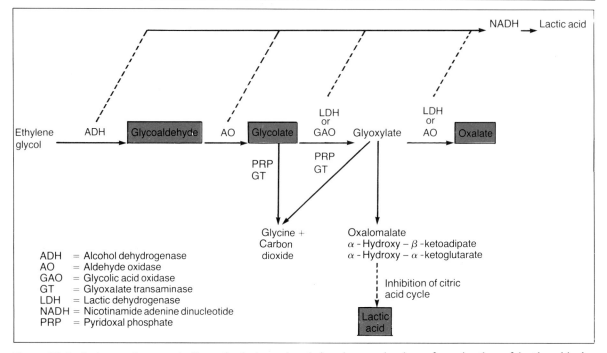

Figure 20.1. *Pathways for metabolism of ethylene glycol showing mechanism of production of lactic acidosis.*

time after ingestion (Table 20.1). The severity of each stage and the progression from one stage to the next depends very largely on the amount of ethylene glycol ingested. Death may occur during any of the three stages.

Diagnosis

Ethylene glycol poisoning should be strongly suspected in the presence of the following:

1. An apparently inebriated patient with no alcohol on the breath.

2. Coma associated with metabolic acidosis and a large anion gap (serum bicarbonate may be <10 mmol/l).

3. Urinalysis demonstrating calcium oxalate (monohydrate or dihydrate) crystalluria, microscopic haematuria, low specific gravity and proteinuria.

4. Gastric lavage fluid may have the appearance of antifreeze solution.

Suspicion of ethylene glycol poisoning may be confirmed by measuring the serum levels of ethylene glycol and oxalic acid. Other abnormalities which may be found on investigation are shown in Table 20.2.

Table 20.1.   Clinical features of ethylene glycol poisoning.

Stage 1 (30 min–12 hr). Gastrointestinal and nervous system involvement

Patient appears intoxicated with alcohol (but no alcohol on breath)
Nausea, vomiting, haematemesis
Coma and convulsions (often focal)
Nystagmus, ophthalmoplegias, papilloedema, optic atrophy, depressed reflexes, myoclonic jerks, tetanic contractions

Stage 2 (12–24 hr). Cardiorespiratory system involvement

Tachypnoea
Tachycardia
Mild hypertension
Pulmonary oedema
Congestive cardiac failure

Stage 3 (24–72 hr). Renal involvement

Flank pain
Costovertebral angle tenderness
Acute tubular necrosis

Table 20.2. Ethylene glycol poisoning: typical laboratory investigations.

Investigation	Abnormality
White cell count	Raised (10—40 x 10^3/μl) — predominantly neutrophils
Serum bicarbonate	Reduced (may be < 10 mmol/l)
Serum calcium	Reduced
Serum potassium	Raised
Urinalysis	Low specific gravity Proteinuria Crystalluria (Ca oxalate) Microscopic haematuria
Cerebrospinal fluid	Compatible with meningoencephalitis

Pathology

In patients who have died within 72 hours of ingestion of ethylene glycol there is considerable cerebral oedema, capillary engorgement and haemorrhage, evidence of chemical meningoencephalitis, Betz cell and Purkinje cell chromatolysis and perivascular and meningeal deposition of calcium oxalate crystals.

It is of interest that rats given regular small doses of ethylene glycol have cerebral oxalate deposits in the brain but no symptoms; whereas rats given the aldehyde derivatives of ethylene glycol may have severe central nervous system symptoms in the absence of crystals. It would appear, therefore, that although the central nervous system symptoms are related to ethylene glycol and its aldehyde derivatives, the deposition of calcium oxalate further impairs cerebral function.

Pathologically the lungs show generalized oedema with early bronchopneumonic changes. Widespread petechial haemorrhages are found in the pleura, lungs, heart and pericardium. Cardiac dilation may occur together with degenerative myocardial changes. Occasionally oxalate crystals have been found in the lung parenchyma.

The proximal tubules may become dilated, and degeneration of tubular epithelium is seen in those patients with renal involvement. Calcium oxalate crystals and fat droplets are found in tubular epithelial cells. Distal tubular degeneration may also be present, although less pronounced than that in the proximal tubules. Glomerular damage is not a prominent feature but increased cellularity, thickened basement membranes and granular deposits in Bowman's membrane are found. Animal experiments suggest that the tubular damage is due to the aldehyde derivatives of ethylene glycol rather than, or as well as, calcium oxalate. Yet it seems that ethylene glycol is most toxic to those animal species which oxidize it most readily to oxalate, despite the small percentage that is actually metabolized along this pathway.

Treatment

Early diagnosis and appropriate therapy can significantly reduce the mortality from ethylene glycol poisoning. Treatment should include:

1. Gastric lavage to prevent further absorption and to confirm the diagnosis.

2. Supportive measures to combat shock and respiratory distress (page 27). Some severely poisoned patients develop the radiological appearance of interstitial pulmonary oedema. This is due to the direct toxic effect of glycol metabolites and, in some cases, to sodium overload as a result of alkali therapy (see below).

3. Correction of the metabolic acidosis with intravenous sodium bicarbonate. Animal work has shown that the LD_{50} for rats poisoned with ethylene glycol and then treated with sodium bicarbonate is over four times that for untreated rats. Parry and Wallach (1974) have suggested that, although correction of the acidosis does not seem to alter the depth of coma in humans, it does enhance survival. In severe cases, as much as 1000 to 2000 mmol of bicarbonate may be needed to correct the acidosis. This inevitably means that a very large sodium load must be given and this, in conjunction with the direct toxic effect of the glycol metabolites, may produce a clinical picture indistinguishable from that of 'shock lung'. It would seem reasonable, therefore, to institute elective mechanical ventilation in all severely poisoned patients to prevent this often fatal complication. In addition, the use of haemodialysis—ultrafiltration techniques will allow the removal of substantial amounts of sodium.

4. Correction of hypocalcaemia with intravenous calcium gluconate.

5. Use of ethyl alcohol as a competitive inhibitor of ethylene glycol metabolism. Ethyl alcohol, the normal substrate of alcohol dehydrogenase, inhibits the oxidation of ethylene glycol by liver alcohol dehydrogenase. It has been suggested that it is necessary to maintain a plasma ethanol level of 1000 to 2000 mg/l to inhibit the breakdown of glycol but, as the affinity of the enzyme alcohol dehydrogenase for ethyl alcohol is many times that for ethylene glycol, a

much lower plasma ethanol level may be sufficient to inhibit glycol metabolism.

The half-life of ethylene glycol is about three hours in humans and, for this reason, an ethanol infusion should be commenced as soon as possible after ingestion of the overdose if it is to be fully effective. It should be continued until ethylene glycol can no longer be detected in the plasma. The amount of ethanol required to maintain a plasma alcohol level of 1000 to 2000 mg/l is dependent upon the patient's previous ethanol intake. A loading dose of 50 g ethyl alcohol orally, followed by an infusion of 10 to 12 g/hr should be satisfactory, but it is necessary to measure the blood alcohol levels regularly. If haemodialysis is employed the infusion rate should be increased to 17 to 22 g/hr because ethanol is readily dialysable. Alternatively ethanol may be added to the peritoneal dialysate fluid in a dose of 1 to 2 g per litre of dialysate.

Pyrazole and 4-methyl pyrazole are potent alcohol dehydrogenase inhibitors which have been used experimentally to reduce mortality in animals poisoned with ethylene glycol. Pyrazole is too toxic to be used clinically but 4-methyl pyrazole has been used experimentally in man to modify ethanol and acetaldehyde metabolism.

6. Dialysis and haemoperfusion. Ethylene glycol and its aldehyde metabolites are removed by dialysis. Oxalate, however, is poorly dialysable. In addition, it may also be necessary to treat the uraemic complications of ethylene glycol poisoning with dialysis and to use haemodialysis—ultrafiltration to correct any sodium overload (see above).

Haemodialysis and haemoperfusion appear to remove very little ethylene glycol but our own work at Guy's Hospital has shown that substantial quantities may be removed by peritoneal dialysis. For example, 141 g ethylene glycol were removed over a 38-hour period from a patient whose initial plasma glycol level was 6.8 g/l.

Conclusions

The ingestion of substantial amounts of ethylene glycol is potentially very serious. In severely poisoned and untreated patients, or in those who present late, the mortality is high. However, a fatal outcome may be prevented by the use of gastric lavage, the application of supportive measures to combat shock, respiratory impairment, acidosis and hypocalcaemia, the use of ethanol as a competitive inhibitor of ethylene glycol metabolism and the active removal of glycol by peritoneal dialysis.

References

Clinical Aspects

Parry MF, Wallach R. Ethylene glycol poisoning. Am J Med 1974; 57:143–50.

Further Reading

Biochemical Mechanisms of Toxicity

Bachman E, Golberg L. Reappraisal of the toxity of ethylene glycol – III. Mitochondrial effects. Food Cosmet Toxicol 1971; 9:39–55.

Chou JY, Richardson KE. The effect of pyrazole on ethylene glycol toxicity and metabolism in the rat. Toxicol Appl Pharmacol 1978; 43:33–44.

Clay KL, Murphy RC. On the metabolic acidosis of ethylene glycol intoxication. Toxicol Appl Pharmacol 1977; 39:39–49.

McChesney EW, Golberg L, Parekh CK, Russell JC, Min BH. Reappraisal of the toxicology of ethylene glycol – III. Metabolism studies in laboratory animals. Food Cosmet Toxicol 1971; 9:21–38.

Clinical Aspects

Ahmed MM. Ocular effects of antifreeze poisoning. Br J Opthal 1971; 55:854–5.

Bove KE. Ethylene glycol toxicity. Am J Clin Pathol 1966; 45:46–50.

Bowie MD, McKenzie D. Diethylene glycol poisoning in children. S Afr Med J 1972; 46:931–4.

Kahn HS. A recovery from ethylene glycol (antifreeze) intoxication: a case of survival and two fatalities from ethylene glycol including autopsy findings. Ann Intern Med 1950; 32:284–94.

Moriarty RW, McDonald Jr RH. The spectrum of ethylene glycol poisoning. Clin Toxicol 1974; 7:583–96.

Pons CA, Custer RP. Acute ethylene glycol poisoning: a clinicopathologic report of eighteen fatal cases. Am J Med Sci 1946; 211:544–52.

Seeff LB, Hendler ED, Hosten AO, Shalhoub RJ. Ethylene glycol poisoning. Medical Annals of the District of Columbia 1970; 39:31–6.

Underwood F, Bennett WM. Ethylene glycol intoxication: prevention of renal failure by aggressive management. J Am Med Assoc 1973; 226:1453–4.

Vale JA, Widdop B. Bluett NH. Ethylene glycol poisoning. Postgrad Med J 1976; 52:598–602.

Wacker WEC, Haynes H, Druyan R, Fisher W, Coleman JE. Treatment of ethylene glycol poisoning with ethyl alcohol. J Am Med Assoc 1965; 194:1231–33.

Walton EW. An epidemic of antifreeze poisoning. Med Sci Law 1978; 18:231–7.

Haemodialysis and Haemoperfusion

Sangster B, Prenen JAC, De Groot G. Case 38 – 1979; ethylene glycol poisoning. New Engl J Med 1980; 302:465.

Underwood F, Bennett WM. Ethylene glycol intoxication: prevention of renal failure by aggressive management. J Am Med Assoc 1973; 226:1453–4.

Chapter 21

J. A. Vale and T. J. Meredith

Paraquat Poisoning

Paraquat (1,1'-dimethyl-4,4'-bipyridylium) is the most important of the bipyridylium herbicides and is marketed in the UK in a variety of formulations as the dichloride salt (Table 21.1). Under the Poisons Rules the water-soluble concentrates may be supplied only to bona fide farmers and horticulturalists.

Table 21.1. Trade names of paraquat-containing preparations in the UK.

25 g/kg	100 g/l	200 g/l
Weedol (granules) also contains diquat	Dexuron also contains diuron	Gramoxone
Pathclear (granules) also contains diquat and simazine	Gramonol also contains monolinuron	Gramoxone S
	Tota-Col also contains diuron	Dextrone X
	Cleansweep also contains diquat	

Note: Paraquat is most widely sold as Weedol and Gramoxone

Use in Agriculture and Horticulture

Paraquat kills plants by acting on the green parts rather than the woody stems. The mechanism of this phytotoxic effect is uncertain, but it may be due to peroxidation of lipid cell membranes following transformation of molecular oxygen into superoxide radicals (O_2^-), hydroperoxy radicals (HO_2^-) or hydrogen peroxide (see below).

Paraquat is inactivated completely and rapidly by contact with clay in the soil – a property which indicates a possible approach to the treatment of paraquat poisoning. In addition, it enables the farmer to kill weeds on the ground and then plant or seed directly through the killed vegetation, thus eliminating, or at least reducing, the necessity for ploughing.

Toxicity

Although paraquat can be absorbed through the skin and bronchial mucosa, serious poisoning has followed only from the ingestion, and rarely the injection, of the herbicide. In the 15-year period following its introduction in 1963, 211 patients died in England and Wales from a paraquat overdose (Figure 21.1). In contrast to earlier years most adult cases are now due to deliberate self-poisoning rather than to accidental ingestion which may occur when the herbicide is decanted into urine or lemonade bottles.

The mechanism whereby paraquat produces lesions in the lungs and other organs has not been elucidated clearly, but it may involve the reduction of paraquat to a radical ion. Histological similarities between changes in the lung following oxygen toxicity and paraquat poisoning have led to the following hypothesis. Paraquat accepts electrons from the mitochondrial electron transport chain with resultant reduction to an unstable free radical (Figure 21.2). This in turn

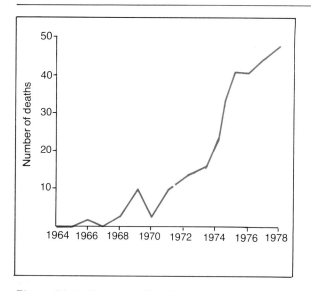

Figure 21.1. *The mortality from paraquat poisoning in England and Wales, 1964–1978.*

damage, probably by peroxidation of cell membrane lipids and oxidation of cellular enzymes. In addition, paraquat stimulates the pentose-phosphate pathway, reduces the level of NADPH and inhibits fatty acid synthesis in the lung. It has therefore been suggested that the primary mechanism of toxicity of paraquat may be the oxidation of NADPH which inhibits vital physiological processes and renders the cell more susceptible to attack from lipid hydroperoxides (Smith et al. 1979).

The lung is particularly sensitive to the above effects, first, because paraquat is concentrated in the lung by an energy-dependent process, and second, because oxygen tensions are higher in the alveolar lining cells of the lung than in any other part of the body.

Clinical Features

Local Effects

can interact with oxygen, with reconversion to paraquat and the generation of a superoxide. Small amounts of superoxide are formed normally whilst breathing air and are rapidly inactivated by the enzyme superoxide dismutase (SOD). However, with increased production of superoxide due to the effects of paraquat, the capacity of SOD is exceeded. As a result, the excess superoxide is free to cause tissue

In its concentrated form paraquat has a strong irritant action on various types of epithelia. Thus, it will cause blistering and soreness of the skin and cracking and loss of the fingernail if the nail bed has been contaminated. Severe inflammation of the cornea and conjunctiva may follow the accidental splashing of

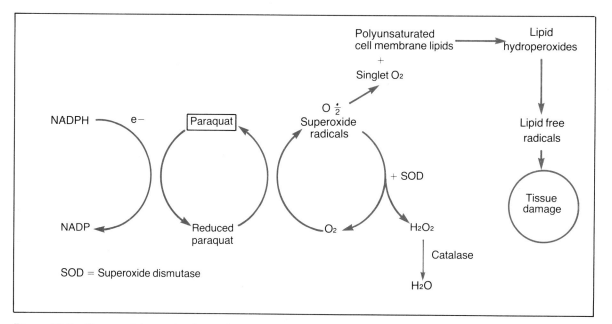

Figure 21.2. *The possible mechanisms of toxicity of paraquat.*

paraquat concentrate into the eyes. The inflammation develops gradually, reaching a maximum after 12 to 24 hours. Although healing may be slow, recovery is usually complete. Inhalation of spray mist or dust sometimes causes nose bleeds and soreness of the throat.

Systemic Effects

Absorption of paraquat from the gut is slow and excretion is dependent on the renal tubular mechanism for active secretion of strong bases. However, tubular function becomes impaired within 24 hours of ingesting paraquat and thus prevents, or at least reduces, the elimination of the herbicide. If a sufficient quantity of the herbicide has been taken — as little as 10 ml of the 20 per cent concentrate may be lethal — death can result within hours or days from single or multiple organ failure. Pulmonary oedema, cardiac and renal failure and hepatic impairment are other common features of paraquat poisoning.

In those who are less severely poisoned abdominal pain, vomiting and diarrhoea are prominent symptoms. Renal failure, mild hepatocellular jaundice and respiratory impairment are frequent associated complications. Most of these effects will be evident within three or four days of ingestion and the final outcome depends invariably on the severity of the lung lesion.

It is probable that the type of lung damage is dose-related. When small amounts of paraquat are swallowed (and the initial plasma paraquat levels are low) there may either be no pulmonary damage or minimal changes associated with only a reduction in gas transfer factor. These changes may well be reversible. With the ingestion of larger amounts of paraquat, sufficient lung damage may occur to cause death from a pronounced alveolar oedema (Figure 21.3) before the development of pulmonary fibrosis — a complication which does not develop unless the patient survives beyond a few days. Pulmonary fibrosis and progressive respiratory failure may occur up to six weeks after ingestion.

Assessment of the Severity of Poisoning

The lack of serious symptoms after the ingestion of a small, but potentially fatal, dose of paraquat is a source of difficulty. In many cases, the degree of severity of poisoning will be apparent on admission to hospital from a consideration of the history of the case and the patient's symptoms. A fatal outcome may be predicted, with a fair degree of certainty, if more than a 'mouthful' of the 20 per cent concentrate has been ingested. In contrast, survival is likely if less than one sachet of 'Weedol' (a granular preparation of paraquat) has been taken.

The diagnosis may be confirmed by performing a simple qualitative urine test [10 ml urine + 2 ml 1 per cent Na dithionite in 1N NaOH gives a blue colour (Berry and Grove 1971)]. Fortunately an accurate radioimmunoassay test has been developed at Guy's Poisons Unit (Levitt 1979) and this is now available at many centres in Britain (Telephone 01-407 7600, Ext. Poisons, for nearest centre). With this test it is possible to predict whether or not a patient is likely to succumb to an overdose of paraquat (Figure 21.4).

Treatment of Local Toxic Effects

The local toxic effects of paraquat should be treated as follows: the skin should be washed with soap and water and any contaminated clothing removed; immediate and copious irrigation of the eyes should be followed by the installation of prophylactic antibiotics. Once the regrowth of corneal and conjunctival epithelium is complete, local steroid treatment will aid the resolution of granulation tissue.

Treatment of Systemic Poisoning Table 21.3

There are a number of possible approaches to the treatment of systemic paraquat poisoning, and these are discussed below. (See Table 21.2.)

The Elimination of the Herbicide from the Gut

Sorbents

It has been shown in animals that Fuller's Earth and Bentonite can remove paraquat from the gut efficiently if given very soon after ingestion. In addition it has been demonstrated in rats that gastric lavage and the administration of Bentonite and purgatives at two- to three-hourly intervals prevent the absorption of paraquat into the lung. Consequently the rats used in these experiments survived a dose of paraquat which would normally be lethal.

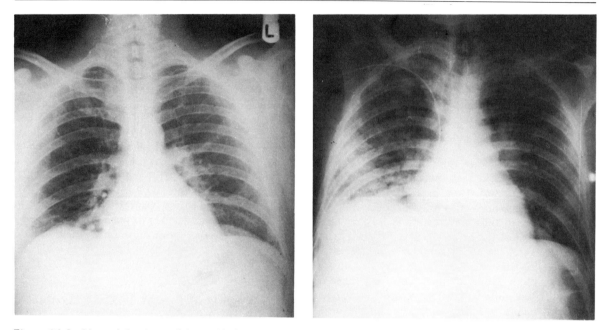

Figure 21.3. *Above left, above right and below. Progressive radiological changes in paraquat poisoning.*

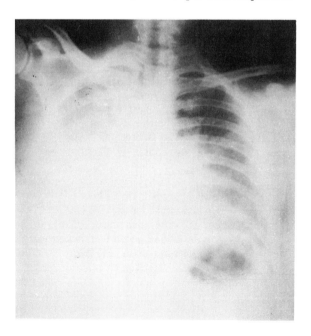

Based on this experience patients at Guy's Hospital have been given a Fuller's Earth/magnesium sulphate mixture after gastric lavage has been performed. (Lavage is unlikely to be of value more than three to four hours after the overdose and may be hazardous if there is oesophageal damage.) Fuller's Earth is preferred to Bentonite as it can be used as a 30 per cent suspension, whereas Bentonite swells in water and can be used only as a 6 per cent suspension.

Magnesium sulphate (5 per cent solution) is included to increase the rate of elimination of the Fuller's Earth—adsorbed paraquat complex from the gut. Fuller's Earth should not be given without a purgative as the gut may become 'blocked' if this sorbent is used alone. The sorbent/purgative mixture is given in a dose of 250 ml four-hourly after a similar amount has been left in the stomach following lavage. This treatment often produces marked diarrhoea, so adequate fluid replacement is essential.

Gut Lavage

An alternative approach is to use whole gut irrigation. Patients are given 4 litres of fluid hourly to empty the gut. However, as 1 to 2 litres of fluid are adsorbed as a result of this technique it is possible that the amount of paraquat absorbed from the gut might be increased. The use of high doses of mannitol in a low volume of fluid may avoid this possibility, but further results are needed before this method is advocated.

Increased Elimination of Paraquat

Forced Diuresis

Forced diuresis has been widely used and, though early reports suggested that the clearance of paraquat was increased, more recent work has not supported this conclusion. This is not suprising as the elimination of paraquat depends more on active tubular secretion than glomerular filtration and, because it is not re-

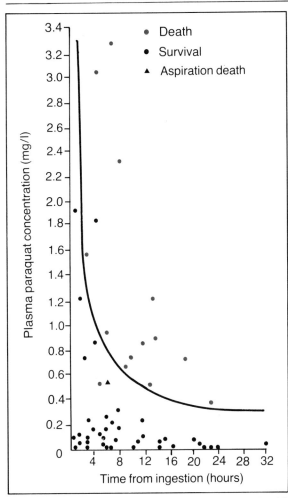

Figure 21.4. *Plasma paraquat concentrations in 44 patients related to time after ingestion and outcome.*

Table 21.2. Management of systemic paraquat poisoning.

Gastric lavage if < 4 hours after overdose

Leave 250 ml of a 30% suspension of Fullers' Earth and a 5% suspension of magnesium sulphate in the stomach

Repeat this dose 4-hourly until the faecal specimens are negative on testing with alkaline sodium dithionite

Consider haemoperfusion if patient presents < 8 hours after the overdose

Haemodialysis

There is very little evidence to suggest that dialysis reduces mortality due to paraquat poisoning, particularly when the paraquat concentrate has been ingested. At low plasma paraquat concentrations (<1 mg/l) charcoal haemoperfusion is much more efficient than haemodialysis (a clearance of 100 ml/min compared with 10 ml/min). At plasma concentrations of >20 mg/l both techniques are equally efficacious with clearances of around 100 ml/min being achieved.

Charcoal Haemoperfusion

We have shown that charcoal haemoperfusion will significantly reduce the mortality in beagle dogs given a normally lethal dose of paraquat (10 mg/kg body weight) and perfused up to 12 hours after being poisoned. Unfortunately similar results have not been obtained in humans, at least not in those who have been severely poisoned (Table 21.3).

absorbed by the tubules, forced diuresis is unlikely to increase the elimination of the herbicide. Moreover, it has been observed that significant quantities of paraquat appear in the urine in the first 24 hours after ingestion. Thereafter, in the majority of cases, very little is excreted; forced diuresis does not appear to increase elimination of paraquat in these circumstances either. In addition, the use of forced diuresis may be hazardous in patients who have rapidly developing renal failure.

Peritoneal Dialysis

Paraquat has been recovered only infrequently and in small amounts in peritoneal dialysate fluid, unless the patient has developed renal failure. Peritoneal dialysis, therefore, has no place in the treatment of systemic paraquat poisoning.

The Use of Low Tension Oxygen Therapy

On the basis of the supposed mechanism of toxicity of paraquat, and the finding that the administration of oxygen to patients poisoned with paraquat seemed to accelerate the lung changes and death, several workers have used rat models to elucidate the value of a low inspired oxygen tension. Douze et al. (1974) found that the mortality in rats poisoned with paraquat was significantly reduced, and similar findings were reported by Rhodes and his co-workers (1976) in America. More recent work by the American group, which was reported in 1978, has shown no advantage. The value of low tension oxygen therapy (with or without positive end expiratory pressure ventilation) has not been established in humans. There is, however, strong evidence that the administration of oxygen, particularly in hypoxic patients, is contraindicated.

Table 21.3. Clinical course of 12 patients poisoned with Gramoxone (20 per cent paraquat).

Sex	10♂ 2♀
Age	16 – 77 yr (mean 41.5 yr)
Amount ingested	30 – 300 ml (mean 105 ml)
Treatment	Gastric lavage and Fullers' Earth (10 min – 3 hr after ingestion; mean 1.7 hr)
	Haemoperfusion (length of perfusion 3 – 36 hr; mean 14.7 hr)
	Mean amount of paraquat removed by haemoperfusion: 96.25 mg paraquat ion (range 8 – 280 mg) N.B. One ml Gramoxone = 200 mg paraquat ion
Outcome	The 12 patients died between 12 hr and 19 days (mean 4.9 days) after ingestion of paraquat
	10 died from multiple organ failure; two died later (13 days; 19 days) from pulmonary fibrosis alone

Administration of Superoxide Dismutase and D-propranolol

Based on the proposed mechanism of toxicity of paraquat, Davies et al. (1977) have administered superoxide dismutase both intravenously and by inhalation for at least one week following the ingestion of paraquat. In addition D-propranalol, which accumulates in high concentrations in the lung, was given in an attempt to prevent uptake of paraquat into the lungs and to displace paraquat already present in the lungs. This regime did not, however, affect the outcome significantly in more than 20 patients who were so treated.

Use of Steroids and Immunosuppressant Drugs

There is at present no antidote for paraquat poisoning. Steroids, immunosuppressive agents (for example, azathioprine) and cytotoxic drugs have been used in treatment but their effectiveness is questionable. Certainly no consistent response seems to be obtained with their use.

Conclusion

The mechanism of toxicity of paraquat has been elucidated, at least partially, in the last few years and a rational approach to therapy has been proposed. However, no treatment at present available will prevent the development of multiple organ failure or pulmonary fibrosis after the ingestion of the paraquat concentrate (Gramoxone and Dextrone). The outcome after the ingestion of small quantities of the granular preparations (Weedol and Pathclear) is likely to be favourable, even without treatment. The widespread availability of a rapid immunoassay method for paraquat estimation enables an accurate prediction to be made about the prognosis.

References

Mechanisms of Toxicity

Smith LL, Rose MS, Wyatt I. The pathology and biochemistry of paraquat. In Oxygen Free Radicals and Tissue Damage. Ciba Foundation Symposium 65; Amsterdam: Excerpta Medica, 1979.

Assessment of the Severity of Poisoning

Berry DJ, Grove J. The determination of paraquat (1,1'-dimethyl-4,4'-bipyridilium cation) in urine. Clin Chem Acta 1971; 34:5–11.
Levitt T. Determinations of paraquat in clinical practice using radioimmunoassay. Proc Anal Div Chem Soc 1979; 16:72–6.
Proudfoot AT, Stewart MS, Levitt T, Widdop B. Paraquat poisoning: significance of plasma paraquat concentrations. Lancet 1979; 2:330–2.

Clinical Features and Treatment

Davies DS, Hawksworth SM, Bennett PN. Paraquat poisoning. Proc Eur Soc Toxicol 1977; 18:21–6.
Douze JMC, Van Dijk A, Gimbrere JSF, Van Heijst ANP, Maes R, Rauws AG. Intensive therapy after paraquat intoxication. Intensivmedizin 1974; 11:241–50.
Rhodes ML, Zavala DC, Brown D. Hypoxic protection in paraquat poisoning. Lab Invest 1976; 35:496–500.

Further Reading

Epidemiology

Fitzgerald GR, Carmody M, Barniville G, O'Dwyer WF, Flanagan M, Silke B. The changing pattern of paraquat poisoning: an epidemiologic study. J Irish Med Assoc 1978; 71:103–8.
Howard JK. Recent experience with paraquat poisoning in Great Britain: a review of 68 cases. Vet Hum Toxicol 1979; 21:Suppl. 213–6.
Warden JA, Rhodes ML. Failure of hypoxia to protect against paraquat toxicity in rats. Am Rev Resp Dis 1978; 117:265.

Mechanisms of Toxicity

Autor AP. Ed. Biochemical Mechanisms of Paraquat Toxicity. New York: Academic Press, 1977.

Haley TJ. Review of the toxicology of paraquat. Clin Toxicol 1979; 14:1–46.

Pasi A. The Toxicology of Paraquat, Diquat and Morfamquat, Bern: Hans Huber, 1978.

Rose MS, Smith LL, Wyatt I. Evidence for energy-dependent accumulation of paraquat into rat lung. Nature 1974; 252: 314–5.

Clinical Features and Treatment

Clark DG. Inhibition of the absorption of paraquat from the gastrointestinal tract by adsorbents. Br J Ind Med 1971; 28: 186–8.

Fairshter RD, Rosen SM, Smith WR, Glauser FL, McRae DM, Wilson AF. Paraquat poisoning. New aspects of therapy. Q J Med 1976; 45:551–65.

Fletcher K. Paraquat poisoning. In: Forensic Toxicology. Ballantyre B, Ed. Bristol: John Wright and Sons, 1974; 86–98.

Higgenbottam T, Crome P, Parkinson C, Nunn J. Further clinical observations on the pulmonary effects of paraquat ingestion. Thorax 1979; 34:161–5.

Okonek S, Hofmann A, Henningsen B. Efficacy of gut lavage, hemodialysis, hemoperfusion in the therapy of paraquat or diquat intoxication. Arch Toxicol 1976; 36:43–51.

Newhouse M, McEvoy D, Rosenthal D. Percutaneous paraquat absorption: an association with cutaneous lesions and respiratory failure. Arch Dermatol 1978; 114:1516–9.

Smith LL, Wright A, Wyatt I, Rose MS. Effective treatment for paraquat poisoning in rats and its relevance to treatment of paraquat poisoning in man. Br Med J 1974; 4:569–71.

Vale JA, Crome P, Volans GN, Widdop B, Goulding R. The treatment of paraquat poisoning using oral sorbents and charcoal haemoperfusion. Acta Pharmacol Toxicol 1977; 41:Suppl.2,109–17.

Vaziri ND, Ness RL, Fairshter RD, Smith WR, Rosen SM. Nephrotoxicity of paraquat in man. Arch Intern Med 1979; 139:172–4.

Chapter 22

R. Goulding

Poisoning due to Pesticides

It may be helpful to outline the principal classes of pesticides according to their economic role:

1. *Rodenticides* are intended to kill rats, mice, moles, etc. (i.e. mammals).
2. *Insecticides* are designed to kill insect and related species that prey on crops, farm stock, etc.
3. *Fungicides* are agents intended to control moulds, fungi, etc., on crops, stored foods, timber.
4. *Herbicides* are used to kill weeds.
5. *Plantgrowth controls* are substances which modify the growth and form of the plants, usually hormonally, without actually killing them.

Since these different agents act in a biochemically specific manner their impact upon man is not at all uniform. Because rats, mice and man share the same physiological attributes, rodenticides ingested by humans are comparatively lethal. In contrast, plant metabolism is very different to that of man and so, generally speaking, the plant pesticides pose relatively little risk to anyone exposed to them.

Pre-Marketing Testing of Pesticides

The use of pesticides in agriculture, horticulture, food storage, timber preservation, etc. is no recent innovation. Years ago quite vicious substances were deployed to such ends – nicotine, strychnine and arsenicals, to name only three.

Since the end of World War II there has been a burgeoning of synthetic chemicals tailored to these needs. Many of these have made an enormous contribution in economic terms to food production. Even so, these chemicals are potentially harmful both to man and to his environment.

Nowadays, it is statutory in many countries for quite demanding pre-marketing toxicity testing to be carried out so that the undesirable consequences of use may be avoided or, at any rate, minimized. The budget for such a pre-marketing testing may be as much as £1,000,000 for a single chemical.

Once a new pesticide has been launched, the practice of graded release has been widely adopted, starting with a small and circumscribed use with close surveillance of all aspects, including worker exposure, and passing on gradually to much wider commercial distribution.

The conditions laid down to ensure safety-in-use are extrapolated largely from the animal findings. Even so, enlightened epidemiological follow-ups (as with drugs) have an important part to play and, in this respect, it is up to every clinician confronted with a case of suspected pesticide poisoning to make a careful and calculated diagnosis to add to the store of knowledge.

So long as the proper guidance on usage has been observed, including protective clothing whenever recommended, serious poisoning from pesticides should never occur, but human misjudgement and carelessness being what it is, accidents are bound to occur. This notwithstanding, the more dramatic cases of pesticide poisoning nearly always present from deliberate misuse, above all in suicidal attempts.

Diagnosis of Pesticide Poisoning

Whether the symptoms appear immediately after the

poisoning episode or, perhaps, years later (and pesticide poisoning is suspected), it is imperative to take a full history as follows:

1. The patient's previous state of health and any antecedent disease.

2. An accurate record of the chemical, or chemicals, which might be aetiologically involved, and the precise manner and extent to which the exposure took place. Usually the trade name is quoted by the patient. However, the officially approved standard name of the main active constituent(s) should also be printed on the label. In the event of doubt, the manufacturers or distributors may be able to help or, in many countries, the poisons information or control service may clarify the issue.

3. The toxicological characteristics of the particular chemical(s) should then be summarized. If the information cannot be found in the literature, poisons centres may assist.

4. A painstaking examination of the patient must then be conducted, with emphasis on those systems which may display the distinctive reactions of the pesticide(s) cited.

5. Finally, it may be necessary to conduct laboratory tests to reinforce the conclusions, e.g. blood cholinesterase for organophosphorus poisoning, blood levels for dinitro compounds, the coagulation profile for some rodenticides, etc. For the majority of farm and garden chemicals, however, there are no such diagnostic investigations.

Only against such a factual background can a reliable diagnosis be made. Too often the symptoms and signs are too vague for a reliable conclusion to be reached.

Skin Reactions to Pesticides

Skin reactions are a common physical complication of pesticide usage. They are mostly due to direct, irritant effects and sometimes to sensitization. The active pesticide principles are not always responsible: the skin reactions are more likely to be caused by the solvents, vehicles, wetting agents and so on that make up the marketed formulation.

Where the likelihood of skin reactions is apparent from animal tests most regulatory agencies, as well as the manufacturers themselves, recommend against skin and mucosal contact and advise on suitable protective precautions.

First-Aid in Cases of Pesticide Poisoning

When the patient is out of reach of a clinic, hospital, or even human habitation, first-aid measures are as follows:

1. Remove the person from any further contact with the chemical, i.e. from a spraying area, a polluted atmosphere, etc.

2. Keep the person at rest.

3. Divest the person of any contaminated clothing and wash any area of affected skin with soap and water or with water alone, the first-aider taking care himself to avoid contact with any noxious material. Then cover the person with unsoiled blankets, or coats, or whatever may be available.

4. If there is any difficulty with breathing or, above all, in the face of respiratory arrest, make sure immediately that the airway is clear and institute assisted ventilation by whatever method is feasible. (The mouth-to-mouth technique is not that of choice if the poison has been taken by mouth.)

5. For poisoning by ingestion the stomach should be emptied as soon as possible. In the field, gastric aspiration and lavage are seldom practicable and induced emesis has to be considered. This should, of course, be abjured if the person is unconscious. Manual simulation of the back of the throat is seldom successful and salt, mustard, etc. are not recommended. Syrup of ipecacuanha is probably the agent of choice, if it is to hand. The benefits of giving activated charcoal by mouth in this situation have yet to be properly appraised.

6. Apart from instances of negligible or insigificant exposure it is prudent to transfer the patient to hospital as soon as possible. The usual rules should be observed in transit – the left lateral and head-down position, with the tongue drawn forward and assisted ventilation if there is any indication that the spontaneous activity is inadequate.

7. For the benefit of the hospital medical staff a note should accompany the patient stating clearly the identity of the suspected agent(s) or, better still, a label or container.

Specific Pesticides

Organophosphorus Insecticides

Nowadays the organophosphorus compounds are the insecticides most widely used throughout the world in crop protection, control of animal infestation, in the domestic domain and for the suppression of the insect vectors of diseases. Chemically and toxicologically they owe their origin to the substances elaborated during World War II for use in chemical warfare — hence their description as 'nerve poisons'. Some of these compounds can in fact cause irreversible damage to the central and peripheral nervous systems; clinical evidence of this has been afforded by the erroneous use of lubricant containing tri-ortho-cresyl phosphate as a foodstuff. A notable epidemic of this type took place in North Africa in 1959. At the present time, no organophosphorus compound possessing this property should be officially released for commercial supply as an insecticide. Screening to detect this propensity should always be introduced beforehand by means of a recognized test with the domestic fowl.

Mode of Action

The biochemical mechanism common to all organophosphorus insecticides is the capacity for depressing the cholinesterase activity of the blood, the brain and other tissues. This is due to chemical binding of the cholinesterase molecule and, within a few hours, this conjugation becomes irreversible. By this means acetylcholine accumulates at the synapses in the autonomic system and, to some extent, at those in the central nervous system, as well as at the autonomic post-ganglionic and skeletal efferent nerve endings. This explains the toxic manifestations.

Symptoms and Signs

The first symptoms are general and may not be recognizable — headache, anorexia, a sense of weakness, exhaustion and a degree of mental confusion. These can proceed to more distinctive changes — vomiting, excessive sweating, conspicuous salivation and cramping abdominal pains. A feeling of constriction in the chest may herald dyspnoea and bronchoconstriction, while more pathognomonically there may be muscle twitchings, first confined to the eyelids, face and neck, but soon extending to the limbs and the rest of the body and culminating in frank convulsions. Of serious import are diarrhoea, tenesmus, urinary incontinence and bronchial constriction, with advancing respiratory embarrassment and coma. The pupils of the eye are classically contracted, but not invariably so, and constitute no index of severity, for this change can come about by topical contact of the chemical with the eyes.

Management

Any patient exhibiting even the slightest indication of organophosphorus poisoning should be kept at complete rest. Of urgent and critical importance is the establishment of a clear airway and adequate ventilation of the lungs. Bronchial suction may be required.

If atropine is to hand, 2 mg by the intramuscular or subcutaneous route should be given immediately or, in advanced cases, intravenously. If there is no prompt relief of distress such injections should be repeated, at intervals of 10 minutes, until it is obvious that a state of continuing 'atropinization' has been achieved and is being maintained. Total doses of as much as 100 mg atropine may be needed.

Because the skin can be a major route of absorption of organophosphorus compounds, contaminated clothing must be removed and the skin washed thoroughly with soap and water. Where the offending material has been swallowed, the stomach should be emptied as soon as possible.

Pharmacologically, the atropine will counteract the acetylcholine excess only at the post-ganglionic and skeletal nerve endings, leaving the abnormal concentrations at the other sites unmodified. That is why, in any severe case, the effort should be made to give, in addition, a cholinesterase reactivator. If this is delayed by more than about 12 hours the blocking of the enzyme becomes irreversible. Such reactivators are pralidoxime (P2S) and toxigonin, though the former is more likely to be procurable. Toxigonin (Obidoxime) is more potent than pralidoxime and crosses the blood—brain barrier. Pralidoxime is given intravenously in a dose of 30 mg/kg body weight every four hours for 12—24 hours depending on the response. Toxigonin is administered intravenously in a dose of 3—6 mg/kg body weight and repeated as above. There is evidence that the two antidotes together are not merely additive in their response, but may be potentiating. After 24 hours the pralidoxome regime, but not the atropine, should be reviewed, for thereafter the effect may be negligible.

In addition, diazepam by intravenous injection is indicated to control convulsions, and there is reason to believe that, in the central nervous system at least, it also assists in correcting the surfeit of acetylcholine.

Laboratory Tests

The urgent therapeutic measures described above

should never wait upon prior laboratory confirmation of the diagnosis. Nevertheless, as soon as convenient, a 5 to 10 ml venous blood sample should be taken from the patient into a dry tube containing anticoagulant, e.g. lithium heparin, not only for diagnostic support but also to judge the severity and progress of the intoxication.

Laboratories capable of performing these investigations are not always within reach, so there may be recourse to more handy and mobile test kits. Difficulties can then arise over the interpretation of the results. Depression of the plasma (pseudo) cholinesterase virtually to zero may reflect no more than excessive exposure and is not necessarily suggestive of clinical poisoning. The level of erythrocyte (true) cholinesterase is more significant. Even so, these levels can be depressed to 60 or 70 per cent of normal without clinical signs, especially if the patient has been handling organophosphorus compounds previously. Another confusing element is the fact that so called 'normal' levels vary from one individual to another.

For workers repeatedly engaged in the manufacture, packing, handling and application of these insecticides it may be useful to monitor their blood cholinesterase status at regular intervals, checking the findings against a pre-exposure level, which is essential. A lowering of the levels may then sound the warning of unacceptable exposure but, in themselves, are no basis for starting active treatment. This must be organized according to the clinical condition of the person under observation.

Carbamates

Chemicals under this generic heading have become increasingly common as commercial insecticides. While quite different in molecular form from the organophosphorus compounds they nevertheless act pharmacologically in the same manner, i.e. by depressing cholinesterase activity. In contrast though, this biochemical conjugation is reversible, so that spontaneous recovery ensues if life is not imperilled meanwhile. Some of these carbamates, however, are intensely toxic so that special formulations, e.g. granules, have been contrived to minimize the risks of exposure.

Symptoms and Signs

These are indistinguishable clinically from those of organophosphorus poisoning, though they may emerge more rapidly or more insidiously.

Management

This should be identical at the outset to that for organophosphorus excess and is equally urgent. Atropine should be administered, usually with good effect, though there is no point in adding pralidoxime or any other cholinesterase reactivator. Blood levels of the enzyme are of less assistance diagnostically and, as long as the vital systems of the body are maintained, recovery is likely to come about spontaneously in about 24 hours.

Bipyridylium Compounds

Besides paraquat, these include diquat and morfamquat. They are used widely throughout the world as total rather than selective weed-killers and they have played a large part in advancing the economics of crop production. At the same time, their toxicity, in human terms, is undeniable. So long as workers respect simple hygienic precautions in handling they will not suffer any harm at all, except occasionally of a minor or local nature. Devastating poisoning in man has come about from swallowing the concentrate, sometimes accidentally, but more often deliberately.

Commercial concentrates are marketed as foul-tasting solutions containing some 10 to 20 per cent of the active component. For home garden use the common formulation is a granule incorporating up to five per cent of the active principle.

Paraquat poisoning is documented in detail in Chapter 21.

Phenoxyacetate and Related Herbicides

Physical operations to eradicate weeds, such as hoeing, burning or repeated cutting, have been progressively supplanted by chemical sprays and applications. Many of the compounds thus employed have a selective biochemical action on certain types of plant growth. Thus the phenoxyacetate herbicides, including 2,4-D and MCPA, exert their main effect upon broad-leaved, dicotyledonous weeds, whilst leaving graminaceous, monocotyledonous crops untouched. For this reason they have been referred to as 'hormonal' weed-killers.

Mode of Action

Since the biochemical pathways in plants are quite different from those found in mammals there is no corresponding toxic mechanism in man, for whom these compounds constitute little risk, despite their widespread use.

Symptoms and Signs

On the skin the concentrated formulations of these phenoxyacetates and similar herbicides may cause mild staining or irritation.

Serious poisoning is rare and occurs only when inordinate amounts have been swallowed deliberately. In such cases, there is hypertension, abdominal pain, vomiting and diarrhoea, proceeding to tachycardia, a fall in blood pressure and sometimes ventricular fibrillation. Convulsions may appear, along with dysarthria, mental confusion and central nervous system depression. Myotonia may present initially, complicating the incoordination and ataxia, and giving way to generalized muscle weakness, loss of tendon reflexes, coma and death.

Management

No specific antidote is known, so reliance must be placed on general supportive measures with the customary removal of contaminated clothing and washing of the skin. After ingestion vomiting is usually prominent; if not, the stomach should be emptied by gastric aspiration and lavage. ECG monitoring is advisable as soon as possible to detect cardiac abnormalities, for which the orthodox antiarrhythmic correction is indicated. While the clinical evidence for promoting excretion of the unchanged chemical via the urine is not impressive, forced alkaline diuresis may be worth while.

Dioxin

Dioxin is one of the most powerful poisons known, but its toxic mechanism remains obscure. In addition to causing chloracne, it has been shown in certain situations, mostly experimental, to be mutagenic and to cause congenital abnormalities. Biochemically it interacts with DNA.

It happens that, by the process of chemical manufacture, a trace of dioxin can, and usually does, persist in the 2,4,5—T that comes onto the market. During the Korean war a form of 2,4,5—T known as 'Agent Orange', possessing a relatively high dioxin content, was used as a jungle defoliant. It is alleged that military personnel and the local populace coming into contact with it were thereby victims of serious disease. There have been numerous anecdotal case reports, together with epidemiological assertions, about abortions and congenitally deformed offspring of women living in an area in which 2,4,5—T has been widely used in forestry. The arguments are not conclusive, but suspicion and anxiety naturally persist, while objective scientific and medical assessment tends to be overwhelmed by sensational reports and 'judgement by the media'. The 2,4,5—T which is currently marketed as a commercial herbicide is monitored to ensure that the dioxin carry-over is minimal. It is difficult medically and pharmacokinetically to see how this could constitute a human hazard, but further investigations and appraisals are proceeding, along with legal hearings in the USA to resolve the problem.

Triazene Herbicides

This group comprises a large number of chemical weed-killers, some of them being used as selective agents and others, e.g. simazine and atrazine, notably in higher concentrations, being employed as total suppressants of vegetation on paths, drives, railway tracks, etc. Their botanical behaviour is directed against plant photosynthesis and, again, their toxic capacity towards mammals, including man, is regarded as of a very low order. They are for the most part non-irritating and non-sensitizing and their occupational hazards are virtually unknown.

Symptoms and Signs

Cases of human poisoning, even from deliberate ingestion, have not been reported. Anyway, most of these materials are fine drug powders which are difficult to swallow in quantity. No clinical picture of systemic toxicity therefore exists.

Management

Where a substantial overdose has been taken only symptomatic treatment can be recommended.

Chlorates

For the total and lasting obliteration of weeds on industrial sites, drives, pathways, etc., the chlorates (sodium and potassium) have been the agent of choice over many decades and are still sometimes preferred to the triazines. Purchased in powder form, the chemical is commonly dissolved in water before application. In the dry state, either prior to dissolving or, equally, after the solution has dried, the chlorates are powerful oxidizing agents and their greatest risk to man is through fire and explosion.

Mode of Action

Percutaneous or respiratory absorption of the chlorates is negligible, so apart from local irritation and combustion, to which reference has already been made, the occupational hazards can almost be dismissed. However, if these chemicals are taken by mouth, by accident or intent, they are highly toxic, a dose of about 15 g being regarded as lethal for an adult and as little as 2 g for a child.

Symptoms and Signs

Upon ingestion there is at once a 'burning' sensation in the mouth and throat, coupled with vomiting, abdominal discomfort, confusion, cyanosis and, characteristically, methaemoglobinaemia. Convulsions, renal damage and anuria may follow.

Management

Prompt emptying of the stomach is essential, followed by a saline purge. Methaemoglobinaemia can be corrected by the intravenous injection of methylene blue — 5 to 25 ml of a one per cent solution. Fluid intake and output should be encouraged prior to the onset of renal damage. Once the kidneys are affected haemodialysis should be mobilized. The first 24 hours is the most dangerous period and, once this has passed, survival is usually attended by complete recovery so long as the kidneys are safeguarded.

Dinitro Compounds

Tragic casualties among workers with dinitro compounds focussed attention upon the occupational hazards of farm chemicals some decades ago. Some of these agents, such as DNOC (dinitro-ortho-cresol), are favoured as 'winter washes' in orchards. As such, the concentration of the solutions sprayed on the trees is relatively low and the weather is seldom warm at this time of the year. Poisoning is then unlikely to arise. Another commercial indication for these dinitro compounds is for weed control and as desiccants on, for example, potato haulm. For this activity more concentrated solutions are essential and, climatically, temperatures in the field are likely to be higher. The risks to personnel are correspondingly intensified.

Mode of Action

The dinitro compounds have been identified biochemically as 'uncouplers' of oxidative phosphorylation, modifying energy transfer at a cellular level. The result is a stimulation of metabolism throughout the body tissues, with the creation of a hypermetabolic state quite independent of the thyroid gland.

Symptoms and Signs

Many of these chemicals are deeply yellow in colour, and staining of the skin should be an alerting sign to excessive exposure, without necessarily being indicative of clinical poisoning. Such appearances call at once for more careful methods of handling.

When the uptake, which usually proceeds occupationally via the skin, is sufficient to provoke toxic manifestations, these will include tiredness, disproportionate sweating and thirst. Thereafter, loss of weight, restlessness, tachycardia and pyrexia occur, which may advance to profound exhaustion, collapse and death from hypermetabolism.

Management

Contaminated clothing should be jettisoned and the skin should be washed thoroughly. Complete rest is dictated and, as there is no specific antidote, support should be given by replenishment of fluid and electrolytes, oxygen administration and cold sponging. For all but the minor cases hospital admission is mandatory. Provided that the vital processes can be preserved throughout the acute phase there is usually complete recovery, for no tissue damage is sustained and the offending chemicals are totally metabolized by the body and eliminated.

Treatment should never be deferred pending laboratory diagnosis, but in some centres it is possible to ascertain the blood dinitro levels using a sample of about 5 ml taken into a dry tube containing anticoagulant. These measurements not only offer diagnostic confirmation but are of value in monitoring workers for excessive exposure and for instituting more effective occupational hygiene.

Pentachlorophenol and Related Pesticides

Related pharmacologically to the dinitro compounds are such herbicides as bromoxynil and ioxynil and also pentachlorophenol, which is still one of the mainstays of timber preservation. With the last-named compound serious and fatal casualties have occurred, the more so if it is used in large volumes and in hot climates where protective clothing can be as unacceptable as it is uncomfortable.

Symptoms and Signs

Apart from the absence of yellow staining of the skin, pentachlorophenol poisoning presents clinically in the same manner as that from dinitro compounds, i.e. a hypermetabolic state. There is no validation of the belief that repeated exposure to pentachlorophenol is the cause of polyneuropathy or similar disorders.

Management

Care of the patient with pentachlorophenol poisoning follows the same rules as those for dinitro poisoning — disposal of clothing, washing of the skin, rest, rehydration, oxygen, cold sponging and general support. Emergence from the acute phase should signal complete recovery.

Laboratory tests are rarely informative, though the analysis of the urine for phenols may be helpful where diagnostic doubt otherwise prevails.

Organochlorine Insecticides

Probably no single group of chemical pesticides has been the subject of more toxicological alarm, publicity and sensation than that of the organochlorine insecticides, among which DDT, aldrin, dieldrin, lindane and endrin are numbered. Chemically and biologically they prove to be remarkably stable and, for this reason, they tend to persist and accumulate in the environment. Anxiety about their ubiquitous and continuing presence, above all in the fauna globally, has led to official phasing-out or even total banning. Today few, if any, inhabitants of this world can be demonstrably free from the presence of at least traces of organochlorines sequestered in their body fat. Whether these tissue stores have ever exerted any harmful effect upon the host remains highly debatable. At the same time, it must be admitted that the record of safety for these chemicals from the standpoint of acute toxicity is well nigh exemplary, the only impressively serious cases having been due to gross, oral misuse.

Symptoms and Signs

The pharmacodynamic effect of the organochlorines is focused upon the central nervous system and is displayed as anxiety and excitement, followed by muscle fibrillations and frank convulsions, with very little obtunding of consciousness. Respiration may be stimulated at first, though subsequently this gives way to respiratory insufficiency and apnoea.

Management

Any percutaneous absorption should be mitigated by disposing of soiled clothing and washing the skin. Whenever substances of this nature have been swallowed, the stomach should be emptied and a saline purge should be administered. Any oleaginous material in the lumen of the gut is likely to encourage absorption so milk, olive oil and like products should not be given.

Convulsions should be controlled promptly by the intravenous injection of diazepam or, in refractory cases, by 'curarisation' and assisted ventilation. A clear airway is a paramount need and, even so, respiratory support may be required, occasionally by way of endotracheal intubation.

So long as the patient is maintained in this manner, gradual and complete recovery is the expected outcome, the offending organochlorine material meanwhile having become redistributed in the body to the adipose tissues where it is beyond the range of toxic influence.

Fungicides — Mercurials

As fungicides, mercurial compounds have been in vogue for many years, both in the organic form — alkyl, alkoxy and aryl derivatives, and as inorganic salts. Toxicologically the two groups have different characteristics.

Inorganic Mercurials

These are valuable commercially for the treatment of onion seed, some bulbs and the roots of brassica plants, as well as for lawns and golf greens. Mercurous chloride ('corrosive sublimate') is readily water-soluble and is highly poisonous, behaving as a protein coagulant and corrosive.

Symptoms and Signs

In contact with the skin and, more so, the mucosa, this salt is highly irritant. If taken by mouth in a dose of as little as 0.5 g, it immediately gives rise to a metallic taste, salivation, vomiting and, above all, a profuse and violent diarrhoea, which is often mucoid and bloody and soon brings about dehydration, exhaustion and collapse. Later on there may be renal damage with albuminia and anuria.

Mercuric chloride (Calomel), being less soluble, is much less pronounced in its action, though large amounts relative to a therapeutic dose may mimic the effects of the mercurous salt.

Management

Urgent supportive measures are called for with prompt

restoration of the fluid and electrolyte status. Gastric aspiration and lavage are pointless. Dimercaprol may be given as an antidote against any systemic hydrargism, while it does very little to abate the gastrointestinal reactions. The dosage required is described on page 34.

Kidney failure may call for haemodialysis.

Organic Mercurials

These still feature as the most reliable fungicides for treating cereal seeds, as canker paints and for bulb treatment. Whenever seed grain is dressed with mercurials a suitable dye should be added so as to impart to the final product a distinctive colour which will deter would-be consumers.

Where large quantities of seed are being dressed, especially in a closed atmosphere, the ambient concentration of organomercurials may attain dangerous levels. Totally enclosed procedures should therefore be adopted so far as is practicable, coupled with efficient ventilation of the premises.

Mode of Action

The aryl mercurials are much less toxic to man than the alkyl or alkoxy compounds. This may be due to their different kinetic distribution within the tissues, the alkyl and alkoxy moieties more readily penetrating the central nervous system where it is believed there is interaction with sulphydryl groupings, particularly on vital enzyme systems.

Symptoms and Signs

On the skin, organic mercurials may be irritant, causing erythema and blistering, the appearance of which is sometimes delayed for some hours. Percutaneous uptake may occur as well.

In the atmosphere, these chemicals may cause acute soreness of the eyes and coughing, with prolonged exposure leading to gastrointestinal symptoms, renal dysfunction and central nervous system damage.

Poisoning from the alkyl and alkoxy mercurials is seen most dramatically when they are ingested, either deliberately or accidentally. For example, in Iraq recently large quantities of dressed grain intended for seed were by misadventure consumed, resulting in tiredness, loss of memory, difficulty in mental concentration and numbness and tingling of the extremities, all of these symptoms evolving gradually. Next there was ataxia, which was either slight or disabling, with dysarthria, and characteristically, constriction of the visual fields or blindness.

Management

The usual procedure described earlier for other pesticides should be followed for soiled clothing and the skin. Blisters should be pricked to release the mercury-containing fluid.

Acute ingestion calls for emptying the stomach. In an effort to minimize the systemic disorders there is usually resort to dimercaprol or, preferably, N-acetyl penicillamine (200 mg by mouth four-times-a-day), though the response to this apparently specific therapy is disappointing overall. The damage seen in the central nervous system is nearly always irreversible.

Dithiocarbamates

For the control of fungal infections on crops, fruit trees, flowers and other products, both commercially and domestically, the dithiocarbamates have gained increasing favour over the past few years. They are of low mammalian toxicity and are rarely incriminated in poisoning, their only disadvantage being that sometimes they cause skin and mucosal irritation. Careless handling of these compounds in factories and in their packing has led to a few instances of systemic toxicity.

Symptoms and Signs

Their mode of action on mammalian tissues is unknown. Direct ingestion has been followed by vomiting and depression of the central nervous system with respiratory paralysis.

Management

As there is no specific remedy, management of poisoning rests on symptomatic treatment, with particular attention being paid to respiratory support.

Arsenicals

The various arsenicals, though largely relied upon in previous decades, have now yielded place to the synthetic farm chemicals. The principal use of arsenicals at the present time is in timber preservation.

Mode of Action

Poisoning from arsenicals comes about by swallowing them, accidentally or deliberately. Occupationally uptake can take place through the skin, or by inhalation, but such incidents nowadays are almost unknown. At a cellular level arsenic reacts with vital sulphydryl enzymes.

Symptoms and Signs

The cardinal features of acute oral arsenical poisoning are a latent period of an hour or two, giving way to abdominal pain, vomiting and, impressively, choleraic diarrhoea, with dehydration and collapse.

Excessive chronic exposure leads to anorexia, diarrhoea, weight loss, peripheral neuritis and a striking pigmentation of the skin, referred to as a 'raindrop' pattern.

Management

For the choleraic state, urgent fluid and electrolyte replacement is obligatory and, in addition, a course of dimercaprol by injection may counteract direct systemic effects.

For chronic poisoning the primary need is to ensure that further exposure is obviated and dimercaprol should also be used.

In cases of acute poisoning, arsenic may be detected analytically in the stomach contents, faeces and blood, but such tests can seldom be marshalled in time to assist in diagnosis and treatment.

Of more value are the specific quantitative assays for arsenic in hair and/or nails, that can be most informative where chronic exposure is suspected. The technique, however, is by neutron activation, facilities for which exist in very few centres. The great virtue of the technique is that, from linear analyses of hair, not only the intensity but also the timing of the arsenic excess can be deduced.

Nicotine

Like arsenic, nicotine has given way progressively to the less toxic pesticide chemicals, so that this alkaloid finds employment today only as 'smokes' or, less frequently, as sprays in horticulture, chiefly under glass.

Mode of Action

Nicotine is highly toxic, a single dose of about 40 mg being fatal to man. Uptake, too, can take place readily through the skin, by inhalation or from the gut.

The effect pharmacologically is upon the autonomic nervous system, first stimulating and then depressing the ganglia.

Symptoms and Signs

The onset of symptoms is nearly always rapid, with nausea, dizziness, vomiting, salivation, hyperpnoea, tachycardia and sweating. These proceed quickly to convulsions, cardiac arrhythmias, coma and death.

Management

Therapeutically there is no means of specifically counteracting the intrusion of nicotine at the autonomic ganglia. Instead, apart from resorting to injection of diazepam for the convulsions, management must be generally supportive.

Rodenticides

Anticoagulants

Today such vicious poisons as phosphorus have been withdrawn from use as rodenticides and red squill has been outlawed. The most widely accepted rodenticides for both commercial and domestic areas are the anticoagulants, primarily warfarin. The animals, by nibbling away at the baits, are soon reduced to an anticoagulant state and succumb to internal haemorrhages. Other animals may be at risk if the baits are equally within their reach, while secondary poisoning may overtake dogs who devour the carcasses of rats and mice with residues of these anticoagulants still in their tissues. In contrast, poisoning in man from these agents is virtually unknown, for the persistent consumption of the baits is a remote possibility — except in a few instances of carefully orchestrated homicide. What is more, for the critical anticoagulant state to be achieved from a single ingestion, the amount of bait needed to be swallowed would be truly deterrent.

Wherever there is fear that an anticoagulant rodenticide may have been taken in toxic quantities the anticoagulant status of the blood should be checked and then, if indicated, vitamin K_1 should be injected as the specific antidote.

Chloralose

Another common rodenticide bait incorporates α-chloralose. Following oral ingestion this acts in the same manner as chloral hydrate, being metabolized to trichlorethyl alcohol, which depresses the central nervous system and, at sufficient levels in the body, brings about coma, respiratory depression and death.

Again, the mass of bait — often as sponge cake — that would have to be ingested as a single dose to exert a toxic effect would be quite disproportionate. Deaths in humans, adults or children, have not been recorded, but cases of relative overdose have had to be treated by the usual supportive measures that have been so successful in ensuring the recovery of patients who have taken an overdose of hypnotic drugs.

Fluoroacetates

These act specifically at a cellular level by interrupting the tricarboxylic acid (citric acid) cycle. A single dose of fluoroacetic acid or its fluoroacetates may be fatal to man. Percutaneous uptake is known to occur, but is not a major route of entry into the body. Poisoning is much more likely to come about from oral ingestion.

Thereafter, a delay of an hour or two may follow before the abrupt onset of anxiety, with muscle twitchings, cardiac irregularities, convulsions, coma and collapse. Terminally, pulmonary oedema may be evident.

There is no specific way of restoring the function of the tricarboxylic acid cycle. Diazepam can be injected for the convulsions, a clean airway must be established with assisted ventilation and it is customary to give a 10 per cent solution of calcium gluconate intravenously. It must be conceded that no treatment seems to avail if anything like a lethal dose has been taken.

Phosphine

This gas, as such, is not purveyed as a rodenticide, but solid magnesium or aluminium phosphide preparations, conveniently in capsule form, are marketed for this purpose. By the action of moisture on these compounds phosphine is released. This is a highly toxic gas with the smell of bad fish. It acts on the gastrointestinal and central nervous systems, giving rise first to abdominal pain, nausea and vomiting and going on to vertigo, gross ataxia, convulsions, coma and death, typically within two hours. Treatment is symptomatic and seldom effective.

Further Reading

General

Mechanisms of toxicity. Br Med Bull 1969; 25:219–309.

Poisonous Chemicals Used on Farms and Gardens. London: Department of Health and Social Security, 1969.

The Safe Use of Poisonous Chemicals on the Farm. London: Ministry of Agriculture, Fisheries and Food, 1975.

Pesticides

Ben-Dyke R, Sanderson DM, Noakes DN. Acute Toxicity Data for Pesticides. Saffron Walden, Essex: Chesterford Park Research Station, 1970.

Matthews GA, Clayphon JE. Safety precautions for pesticide application in the tropics. Pans 1973; 19 (No. 1):1–12.

Modern Trends in the Prevention of Pesticide Intoxication. Copenhagen: WHO, 1972.

Pesticide Safety Precautions Scheme Agreed Between Government Departments and Industry. London: Ministry of Agriculture, Fisheries and Food, 1971.

Safe Use of Pesticides. Geneva: International Labour Office, 1979.

Seminar on Health Hazards of Pesticides. Alexandria: WHO, 1973.

Tordoir WF, Heemstra EAH van (Eds). Field Worker Exposure during Pesticide Application. Amsterdam: Elsevier, 1980.

Organophosphorus Poisoning

Hierons R, Johnson MK. Clinical and toxicological investigations of a case of delayed neuropathy in man after acute poisoning by an organophosphorus pesticide. Arch Toxicol 1978; 40:279–84.

Milby TH. Prevention and management of organophosphate poisoning. J Am Med Assoc 1971; 216:2131–3.

Namba T, Nolte CT, Jackrel J, Grob D. Poisoning due to organophosphate insecticides. Am J Med 1971; 50:475–92.

Nelson DL, Crawford CR. Organophosphorus compounds: the past and the future. Clin Toxicol 1972; 5:223–30.

Ottevanger CF. An Epidemiological and Toxicological Study of Occupational Exposure to an Organophosphorus Pesticide. Rotterdam' Phoenix and Den Oudsten BV, 1976.

Peoples SA, Maddy KT. Organophosphate pesticide poisoning. West J. Med 1978; 129:273–7.

Vale JA, Scott GW. Organophosphorus poisoning. Guy's Hospital Reports 1974; 123:13–25.

Phenoxyacetate Herbicide Poisoning

Kohli JD, Khanna RN, Gupta BN, Dhar MM, Tandon JS, Sircar KP. Absorption and exretion of 2,4-dichlorophenoxyacetic acid in man. Xenobiotica 1974; 4: 97–100.

Young JF, Haley TJ. Pharmacokinetic study of a patient intoxicated with 2,4-dichlorophenoxyacetic acid and 2-methoxy-3,6-dichlorobenzoic acid. Clin Toxicol 1977; 11: 489–500.

Chlorate Poisoning

Bloxham CA, Wright N, Hoult JG. Self-poisoning by sodium chlorate – some unusual features. Clin Toxicol 1979; 15: 185–8.

Helliwell M, Nunn J. Mortality in sodium chlorate poisoning. Br Med J 1979; 1:1119.

Kennedy AC, Luke RG. Sodium chlorate poisoning. Br Med J 1967; 3:801.

Knight RK, Trounce JR, Cameron JS. Suicidal chlorate poisoning treated with peritoneal dialysis. Br Med J 1967; 3: 601–2.

Stoodley BJ, Rowe DJF. Haematological complications of chlorate poisoning. Br Med J 1970; 2:31–2.

Pentachlorophenol Poisoning

Pentachlorophenol and Sodium Pentachlorophenate. American Industrial Hygiene Association: Hygienic Guide Series.

Mercury Poisoning

Amin-Zaki L, Majeed MA, Clarkson TW, Greenwood MR. Methylmercury poisoning in Iraqui children: clinical observations over two years. Br Med J 1978; 1:613–6.

Gerstner HB, Huff JE. Selected case histories and epedimiologic examples of human mercury poisoning. Clin Toxicol 1977; 11:131–50.

Marsh DG. Organic mercury: methylmercury compounds. In, Handbook of Clinical Neurology: Intoxications of the Nervous System (part 1). Vinken PJ, Bruyn GW (Eds). Amsterdam: North Holland Publishing Co, 1979.

Pieter Kark RA. Clinical and neurochemical aspects of inorganic mercury intoxication. In, Handbook of Clinical Neurology: Intoxications of the Nervous System (part 1). Vinken PJ, Bruyn GW (Eds). Amsterdam: North Holland Publishing Co, 1979.

Shiraki H. Neuropathological aspects of organic mercury intoxication, including Minamorta disease. In, Handbook of Clinical Neurology: Intoxications of the Nervous System (part 1). Vinken PJ, Bruyn GW (Eds). Amsterdam: North Holland Publishing Co, 1979.

Fluoroacetate Poisoning

Reigart, JR, Breggeman JL, Keil JE. Sodium fluoroacetate poisoning. Am J Dis Child 1975; 129:1224–6.

Chapter 23

J. A. Vale and T. J. Meredith

Poisoning due to Aliphatic, Aromatic and Chlorinated Hydrocarbons

Aliphatic Hydrocarbons

The aliphatic series of hydrocarbons includes both saturated and unsaturated compounds which are derived almost exclusively from petroleum or petroleum processing. The saturated series is composed of gases (methane, ethane, propane and butane), liquids and solids. Unsaturated aliphatic hydrocarbons are byproducts of the petrochemical industry and are essential to the synthesis of many plastics and synthetic rubbers. Ethylene, propylene and butadiene, isoprene and acetylene all have weak anaesthetic properties at high concentrations.

Saturated Aliphatic Hydrocarbons

Methane

This hydrocarbon is the principal constituent of natural gas and is inert, in marked contrast to the toxic carbon monoxide-containing manufactured gas which it has now replaced in most households in Europe and North America. Methane may produce asphyxia in poorly ventilated areas or, if the concentration is high enough, an explosion. Both asphyxia and explosion have occurred in coal mines following the accumulation of methane ('marsh gas' or 'fire damp').

Aliphatic Hydrocarbon Mixtures

The mixtures which are commercially available include petroleum ether, benzine (not benzene), petroleum naphtha, gasoline and paint thinner. Higher boiling point mixtures including kerosene, jet fuels and lubricating oils. Such mixtures may also contain aromatic hydrocarbons such as benzene which is far more toxic than the qualitatively predominant aliphatic hydrocarbons. The precise composition of these mixtures will reflect the origin of the petroleum, molecular modifications effected at the refineries and the addition of other materials such as anti-oxidants, 'anti-knock' compounds, corrosion inhibitors, combustion improvers and dyes.

In 1962, an extensive cooperative study of accidental poisoning due to petroleum distillate products was reported. The investigation was coordinated by the American Academy of Pediatrics in the United States Public Health Service. Of the 760 cases reported, 55 per cent were due to paraffin (kerosene) as were the two reported deaths. Pulmonary complications occurred in 42 per cent. Spontaneous or induced vomiting resulted in a higher incidence of pulmonary complications (49 per cent) than occurred in those not vomiting (34 per cent). Nervous system complications occurred in 31 per cent and appeared to be related to the quantity ingested.

Petroleum distillate products cause nearly 100 accidental deaths per year in the USA; most of these deaths are in children under five years of age. It has been estimated that nearly 28,000 non-fatal poisonings due to petroleum distillate products occur annually in children under five years of age (Subcommittee on Accidental Poisoning, 1962). The incidence in Great Britain is small in comparison and deaths are rare.

Acute Poisoning due to Petrol (Gasoline)

The inhalation of high concentrations of petrol, such as are encountered by workmen cleaning storage tanks, may cause immediate death. It is possible that these hydrocarbons sensitize the myocardium so that circulating levels of adrenaline (epinephrine) may precipitate ventricular fibrillation (Reinhardt et al. 1971). In addition, high concentrations of gasoline vapour may lead to death from acute respiratory failure.

Clinical Features

Headache, blurred vision, dizziness, nausea and vomiting.
Incoordination, restlessness, excitement, confusion, disorientation, hallucinations.
Ataxia, tremor, delirium, coma.

Note: Patients who are intoxicated with aliphatic hydrocarbons predominantly lapse into coma and become areflexic, whereas those poisoned with aromatic hydrocarbons develop coma, motor unrest and hyperreflexia.

Treatment

1. Avoid gastric lavage and emesis because of the risk of chemical pneumonitis.

2. Supportive measures.

Chronic Poisoning due to Petrol (Gasoline)

Chronic exposure to petrol (gasoline) vapour, such as occurs in men engaged in cleaning out storage tanks or in children who habitually sniff gasoline, may lead to organic lead poisoning. Tetraethyl lead (the anti-knock additive) is non-toxic and is converted in the liver to triethyl lead. In addition, it is possible that triethyl lead can be further degraded to inorganic lead (Robinson 1978). Symptoms appear after a latent period of about one week following exposure.

Clinical Features

Nausea, vomiting, diarrhoea.
Insomnia, irritability, restlessness, anxiety.
Hypothermia, relative bradycardia, hypotension.
Muscle weakness, brisk reflexes, extensor plantar responses, tremor, chorea, convulsions, myoclonus, encephalopathy.
Loss of short-term memory, mania, suicidal tendencies.

Poisoning due to Paraffin (Kerosene)

Kerosene is relatively non-toxic by the oral route.

The fatal oral dose for an adult is probably at least 100 ml. The morbidity is due to aspiration, which occurs at the time of ingestion or during treatment, as a result of low surface tension and high vapour pressure — even a few millilitres of paraffin entering the respiratory passages will spread through the lungs and produce severe chemical pneumonitis.

Clinical Features

Transient euphoria (after inhalation).
Burning sensation in the mouth, throat and chest, headache, nausea, vomiting, diarrhoea (may be bloody).
Tinnitus, weakness, restlessness, muscular incoordination, confusion, disorientation and convulsions.
Drowsiness and coma.
Respiratory failure.
Ventricular fibrillation (rarely).

Treatment

1. Avoid gastric lavage and emesis because of the risk of chemical pneumonitis.

2. Absorption can be slowed by giving olive oil orally, although this may be hazardous in itself.

3. Supportive measures.

Note: There is no definitive evidence that steroids reduce the degree of pneumonitis.

References

Reinhardt CF, Azar A, Maxfield ME, Smith PE, Mullin LS. Cardiac arrhythmias and aerosol 'sniffing'. Arch Environ Health 1971; 22:265–79.
Robinson RO. Tetraethyl lead poisoning from gasoline sniffing. J Am Med Assoc 1978; 240:1373–4.
Sub-committee on accidental poisoning: cooperative kerosene poisoning study. Pediatrics 1962; 29:648–74.

Further Reading

Arena JM. Emergency treatment of hydrocarbon products ingestion. J Am Med Assoc 1973; 226:213.
Baldachin BJ, Melmed RN. Clinical and therapeutic aspects of kerosene poisoning: a series of 200 cases. Br Med J 1964; 2:28–30.
Foley JC, Dreyer NB, Soule AB, Woll E. Kerosene poisoning in young children. Radiology 1954; 62:817–29.
Gershen-Cohen J, Bringhurst LS, Byrne RN. Roentgenography of kerosene poisoning (chemical pneumonitis). J Roentgenology 1953; 69:557–62.
Goldfrank L, Kirstein R, Bresnitz E. Gasoline and other hydrocarbons. Hosp Physician 1979; 15:32–8.
Hansen KS, Sharp FR. Gasoline sniffing, lead poisoning and myoclonus. J Am Med Assoc 1978; 240:1375–6.
Poklis A, Burkett CD. Gasoline sniffing: a review. Clin Toxicol 1977; 11:35–41.

Aromatic Hydrocarbons

The aromatic series of compounds is based upon benzene and molecules which incorporate one or more benzene rings. The petrochemical industry provides the major source of aromatic hydrocarbons, which include, in addition to benzene itself, toluene and xylenes, diphenyl and diphenyl oxide and naphthalene. Toluene and the xylenes have, relative to benzene, much lower toxicity and volatility.

Certain industrial solvent mixtures containing predominantly toluene or xylene have been reported to cause bone marrow failure. However, it is now thought that these mixtures were contaminated with benzene and that this compound was the cause of the bone marrow depression as animal studies have failed to demonstrate a convincingly myelotoxic effect of toluene or xylene.

Benzene

Benzene is a colourless, volatile liquid with a pleasant odour. It is a common ingredient in many paints and varnish removers and some gasolines. It is also the primary raw material for styrene (used in the production of synthetic rubber), for phenol, for nylon intermediates and for synthetic detergents of the alkylauryl sulphonate type.

Acute Poisoning due to Benzene

Acute poisoning results when benzene is ingested or inhaled with suicidal or parasuicidal intent, and is also encountered when workmen enter storage tanks for the purpose of cleaning.

Clinical Features

Dizziness, weakness, euphoria, headache.
Nausea and vomiting.
Visual blurring, tremors, ataxia.
Chest tightness, respiratory depression, cardiac arrhythmias, coma and convulsions.

Treatment

1. Remove from exposure if inhaled.

2. Emesis or gastric lavage if patient presents soon after ingestion (great care should be exercised to avoid aspiration).

3. Intensive supportive therapy.

Chronic Poisoning due to Benzene

The toxic effects of chronic poisoning may not become apparent for months or years after the initial contact and, indeed, may appear after all exposure has ceased.

Clinical Features

Headache, anorexia.
Drowsiness, nervousness, pallor.
Anaemia (including aplastic anaemia), petechiae, abnormal bleeding, leukaemia.
Encephalopathy, tremulousness, emotional instability and cerebral atrophy.
Chromosome abnormalities, lymphomas.

Treatment

1. Remove patient from contaminated environment.

2. Treat anaemia with repeated blood transfusions.

In chronic poisoning a steady decrease in the cellular elements of the blood or bone marrow indicates a poor outcome. However, patients have recovered after as much as a year of almost complete absence of formation of new blood cells.

Further Reading

Committee on Toxicology of the National Research Council: Health effects of Benzene – a review. Washington DC: US Department of Commerce, National Technical Information Service PB 254 388 pp1–23, 1976.

National Institute of Occupational Safety and Health Criteria Document: Toluene. Washington DC: US Department of Health, Education and Welfare, 1973.

National Institute of Occupational Safety and Health Criteria Document: Benzene. Washington DC: US Department of Health, Education and Welfare, 1974.

National Institute of Occupational Safety and Health Criteria Document: Xylene. Washington DC: US Department of Health, Education and Welfare, 1975.

Forni A, Pacifico E, Limonta A. Chromosome studies in workers exposed to benzene or toluene or both. Arch Environ Health 1971; 22:373–8.

Haley TJ. Evaluation of the health effects of benzene inhalation. Clin Toxicol 1977; 11:531–48;

Hakkinen I, Siltanen E, Hernberg S, Seppalainen AM, Karli P, Vikkula E. Diphenyl poisoning in fruit paper production. Arch Environ Health 1973; 26:70–4.

Knox WJ, Nelson JR. Permanent encephalopathy from toluene inhalation. New Engl J Med 1966; 275:1494–6.

Pagnotto LD, Elkins HB, Brugsch HG. Benzene exposure in the rubber coating industry – a follow up. Am Ind Hyg Assoc J 1979; 40:137–46.

Vianna NJ, Polan A. Lymphomas and occupational benzene exposure. Lancet 1979; i:1394–5.

Vigliani EC, Forni A. Benzene and leukaemia. Environ Res 1976; 11:122–7.

Winek CL, Collom WD. Benzene and toluene fatalities. J Occup Med 1971; 13:259–61.

Chlorinated Hydrocarbons

Chlorinated hydrocarbons have a widespread and essential role in the chemical industry and in a variety of manufacturing operations, including the production of plastics and pesticides. These compounds are also used as solvents (dry cleaning and surface degreasing agents) and as vehicles for paints, varnishes and other industrial coatings. The more important chlorinated hydrocarbons include: tetrachloromethane (carbon tetrachloride), 1,1,1-trichloroethane (methyl chloroform), trichloroethylene, tetrachloroethylene (perchloroethylene) and trichloromethane (chloroform).

Carbon Tetrachloride

Carbon tetrachloride is a chlorinated hydrocarbon chemically related to chloroform. For many years it was used in such products as cleaners, grease solvents, fire extinguishers and dry shampoo, and in medicine as an anaesthetic and antihelminthic agent. Many of these uses have now been abandoned because of its extreme toxicity. In 1970, the US Food and Drug Administration banned its sale in any product used in the home.

Carbon tetrachloride is readily absorbed from the lungs and GI tract and, to a lesser extent, from the skin. Poisoning may be acute or chronic. Acute poisoning may result from inhalation of the vapour while the chemical is being used in a poorly ventilated area, or from the inhalation or the ingestion of the liquid with suicidal or parasuicidal intent. Chronic intoxication is usually due either to industrial exposure or 'sniffing' (see below).

Acute Poisoning due to Carbon Tetrachloride

The clinical features are similar whether poisoning is due to inhalation or ingestion, except that GI symptoms, including haematemesis and abdominal pain, are more severe, and the possibility of hepatic damage is greater when carbon tetrachloride is ingested. Hepatorenal damage may be delayed for up to two to three days after exposure and may occur in the absence of nervous system involvement.

Clinical Features

Irritation of eyes, nose and throat (if inhaled).
Nausea, vomiting, diarrhoea, abdominal colic, haematemesis.
Headache, dizziness, stupor, convulsions, unconsciousness.
Bradycardia, hypotension, cardiac arrhythmias including ventricular fibrillation.
Respiratory depression.
Subsequently, renal tubular necrosis, hepatic necrosis and fatty infiltration, cerebellar damage, optic neuritis, adrenal cortical necrosis, pancreatitis, pulmonary oedema, aplastic anaemia, haemolytic anaemia.

Chronic Poisoning due to Carbon Tetrachloride

Continued exposure to concentrations of carbon tetrachloride in excess of 100 p.p.m. may result in symptoms of chronic intoxication. (The minimal concentration detectable by odour is 80 p.p.m.) The maximal safe atmospheric concentration of carbon tetrachloride has been set at 10 p.p.m. for 8 hours of exposure (National Institute of Occupational Safety and Health Criteria Document: Carbon Tetrachloride).

Clinical Features

Nausea, vomiting, anorexia, abdominal pain, weight loss, pancreatitis.
Fatigue, apathy, mental confusion, loss of memory, depression.
Paraesthesiae, loss of peripheral colour vision.
Hepatorenal damage.

It has been suggested that if persons damaged by exposure to solvents are exposed again, even to low concentrations, then a fever of short duration, together with severe depression and fatigue, may occur (Capurro and Capurro 1979). (See also solvent abuse below)

Treatment

1. If carbon tetrachloride has been inhaled, the patient should be removed to fresh air. Remove any contaminated clothing.

2. Gastric lavage if patient is seen soon after ingestion.

3. Supportive measures.

4. Treat cardiac arrhythmias.

5. Treatment for acute renal and hepatic failure.

6. The value of haemoperfusion has not been established though the outcome in one case has been reported (Schwarzbeck and Kosters 1976).

Patients who have been chronically exposed to carbon tetrachloride should be removed from the contaminated environment and treated as indicated for acute poisoning.

References

Bagnasco FM, Stringer B, Muslim AM. Carbon tetrachloride: radiographic changes. New York State J Med 1978; 78: 646–7.

Capurro PU, Capurro C. Solvent exposure and mental depression. Clin Toxicol 1979; 15:193–5.

Schwarzbeck A, Kosters W. Extracorporeal haemoperfusion in acute carbon tetrachloride intoxication. Arch Toxicol 1976; 35:207–11.

Further Reading

Dawborn JK, Ralston M, Weiden S. Acute carbon tetrachloride poisoning: transaminase and biopsy studies. Br Med J 1961; 2:493–4.

Folland DS, Schaffner W, Ginn HE, Crofford OB, McMurray DR. Carbon tetrachloride toxicity potentiated by isopropyl alcohol: investigation of an industrial outbreak. J Am Med Assoc 1976; 236:1853–6.

Luse SA, Wood WG. The brain in fatal carbon tetrachloride poisoning. Arch Neurol 1976; 17:304–12.

National Institute of Occupational Safety and Health Criteria Document: Carbon tetrachloride. Washington DC: US Department of Health, Education and Welfare, 1975.

Oettingen WF von. The Halogenated Hydrocarbons: Toxicity and Potential Dangers. Public Health Service Publication No. 414. Washington DC: US Government Printing Office, 1955.

Recknagel RO. Carbon tetrachloride hepatotoxicity. Pharm Rev 1967; 19:145–208.

Sesame HA, Castro JA, Gillette JR. Studies on the destruction of liver microsomal cytochrome P_{450} by carbon tetrachloride administration. Biochem Pharmacol 1968; 17: 1759–68.

Stevens H, Forster FM. Effects of carbon tetrachloride on the nervous system. Arch Neurol Psychiat 1953; 70:635–49.

Straus B. Aplastic anaemia following exposure to carbon tetrachloride. JAMA 1954; 155:737–9.

Trichloroethylene

Trichloroethylene is a colourless volatile liquid which is widely used as an industrial solvent, particularly in metal degreasing and extraction processes. It is rapidly absorbed and excreted via the lungs, and is metabolized in the liver. The principal metabolite, trichloroacetic acid, may appear in the urine for several weeks after exposure. Because of its use as an anaesthetic the acute effects of the inhalation of trichloroethylene have been extensively studied. Rarely, trichloroethylene may be ingested with suicidal intent; more usually, it is inhaled either accidentally or for 'kicks'. Sudden death in workers exposed to trichloroethylene has been described and is thought to be due to sensitization of the heart to circulating catecholamines with resultant ventricular arrhythmias.

Acute Poisoning due to Trichloroethylene

Clinical Features

Dizziness, headache, nausea, vomiting, excitement, loss of consciousness (recovery is usually rapid). Ventricular tachycardia and fibrillation.

Note: At high concentrations unconsciousness may occur without preceding excitement.
Nausea and vomiting may persist for several hours.

Treatment

1. Move to fresh air.
2. Remove contaminated clothing.
3. Supportive measures.

Chronic Poisoning due to Trichloroethylene

Clinical Features

Nausea, anorexia, fatigue, weight loss.
Visual impairment (conjunctivitis, optic atrophy).
Cranial nerve palsies, ataxia, impairment of intellectual function.
Painful joints.
Dermatitis and eczema.

Note: Recent evidence suggests that this compound is not carcinogenic (Henschler et al. 1980).

Treatment

Remove the patient from the contaminated environment.

References

Henschler D, Romen W, Elsasser HM, Reichert D, Eder E, Radwan Z. Carcinogenicity study of trichloroethylene by long term inhalation in three animal species. Arch Toxicol 1980; 43:237–48.

Further Reading

Alapin B. Trichloroethylene addiction and its effects. Br J Addict 1973; 68:331–5.

Anonymous. Hazards of working with trichloroethylene. Br Med J 1974; 4:525.

Feldman RG. Trichloroethylene. In, Handbook of Clinical Neurology: Intoxications of the Nervous System (part 1). Eds Vinken PJ, Bruyn GW. Amsterdam: North Holland Publishing Co, 1979.

Kimmerle G, Eben A. Metabolism, excretion and toxicology of trichloroethylene after inhalation. 2. Experimental human exposure. Arch Toxicol 1973; 30:127–38.

National Institute of Occupational Safety and Health Criteria Document: Trichloroethylene. Washington DC: US Department of Health, Education and Welfare, 1973.

Messite J. Trichloroethylene. J. Occup Med 1974; 16:194–7.

Mitchell ABS, Parsons-Smith BG. Trichloroethylene neuropathy. Br Med J 1969; 1:422–3.

Salvini M, Binaschi S, Riva M. Evaluation of the psychophysiological functions in humans exposed to trichloroethylene. Br J Ind Med 1971; 28:293–5.

Smith GF. Trichloroethylene: a review. Br J Ind Med 1966; 23:249–62.

1,1,1-Trichloroethane

This halogenated aliphatic hydrocarbon is widely used as a solvent, particularly in the cold cleaning of metal surfaces. 1,1,1-trichloroethane is thought to have a low toxicity. Few deaths have been recorded in the literature and most were thought to be accidental (Caplan et al. 1976).

Clinical Features

Dizziness, nausea, coma, respiratory depression.

Treatment

1. Move to fresh air.
2. Remove contaminated clothing.
3. Supportive measures.

References

Caplan YH, Backer RC, Whitaker JQ. 1,1,1-trichloroethane: report of a fatal intoxication. Clin Toxicol 1976; 9:69–74.

Further Reading

Kay RW. Survey of toxic hazards during vapour degreasing with trichloroethylene and 1,1,1-trichloroethane. Ann Occup Hyg 1973; 16:417–9.

National Institute of Occupational Safety and Health Criteria Document: 1,1,1-Trichloroethane. Washington DC: US Department of Health, Education and Welfare, 1976.

Parker JC, Casey GE, Bahlman LJ, Leidel NA, Rose D, Stein HP, et al. Chloroethanes: review of toxicity. Am Ind Hyg Assoc 1979; 40:A46–60.

Stewart RD. The toxicology of 1,1,1-trichloroethane. Ann Occup Hyg 1968; 11:71–9.

Travers H. Death from 1,1,1-trichloroethane abuse: case report. Milit Med 1974; 139:889–90.

Tetrachloroethylene (Perchloroethylene)

Tetrachloroethylene is an organic solvent used industrially in dry-cleaning and degreasing operations. Tetrachloroethylene can be absorbed via the GI tract, the lungs or through intact skin. Following absorption tetrachloroethylene is excreted via the lungs or metabolized in the liver to trichloroacetic acid which is excreted in the urine.

Its toxicological properties parallel very closely those associated with trichloroethylene (see above); treatment is similar.

Further Reading

Lukaszewski T. Acute tetrachloroethylene fatality. Clin Toxicol 1979; 15:411–5.

National Institute of Occupational Safety and Health Criteria Document: Tetrachloroethylene. Washington DC: US Department of Health, Education and Welfare, 1976.

Stewart RD. Acute tetrachloroethylene intoxication. J Am Med Assoc 1969; 208:1490–2.

Solvent Abuse

Solvent abuse may be defined as the intentional inhalation of volatile organic chemicals other than the conventional anaesthetic gases. This definition includes the inhalation of vapours of organic solvents (either pure or in combination with other non-volatile ingredients), hydrocarbon mixtures such as lighter fluid and petrol, and aerosol propellants.

Contrary to popular belief, solvent 'sniffing' is by no means a recent phenomenon, nor without harm. The misuse of nitrous oxide, ether and chloroform by adults was fashionable as early as the 19th century. Since 1970, there have been about 50 deaths in Great Britain due to this cause.

Most 'sniffers' are male and adolescent and indulge in the habit as a group activity. Some young 'sniffers' progress to regular and heavy drinking within a short time of becoming addicted or habituated to solvents. When a group of abusers was questioned (Hayden et al. 1976) about the subjective experience of solvent abuse most agreed that marijuana provided somewhat similar effects, even though vivid hallucinations were an added effect of solvent use. The solvents were either 'bagged' (sprayed into a plastic bag and then inhaled until the patient passed out) or 'huffed' (sprayed onto a cloth held to the mouth).

Diagnosis

The diagnosis should be suspected if groups of adolescents or individuals behave as if they are drunk. The hair, breath or clothing may smell of solvent and the clothing is often stained. Unexplained listlessness, anorexia and marked moodiness are suggestive of abuse.

Pathology

Fortunately, gross pathological changes are rare, though they have been described in solvent abusers (Hayden et al. 1976). Since benzene has been replaced by toluene in many commercial products, most serious illness arises today from inhalation of chlorinated hydrocarbons or saturated hydrocarbons (e.g. hexane), or from the cardiac toxicity of the fluorocarbon aerosol propellants.

A study by Bass (1970) of 110 cases of sudden death without plastic bag suffocation, showed that trichloroethylene and fluorinated hydrocarbons were most frequently involved. Autopsy revealed no anatomical abnormalities that could explain the sudden deaths. Animal experiments have now indicated that death occurs due to ventricular fibrillation or asystole subsequent to slowing of the sinoatrial pacemaker. In addition, the myocardium may be sensitized by the hydrocarbons to the action of endogenous catecholamines (Reinhardt et al. 1971).

The features of chronic gasoline sniffing are described above on page 154.

References

Bass M. Sudden sniffing death. J Am Med Assoc 1970; 212: 2075–9.

Hayden JW, Comstock EG, Comstock BS. The clinical toxicology of solvent abuse. Clin Toxicol 1976; 9:169–84.

Reinhardt CF, Azar A, Maxfield ME, Smith PE, Mullin LS. Cardiac arrhythmias and aerosol 'sniffing'. Arch Environ Health 1971; 22:265–79.

Further Reading

Oliver JS, Watson JM. Abuse of solvents 'for kicks'. Lancet 1977; i:84–6.

Watson JM. Clinical and laboratory investigations in 132 cases of solvent abuse. Med Sci Law 1978; 18:40–3.

Chapter 24

T. J. Meredith and J. A. Vale

Poisoning due to Household Products

It is widely believed that household products contain an enormous variety of toxic chemicals, so the ingestion of these substances by children is a frequent cause for alarm among parents and doctors alike. The extent of this concern is reflected by the number of enquiries made to poisons information centres. In the UK, the National Poisons Information Service (NPIS) supplies information only to, members of the medical profession. Nevertheless, in 1978 nearly 26,000 enquiries were made to the London centre of the NPIS and 28 per cent of these concerned household products, of which 69 per cent involved children under the age of five years. The statistics in America are similar even though 'poison control centers' deal with members of the public as well as with medical practitioners (Table 24.1).

So-called poisoning due to household products is more often the result of accidental than deliberate ingestion, and it is young children who are most 'at risk'. It is unusual, though, for these substances to be the cause of serious poisoning when ingested accidentally by young children. Indeed, true poisoning probably occurs only in one third of reported poisoning incidents, and the number of substances which are

capable of causing lasting harm are very few. Certain corrosive agents in particular, however, may cause complications, and these are discussed later in this chapter. Thus it becomes important to distinguish between the toxicity, or potential toxicity, of a household product and the hazard that it presents. The toxicity may be high, but the hazard is usually low. The accidental consumption of household products is rarely followed by death (Table 24.1), although adults intent on suicide may sometimes swallow massive quantities with fatal consequences.

The social and psychological background to self-poisoning and poisoning in children are discussed in Chapter 9. Poisoning due to household products differs in no important respects. It is interesting, though, that this form of poisoning occurs more commonly in summer than in winter, and that the number of incidents increases between the hours of 8.00 and 9.00 a.m. (perhaps when parents are particularly busy). Unfortunately household products are too often stored within easy reach of children, for example, beneath the kitchen sink. Although some products are normally kept locked away, a recent survey showed that over half of the reported cases of poisoning

Table 24.1.   Analysis of poisons enquiries in America and the UK.

Source of information	Total number of enquiries	Enquiries concerning household products (percentage of total)	Deaths due to household products
NCPCC[1] (America, 1976)	147,277	48,352 (30%)	21
NPIS[2] (London, 1978)	25,806	7,343 (28%)	6

[1] National Clearing House for Poisons Control Centers
[2] London Centre of National Poisons Information Service

involve substances which are not in their normal place of storage at the time of the incident. Furthermore these same substances are often transferred to improper containers. A typical example is that of white spirit (turpentine substitute), which is often decanted into a jam-jar, or other wide-necked container, for the purpose of cleaning paint brushes.

General Management of Poisoning due to Household Products

The principles of treatment of a patient suspected of swallowing a household substance are the same as those for any other form of poisoning. It is important to determine, so far as is possible, the quantity which may have been ingested and the toxicity of the product concerned. This latter information may, if necessary, be obtained from the NPIS. Certain factors will modify the toxicity of a given substance and may determine the need for gastric lavage or the administration of an emetic syrup (Table 24.2).

Table 24.2.   Factors which tend to raise or lower the toxicity of household products.

Factors which raise toxicity	Factors which lower toxicity
Liquid	Solid or semi-solid
Pellets	Powdered (unless caustic)
Pleasant flavour	Unpleasant flavour
Large volume	Small volume
Low viscosity (petroleum products)	High viscosity
Method of dispensing or packaging.	

Liquids and pellets are more likely to be ingested in large quantities than powders, solids or semi-solids. Flavour has little to do with whether or not a substance is ingested, but it will influence the amount swallowed. Some substances, such as perfume, are packaged in such small volumes that a toxic dose cannot be obtained from a single container. However, the aspiration of even small quantities of a petroleum distillate, such as turpentine substitute, may be followed by a severe chemical pneumonitis because the low volatility enables the substance to spread rapidly throughout the lungs. Finally the form in which the product is dispensed or packaged is important; a

substance marketed in aerosol form is usually less likely to be ingested in large amounts than a liquid in an ordinary bottle.

Cleaning Products

This group of household products (Figure 24.1) contains some of the more toxic substances: bleach, oven-cleaners and dishwashing machine powders. The majority of incidents involve children aged between one and five years (Figure 24.2). Kettle descalers and drain cleaners are responsible for the most serious cases of poisoning due to ingestion of household products, although rarely are they ingested accidentally.

Poisoning due to Household Bleach

Clinical Features

Household bleach is a three to six per cent sodium hypochlorite solution. When ingested, it may cause a burning sensation in the mouth, throat and oesophagus, accompanied by a sensation of thirst. Vomiting and abdominal discomfort can also occur. The corrosive and irritative properties of bleach may result in pharyngeal and laryngeal oedema. Hypochlorous acid is formed in the stomach by the reaction of bleach

Figure 24.1. *An analysis of 134 cases reported to the London Centre of the National Poisons Information Service in the four month period November 1978 to February 1979.*

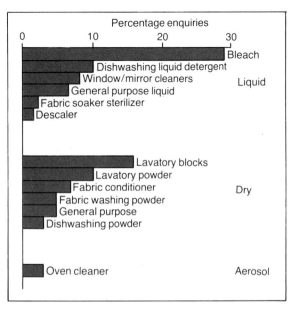

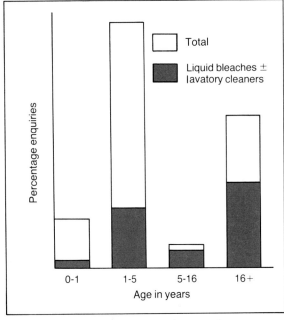

Figure 24.2. *Household cleaning products — age distribution of 'poisoning' incidents. (Reported to NPIS November 1978—February 1979).*

with gastric acid and this further increases the gastric irritation. Free chlorine gas is generated by this reaction in the stomach and this, if inhaled, may cause coughing and pulmonary oedema.

Treatment

When, as is commonly the case, only small quantities of bleach have been ingested, liberal fluids by mouth together with the use of demulcents are all that are required. Gastric lavage is indicated if more than a few mouthfuls have been swallowed, especially if there is evidence of local reaction in the mouth. The use of a 2.5 per cent sodium thiosulphate solution has been advocated for this purpose, but there is no good evidence that this has any special advantage. In fact, serious problems have only followed the ingestion of substantial quantities of bleach, which rarely happens except by deliberate intent.

Poisoning due to Mixture of Bleach with other Cleaning Agents

In some circumstances household bleach may be responsible for the evolution of substantial amounts of poisonous gas. This occurs when several cleaning agents are mixed together in the lavatory bowl. Hypo-

chlorite bleach mixed with ammonia produces chloramine gas which causes nausea and respiratory irritation. More dangerous, though, is the combination of bleach and powder lavatory cleaners, which themselves normally evolve chlorine; not only is chlorine gas formed but also oxides of sulphur, and the combination of these may result in severe respiratory irritation and even pulmonary oedema.

Poisoning due to Corrosive Agents

In contrast to the majority of household chemicals, there are a number of concentrated acid and alkali solutions which constitute a real and serious danger of poisoning.

The majority of oven-cleaners are made from 30 per cent solutions of caustic soda (sodium hydroxide). Inhalation may occur if the aerosol form is sprayed into a hot oven, and the ingestion of any quantity is dangerous.

Kettle descalers consist of concentrated formic acid and are used to remove the deposits of calcium carbonate which accumulate inside kettles in hard-water areas.

Dishwashing machine powders represent a further important exception to the generally low toxicity of household products. The accidental ingestion of these granular powders is uncommon in this country, but occurs more frequently in America and Scandinavia where the use of dishwashing machines is relatively commonplace. The silicates and metasilicates in these powders are very caustic, and lesions similar to those that follow the ingestion of caustic soda may occur.

Drain cleaners are not often used in this country but may consist almost wholly of sodium hydroxide, in either liquid or granular form. Less commonly, drain cleaners contain sulphuric acid, and although hydrogen sulphide (with its characteristic smell of 'rotten eggs'), may result from the reaction between dilute sulphuric acid and iron sulphide present in sewage, this has not proved to be a real problem in this country. However, a number of fatalities have been reported in America.

Car battery acid (concentrated sulphuric acid) is occasionally ingested deliberately by adults with serious consequences.

Clinical Features

All the above-mentioned chemicals cause considerable damage when they come into contact with tissues. Typically acids spare the oesophagus when ingested because of rapid transit and the resistance of the squamous epithelium, although damage does occur in about 20 per cent of cases. Acid flows along the lesser curvature of the stomach to the prepyloric region to cause almost instantaneous coagulative necrosis of one or more layers of the wall of the stomach (Figure 24.3). Alkalis react with protein to form proteinates in a similar manner to acids, but saponification of tissue fat also occurs, resulting in soft, necrotic and deeply penetrating ulcers. In contrast to acids, alkalis damage the oesophagus and spare the stomach because of the protective effect of gastric acid. It has been shown experimentally that a concentrated solution of alkali need be in contact with the oesophageal mucosa for only ten seconds for necrosis of the entire oesophageal wall to occur.

Ingestion of concentrated acid and alkali is quickly followed by ulceration of the alimentary mucosa with lesions in the mouth, oesophagus and stomach. Oesophageal damage can occur in the absence of visible oral ulceration. The pain from these ulcers may be severe and opiates are often necessary to achieve satisfactory relief of pain. Gastric lavage and emesis are contraindicated, but demulcents may be used. Serious and immediate complications that can arise include laryngeal and glottal oedema, and perforation of the oesophagus or stomach. Formic acid may also cause acute renal failure. Oesophageal stricture formation may occur as a late complication of ingestion of alkalis (Figure 24.4). Late compli-

cations following the ingestion of corrosive acids include antral and pyloric stenosis, achlorhydria and protein-losing gastroenteropathy.

Treatment

Endoscopy should be performed on children at risk from serious oesophageal damage following the ingestion of alkalis — suggested by visible lesions in the mouth, severe retrosternal or epigastric pain, or if the ingested agent has a very high pH, e.g. $> pH\ 12$.

Figure 24.4. *Alkali ingestion. This postmortem specimen taken from an elderly lady who died from inhalation pneumonia shows stricture formation in the lower third of the oesophagus. This occurred several months after the ingestion of a concentrated sodium hydroxide solution and required regular dilatation until the time of her death. Courtesy of the Curator of the Gordon Museum, Guy's Hospital.*

Figure 24.3. *Corrosive acid ingestion. The stomach of a young man who ingested kettle descaler (concentrated formic acid) showed widespread coagulative necrosis at postmortem. The area immediately below the oesophagus was spared because the acid was ingested whilst the patient stood in an upright position. (Courtesy of the Curator of the Gordon Museum, Guy's Hospital.)*

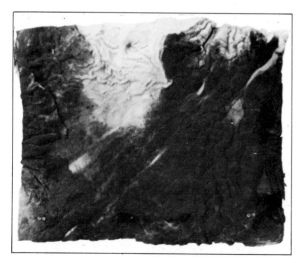

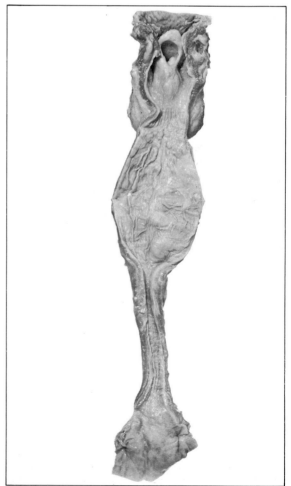

Antibiotics should be administered and steroids are given to reduce the initial oedema and subsequent inflammation and stricture formation, although there is no good evidence for their value in full-thickness lesions.

Until recently the management of the ingestion of corrosive acids has been medical. However, it has become evident that the majority of patients who ingest significant quantities of acid subsequently undergo an operation, if not because of immediate complications then because of the late development of antral or pyloric stenosis. Patients who ingest concentrated acid, and in whom signs of sepsis or peritonitis develop, should have an exploratory laparotomy. Non-viable or marginally viable stomach should be removed and a 'second-look' procedure considered. The current management of the ingestion of corrosive acid is summarized in Table 24.3.

It must be emphasized, though, that the ingestion of large amounts of corrosive materials is exceedingly rare in the UK, and usually occurs only by deliberate intent.

Poisoning due to Surfactants

Many of the remaining cleaning products, and some cosmetics as well, contain chemicals called surfactants. The surfactant used in a particular cleaning product will largely determine the toxicity of the product. Surfactants are molecules which possess both hydrophilic and lipophilic groups. Thus when water, for example, makes contact with an oily medium, surfactant molecules will orient themselves so that the hydrophilic groups extend into the aqueous phase and the lipophilic groups extend into the oily phase. A consequence of this behaviour is the formation of spherical aggregates of surfactant molecules called micelles (Figure 24.5). The hydrophilic portions of the surfactant molecules become directed outwards while the lipophilic portions face inwards toward the centre of the micelle. The provision of a central core of lipid protected from water by the layer of hydrophilic groups allows fat-soluble substances to become dissolved in an aqueous medium.

There are three types of surfactant, each with a different degree of toxicity as follows:

1. Anionic surfactants, which have a negative electrical charge on the lipophilic portion of the molecule.

2. Cationic surfactants, which have a positive electrical charge on the lipophilic portion of the molecule.

3. Non-ionic surfactants, which have no charge at all on the lipophilic group.

Table 24.3.   Management of ingestion of corrosive acid.

Intravenous fluids or blood transfusion for shock and haematemesis
Correction of acid—base balance

No gastric lavage

Antibiotics
No steroids unless aspiration has occurred (steroids may mask abdominal signs, and there is no evidence for their value in third degree burns)

Contrast radiography using water-soluble agent within one hour of ingestion. Endoscopy to the most proximal area of damage (to avoid perforation) within 24 hours and repeat daily

If evidence of second or third degree oesophageal or gastric burns and peritoneal signs are present, then proceed to laparotomy.

If perforation has not occurred by the seventh day, then proceed to laparotomy with a view to antrectomy or pyloroplasty

Figure 24.5. *Micelle formation. Surfactant molecules form micelles in an aqueous environment and these allow fat-soluble substances to be solubilized in the central lipid core. Anionic surfactant molecules are shown here in diagrammatic form with negative electrical charges on the hydrophilic groups.*

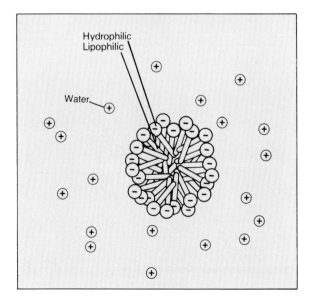

Clinical Features

Anionic detergents irritate the skin by the removal of natural oils and cause redness, soreness and even a papular dermatitis. Ingestion may cause mild gastro-intestinal irritation with nausea, vomiting and diarrhoea. In contrast, non-ionic detergents irritate the skin only slightly and appear to be completely harmless if ingested. Those categories of cleaning products which contain anionic and/or non-ionic surfactants are shown in Table 24.4.

Treatment

The only treatment normally necessary if any of these substances are ingested accidentally is the administration of liberal fluids by mouth together with a demulcent.

Cationic detergents are considerably more toxic than the other two forms of surfactant and they are rarely found in household cleaning materials, although they may occasionally be found in certain disin-fectants.

Other Cleaning Products

Poisoning due to Disinfectant and Antiseptic Solutions

Disinfectant and antiseptic solutions used to contain phenol, but this is now usually replaced by small quantities of either chlorophenol or chloroxylenol. These compounds are less toxic than phenol, but can nevertheless be hazardous if ingested in very large quantities. More importantly, however, disinfectants

---

Table 24.4. Cleaning products containing anionic and/or non-ionic surfactants.

Carpet shampoo

Dishwashing liquid

Dishwashing rinse aid (for dishwashing machines)

Fabric rinse conditioner

Fabric washing powder and flakes

General purpose household cleaning liquids and powders

Scouring liquids, creams and powders

---

may consist of up to 40 per cent isopropyl alcohol which has double the potency and toxicity of ethyl alcohol.

Clinical Features

In addition to local irritation in the mouth and throat, ingestion of disinfectant is accompanied by central effects which include depression of respiration, drowsiness, stupor and even coma. As much as 15 per cent of isopropyl alcohol is converted to acetone in the body and, for this reason, urinalysis may reveal ketonuria.

Treatment

The fatal dose of isopropyl alcohol can be as little as 100 ml in an adult, so gastric lavage should be performed if more than a mouthful is swallowed. Supportive care is necessary for the central depressant effects and, in very severely poisoned patients, the isopropyl alcohol may be removed by haemodialysis.

It should be emphasized though that nowadays the *accidental* swallowing of the popular disinfectants hardly ever entrains any harm.

Cleaning Materials containing Petroleum Products

Window and mirror cleaners contain, as well as isopropyl alcohol, a variety of petroleum products which are dangerous if aspirated into the lungs. Wax-based polishes and metal polishes both contain white spirit, another petroleum product, which in metal polish may form 60 to 80 per cent of the product.

Lavatory Deodorants and Sanitizers

Lavatory deodorants and sanitizers contain dichloro-benzene, a chemical which may exist as one of two isomers. Orthodichlorobenzene is considerably more toxic than paradichlorobenzene, and causes kidney and liver damage. Paradichlorobenzene, therefore, is the substance usually incorporated into lavatory deodorant blocks and this, when ingested, causes nausea, vomiting, diarrhoea and abdominal cramps. Purgation is necessary only if less than a gram has been swallowed; otherwise gastric lavage should be performed.

Cosmetic Agents

Poisoning due to Cosmetic Agents

Cosmetic agents account for more than 15 per cent of enquiries made to the NPIS concerning household products.

Perfumes

Perfumes contain a mixture of essential oils and alcohol (95 per cent ethyl alcohol and 5 per cent methyl alcohol). Probably because of their small containers, it is unusual for perfume to cause serious poisoning. 'Burning' of the mouth and throat, as well as dizziness and tremors, may occur on ingestion. If more than 30 ml is ingested by an adult (and correspondingly less by a child) gastric lavage or emesis is indicated; otherwise dilution with oral fluids is the only necessary treatment.

Nail Polisher and Remover

Nail polish contains a mixture of solvents together with colouring matter. Acetone is the principal constituent of nail polish remover. The ingestion of either product will result in symptoms similar to those caused by perfume, and gastric lavage is necessary only if more than a mouthful has been taken.

Other Preparations

After shave lotion, cologne, antiperspirants, deodorants, hair tonic, sun-tan oil and toilet water all contain significant amounts of ethyl alcohol. Ingestion of any of these preparations will cause a sensation of 'burning' in the mouth and throat and, occasionally, vomiting and drowsiness. The small containers in which these substances are sold usually prevent the consumption of very large quantities. The only treatment usually required, therefore, is the administration of liberal oral fluids although, when large amounts are ingested, an emetic syrup or the use of gastric lavage may become necessary.

Children may develop hypoglycaemia after drinking alcohol, and this can be severe enough to cause convulsions and/or coma. This more serious form of poisoning usually besets children who have drunk sherry, whisky or some other alcoholic drink, rather than following the ingestion of cosmetic products.

Conclusion

It is apparent that the vast majority of household products are not in fact hazardous when swallowed in small quantities by young children. An awareness of this is important for those who have to treat such children, and who have to decide whether or not they require admission to hospital. Gastric lavage should almost never have to be performed in a young child who has swallowed a household product, and only occasionally should the administration of an emetic syrup be necessary. If the child is asymptomatic, and the mother sensible, then in many instances he or she could reasonably be observed overnight at home rather than in hospital. It must be remembered, however, that certain products, such as bleach, become hazardous when ingested in large quantities, usually deliberately by adults, even though they are relatively non-toxic in small amounts. Some substances are dangerous whatever the quantity ingested; kettle descalers, drain cleaners, dishwashing machine powders and battery acid are examples.

Further Reading

Household Products

Goulding R, Ashforth GK, Jenkins H. Household products and poisoning. Br Med J 1978; 1:286–7.

Goulding R, Durham P, Edwards JN. Ingestion of household cleaning products. Br Med J 1980; 280:938.

de Jong AL. Detergent products, what are the ingredients? Why? And how do they react? Vet Hum Toxicol 1979; 21: Suppl. 22–5.

Lawrence RA, Haggerty RJ. Household agents and their potential toxicity. Modern Treatment 1971; 8:511–27.

Lovejoy FH, Flowers J, McGuigan M. The epidemiology of poisoning from household products. Vet Hum Toxicol 1979; 21:Suppl. 33–4.

Temple AR, Veltri JC. Outcome of accidental ingestions of soaps, detergents and related household products. Vet Hum Toxicol 1979; 21:Suppl.31–2.

Velart J. Household products containing acids, alkalis or detergents: toxic effects and their treatment. Vet Hum Toxicol 1979; 21:Suppl. 35–6.

Corrosive Gastric and Oesophageal Injury

Chodak GW, Passaro E. Acid ingestion: need for gastric resection. J Am Med Assoc 1978; 239:225–6.

Cochran ST, Fonkalsrud EW, Gyepes MT. Complete obstruction of the gastric antrum in children following acid ingestion. Arch Surg 1978; 113:308–10.

Di Costanzo J, Noirclerc M, Jouglard J, Escoffier JM, Cano N, Martin J, et al. New therapeutic approach to corrosive burns of the upper gastrointestinal tract. Gut 1980; 21:370–5.

Haller JA, Bachman K. The comparative effect of current therapy on experimental caustic burns of the esophagus. Pediatrics 1964; 34:236–45.

Harness J. Diagnosis and treatment of acid gastric burns. New Physician 1976; 25:70–4.

Krenzelok EP, Clinton JE. Caustic esophageal and gastric erosion without evidence of oral burns following detergent ingestion. J Am Coll Emer Phys 1979; 8:194–6.

Naik RB, Stephens WP, Wilson DJ, Walker R, Lee HA. Ingestion of formic acid containing agents – report of three fatal cases. Postgrad Med J 1980; 56:451–6.

Nicosia JF, Thornton JP, Folk FA, Saletta JD. Surgical management of corrosive gastric injuries. Ann Surg 1974; 180:139–43.

Walker AP. Oesophageal corrosion: methodology, animal data and extrapolation to man. Vet Hum Toxicol 1979; 21: Suppl. 26–30.

Chapter 25

J. A. Vale and T. J. Meredith

Poisoning due to Marine Animals

In many parts of the world poisonous fish are common and dangerous. Vertebrate fish containing toxins capable of causing human illness are divided into three categories based on the location of the toxin as follows:

1. Ichthyosarcotoxic fish contain toxins in their musculature, skin or mucus and are responsible for most cases of fish poisoning.

2. Ichthyo-otoxic fish have toxin in their gonads.

3. Ichthyohaemotoxic fish contain toxin in their blood.

Ciguatera, scombroid and puffer-fish poisoning are the commonest types of ichthyosarcotoxic fish poisoning worldwide.

Shellfish (e.g. mussels, clams, oysters), growing in the open sea, may become poisonous (and cause paralysis when ingested) if they feed on certain dino-flagellates such as *Gonyaulax catenalla* and *Gonyaulax tamarensis*. Alternatively shellfish may cause a milder neurotoxic illness if they become contaminated with toxin derived from another dinoflagellate, *Gymnodinium breve*.

Ciguatera Fish Poisoning ('Cigua' (Spanish) — poisonous snail)

Over 400 fish species have been reported as ciguatoxic, though barracuda, red snapper, amberjack and grouper are most commonly implicated. Ciguatoxic species are particularly common around the coral reefs of the Pacific Islands and the Caribbean. The distribution of affected fish is variable and unpredictable. Fish caught off one beach may be toxic but, if caught off another a few yards away, fish of the same species may be innocuous.

Toxicity

Ciguatera fish contain ciguatoxin which is a lipid-soluble, heat-stable compound which inhibits human red cell cholinesterase in vitro. The mechanism of toxicity in man, however, appears to involve more than just inhibition of cholinesterase activity.

Clinical Features

The onset of symptoms may occur from a few minutes to 30 hours after ingestion of toxic fish. Typically they appear between one and six hours and include abdominal cramps, nausea, vomiting and watery diarrhoea. In some cases initial symptoms, such as numbness and paraesthesiae of the lips, tongue and throat, may occur. Other features described include malaise, dry mouth, metallic taste, myalgia, arthralgia, blurred vision, photophobia and transient blindness (Halstead 1967).

In more severe cases hypotension, cranial nerve palsies and respiratory paralysis may occur. The mortality in these cases may be as high as 12 per cent.

Treatment

Treatment is principally symptomatic, although in a few patients atropine has improved some of the cardiovascular and gastrointestinal manifestations.

Scombroid Fish Poisoning

Scombroid fish have dark meat and migrate; they include mackerel, tuna, bonito and skipjack.

Toxicity

The flesh of scombroid fish has a high free histidine content which is normally metabolized to α-ketoglutarate. Many bacteria, particularly *Proteus spp.*, decarboxylate histidine to histamine and, if fish become contaminated with these organisms, large amounts of histamine accumulate in the flesh (Taylor et al. 1978).

Clinical Features

The precise role of histamine in the pathogenesis of the clinical syndrome is uncertain but the clinical picture is compatible with a histamine reaction. The illness is characterized by flushing, headache, dizziness, burning of the mouth and throat, abdominal cramps, nausea, vomiting and diarrhoea. Symptoms begin within a few minutes to a few hours after the fish is ingested. The mean incubation period in 27 reported outbreaks was 30 minutes (Hughes and Merson 1976). The illness is short-lived; the mean duration in the reported outbreaks was four hours. In one outbreak of over 400 cases no patients died and only one death has been reported in the last century. Though the clinical picture is suggestive of an acute allergic reaction sensitization does not occur and victims may eat similar fish subsequently without ill-effect.

Treatment

Treatment is symptomatic. The only effective preventive measure is to keep raw fish either on ice or frozen, and to process fish whilst still chilled. Cooking, canning, soaking, smoking, salting and autoclaving have no effect on the amount of activity of histamine present in the fish.

Shellfish Poisoning

Paralytic shellfish poisoning is caused by bivalve molluscs contaminated with the neurotoxins produced by one of the toxic dinoflagellates *Gonyaulax catenalla* or *Gonyaulax tamarensis*.

Toxicity

The neurotoxin produced by *G. catenella* is known as saxitoxin and is a heat-stable compound which is thought to block the propagation of action potentials in nerve and muscle (Kao and Nishiyama 1965).

Clinical Features

The illness is characterized by paraesthesiae of the mouth, lips, face and extremities, often accompanied by nausea, vomiting and diarrhoea. In more severe cases, dysphonia, dysphagia, muscle weakness of paralysis, ataxia and respiratory depression may occur (Halstead 1965). In a large outbreak in North-East England in 1968, paraesthesiae, weakness of the extremities and a 'feeling of floating' were the most common symptoms (McCollum et al. 1968).

Treatment

Treatment should consist of measures to remove unabsorbed toxin from the intestinal tract, and symptomatic and supportive measures as required.

Neurotoxic Fish Poisoning

Toxicity

Gymnodinium breve produces at least two heat-stable neurotoxic substances which appear to act by stimulating post-ganglionic cholinergic nerve fibres.

Clinical Features

Within three hours after ingestion of shellfish contaminated by the above toxins, paraesthesiae, reversal of hot and cold temperature sensation, nausea, vomiting, diarrhoea and ataxia occur (Hughes and Merson 1976). This illness appears to be milder than that caused by paralytic shellfish poisoning.

Treatment

The illness is self-limiting and treatment is symptomatic.

Stings from Marine Animals

Fish

Several species of fish which are found in British coastal waters have venomous spines in their fins. They include weever fish (*Trachinus draco* and *Trachinus vipera*), short spined cottus, spiny dogfish and the stingray (*Urobatis halleri*). Bathers and fishermen may be stung if they tread on or handle these species.

Clinical Features

The immediate result of a sting is intense local pain, swelling, bruising, blistering, necrosis and, if the poisonous spine is not removed, chronic sepsis (though this is unusual). Occasionally systemic symptoms including hypotensive collapse, vomiting, diarrhoea and tachycardia occur.

Treatment

Local symptoms may be relieved by immersing the affected part in very hot water. This action relieves the pain by denaturing the thermolabile toxin.

Jelly Fish

Most of the jelly fish found in British coastal waters are non-toxic as their stings cannot penetrate human skin. An exception is the Portuguese Man-of-War (*Physalia*), whose sting contains a toxic peptide, phospholipase A and a histamine-liberating factor.

Clinical Features

The main effect of a *Physalia* sting is local pain but myalgia, griping abdominal pain, nausea, dyspnoea, cyanosis and even death have occurred (in some cases within minutes).

Treatment

Treatment includes analgesia, antihistamine creams and the removal of any tentacles still adherent to the bather using adhesive tape. (The tentacles should not be brushed off with a bare hand as they may still be capable of delivering a sting for many hours after removal from the water).

Sea Urchins

The hollow spines of some sea urchins have glands which produce acetylcholine, tetramine and a neurotoxin. The latter may cause weakness of the facial muscles, lips and tongue. Treatment is supportive.

References

Halstead, BW. Poisonous and Venomous Marine Animals of the World (3 Vols). Washington: Government Printing Office, 1965–1970.

Hughes JM, Merson MH. Fish and shellfish poisoning. New Engl J Med 1976; 295:1117–20.

Kao OY, Nishiyama A. Actions of saxitoxin on peripheral neuromuscular systems. J Physiol (Lond) 1965; 180:50–66.

McCollum JPK, Pearson RCM, Ingham HR, Wood PC, Dewar HA. An epidemic of mussel poisoning in North East England. Lancet 1968; ii:767–70.

Taylor SL, Gutherty LS, Leatherwood M, Tillman F, Lieber ER. Histamine production by foodborne bacterial species. J Food Safety 1978; 1:173–87.

Further Reading

Acres J, Gray J. Paralytic shellfish poisoning. Can Med Assoc J 1978; 119:1195–7.

Bagnis R, Kuberski T, Laugier S. Clinical observations on 3009 cases of ciguatera (fish poisoning) in the South Pacific. Am J Trop Med Hyg 1979; 28:1067–73.

Clark RB. Biological causes and effects of paralytic shellfish poisoning. Lancet 1968; ii:770–2.

Editorial. Fish poisoning. Lancet 1979; ii:1059–60.

Gilbert RJ, Hobbs G, Murray CK, Cruickshank JG, Young SEJ. Scrombrotoxic fish poisoning: features of the first 50 incidents to be reported in Britain (1976–9). Br Med J 1980; 281:71–2.

Greenwood PH. The stinging weever fishes. Practitioner 1975; 215:223–5.

Hashimoto Y. Marine Toxins and Other Bioactive Marine Metabolites. Tokyo: Japan Scientific Press, 1979.

Morse EV. Paralytic shellfish poisoning: a review. J Am Vet Med Assoc 1977; 171:1178–80.

Southcott RV. Marine toxins. In Handbook of Clinical Neurology (Vol 37): Intoxication of the nervous system (Part II). Ed. Vinken PJ, Bruyn GW. Amsterdam: North Holland, 1979.

Chapter 26

G. Kazantzis

The Acute and Chronic Effects of Heavy Metal Poisoning

The effects of ingestion of a metallic compound are more often seen in the general or domestic environment, whilst the effects of absorption by inhalation are usually seen in an occupational setting. The accidental, suicidal or homicidal ingestion of a toxic metal compound gives rise to acute syndromes, usually affecting the gastrointestinal tract in the first instance, but which may secondarily involve the renal, cardiovascular, nervous or haemopoietic systems. Long-term, low-level exposure by ingestion may result from the contamination of food or drink by metals which have cumulative properties in the body.

High-level inhalational exposure usually results from an accident at work, whilst the control of long-term, low-level inhalation exposure forms a large part of industrial hygiene practice. However, such exposure may also occur in the general environment, e.g. inhalation exposure to lead from leaded petrol. Whilst acute exposures are more likely to primarily involve the respiratory system, chronic exposures may affect any organ system. The effect produced is determined not only by the dose, route and pattern of exposure, but also by the chemical and physical form of the metal. Other important factors are individual susceptibility, nutritional and immunological status, presence of intercurrent disease and interaction with other chemicals in the environment.

Acute Clinical Effects

Gastrointestinal Effects

Acute gastroenteritis follows the ingestion of a sufficient quantity of most metals in the form of soluble salts. This may result from the contamination of food or drink, giving rise to 'food poisoning' involving a number of people. Vomiting and diarrhoea may be followed by circulatory collapse and the involvement of other systems.

The ingestion of *mercuric chloride* may give rise to a bloody diarrhoea with mucosal shreds resembling fulminating ulcerative colitis, and this may be followed by the oliguria or anuria of acute renal tubular necrosis.

Acute gastroenteritis has followed the ingestion of the soluble compounds of *arsenic, antimony, cadmium, copper, iron, thallium, zinc* and other metals.

Respiratory Effects

An acute chemical pneumonitis or pulmonary oedema may follow the inhalation of a number of freshly formed metal fumes. The inhalation of *cadmium oxide fume* may give rise to acute symptoms some hours after an apparently innocuous exposure and other metals such as *arsine* and *nickel carbonyl* may do the same.

Respiratory symptoms with rigors and fever may follow some hours after the inhalation of freshly formed *zinc* or *brass fume*, or the fume of other metallic oxides, giving rise to metal fume fever or brass founder's ague.

Cardiovascular Effects

Cardiac arrhythmias, including ventricular fibrillation, may be responsible for a fatal termination following poisoning by *antimony, barium* or *lithium salts*.

Cobalt used as an additive in beer was responsible for a specific cardiomyopathy in heavy drinkers in Canada.

Central Nervous System Effects

A grand mal type of convulsive attack may be the first indication of acute *lead* poisoning, especially in a child, and this may terminate in coma or death. Convulsions may also follow the absorption of *barium, iron, lithium, thallium* and *organic tin compounds.*

An acute psychosis may be the presenting feature in a worker exposed to *tetraethyl lead*, the anti-knock additive in petrol.

Renal Effects

Oliguria and anuria have already been mentioned as occurring following ingestion of inorganic mercuric compounds such as *mercuric chloride* or corrosive sublimate. Such an effect may also follow the ingestion of *iron salts* by children.

Renal failure may be the sequel to the absorption of a number of other metal salts including *antimony, arsenic, copper* and *uranium.*

Haemopoietic Effects

An acute haemolytic anaemia associated with oliguric renal failure may be the presenting feature following the inhalation of *arsine gas*. Arsine is formed when nascent hydrogen is produced in the presence of arsenical compounds, which may only be trace impurities. It may be encountered in a variety of industries, in particular in scrap metal refineries where metallic dross comes into contact with water, in electrolytic processes, in the smelting of arsenical ores and in the manufacture of zinc chloride and sulphate. The diagnosis can only be made where the condition is suspected.

Chronic Clinical Effects

Gastrointestinal and Hepatic Effects

Chronic gastrointestinal symptoms may, in fact, be repeated mild acute attacks of poisoning, as has

occurred, for example, in persons repeatedly ingesting canned fruit juice contaminated with *tin* or *zinc*, or drinking water contaminated with *copper salts.*

Repeated attacks of intestinal colic with constipation may be caused by occupational or environmental exposure to *lead.*

A gastroenteritis followed by neuropathy with skin pigmentation should alert to the possibility of *arsenic* poisoning, whilst a gastroenteritis followed by neuropathy with the subsequent development of alopecia is the classical clinical picture of *thallium* poisoning.

A number of metals are hepatotoxins which produce effects ranging from an increase in liver enzyme levels to clinical jaundice and eventually cirrhosis. *Copper* and *iron* deposition in the liver lead to eventual cirrhosis, as seen in Wilson's disease and haemochromatosis, as can occupational *arsenic* exposure.

Respiratory Effects

Non-caseating granuloma formation followed by pulmonary fibrosis may result from occupational, or even environmental, exposure (Salem sarcoid) to *beryllium fume* or *dust*. Progressive dyspnoea may be the first manifestation of this condition many years after exposure has ceased.

Progressive dyspnoea, with the functional and radiological changes associated with emphysema, has been seen in workers exposed to *cadmium fume* or *dust*. Breathlessness due to pulmonary fibrosis has been seen in workers exposed to the dusts of *tungsten* and *titanium carbides*, with *cobalt* used as a binder. The active agent in hard metal disease, as it is called, is almost certainly the cobalt.

Sensitization to *chromate dust, vanadium pentoxide* and to *organic salts of platinum* has given rise to asthma. Once sensitization to platinum has occurred an asthmatic attack may be triggered by exposure to a minute concentration in the atmosphere, with both an immediate and a delayed reaction.

Nervous System Effects

Lead encephalopathy may be followed by permanent brain damage with cortical atrophy and hydrocephalus. The relationship between low-level, long-term lead exposure and behavioural disturbances in childhood has been considered in Chapter 28.

Manganese workers, in particular miners, have developed parkinsonism with degenerative changes in the basal ganglia.

Degenerative changes with a striking focal distribution, affecting mainly the granular layer in the cerebellum and the occipital lobes of the cortex, have followed the absorption of alkyl mercury compounds.

The characteristic clinical features of *methyl mercury* poisoning are circumoral and peripheral paraesthesiae, ataxia, dysarthria and concentric constriction of the visual fields leading, in more severe cases, to blindness.

Exposure to *inorganic mercury vapour* produces a very different clinical picture, the neurological features consisting of tremor of the hands, eyelids and tongue and a combination of behavioural and personality changes known as erethism. This consists of an abnormal, labile emotional state, nervousness, irritability and insomnia but, in a severe case, a frank psychosis may develop. The term 'mad as a hatter' referred initially to the hatters' trade, where rabbit fur was stirred in vats of hot mercuric nitrate to make felt; the workers inhaling the mercury vapour evolved in the heating process eventually went mad.

Peripheral Neuropathy

A diagnosis of peripheral neuropathy should always be followed by a careful search for evidence of exposure to a neurotoxic agent. Amongst the metals, *lead* exposure can give rise to motor neuropathy involving predominantly the most used units, such as the extensors of the hands.

The peripheral neuropathy which may follow acute *arsenical* poisoning is more often mixed motor and sensory, with a 'glove and stocking' distribution.

Those who survive the acute effects of *thallium* poisoning are likely to develop later a mixed neuropathy with ptosis, retrobulbar neuritis or facial paralysis. In one fatal case, where a psychotic fellow-worker who considered himself an amateur toxicologist dosed the morning tea with thallium to observe its effects, the presentation was that of a Guillain–Barre polyneuritis. *Bismuth* and *antimony salts* have also given rise to polyneuropathy.

Renal Effects

Proteinuria and the Nephrotic Syndrome

Proteinuria has been observed in workers exposed to *mercury vapour* and *inorganic mercury compounds*. In rare cases this has been heavy, giving rise to a nephrotic syndrome. Electron microscopy and immunofluorescent studies suggest that an immunological reaction is involved, with the deposition of antigen–antibody complexes on the glomerular basement membrane. *Gold* also gives rise to proteinuria and the nephrotic syndrome, but only following therapeutic administration in organic form in the treatment of rheumatoid arthritis. Immunofluorescent studies have shown complexes of immunoglobulin and complement.

Glomerular Nephropathy

Prolonged exposure to *lead* may result in nephropathy with interstitial fibrosis. Lead poisoning in childhood has been associated in Australia with chronic nephritis in early adult life and the subsequent development of gout. Lead poisoning should also be considered in the differential diagnosis of glycosuria in children. *Uranium* and *bismuth compounds* have also given rise to nephropathy.

Tubular Dysfunction

Cadmium is a cumulative metal in the body, the target organ following long-term, low-level exposure being the kidney. A mild, low molecular weight or tubular proteinuria has been observed in cadmium workers together with other evidence of renal tubular dysfunction, including renal glycosuria and amino aciduria, hypophosphataemia and hypercalciuria, with defects in water concentration and urinary acidification. The excretion of the low molecular weight protein β_2-microglobulin may be greatly increased and is considered to be the earliest indicator of an effect.

In Japan an increased prevalence of a severe form of osteomalacia, known as itai–itai or ouch–ouch disease, and limited to one geographical area, has been associated with a high intake of cadmium from locally grown rice and from water. The condition, first recognized after World War II, affected mainly multiparous post-menopausal women. The subjects with itai–itai disease showed evidence of renal tubular dysfunction, which epidemiological studies have shown to be more widely distributed in the endemic area. The aetiology of itai-itai disease, in a population which experienced nutritional deficiencies after the war, is still not fully elucidated, but, if not the sole causal agent, cadmium is likely to be an important determinant of the condition. The source of pollution of the river water which irrigated the rice fields was a zinc and cadmium mine upstream from the affected area. A few cases of osteomalacia have been described in cadmium workers. (Kazantzis 1979).

Haemopoietic Effects

The anaemia of chronic *lead* poisoning, which results from decreased haemopoiesis together with increased red cell destruction, has been covered in Chapter 28. Chronic *arsenic* poisoning is also associated with dyshaemopoietic anaemia with leukopenia. *Organo-gold* therapy has given rise to aplastic anaemia, granulocytopenia and thrombocytopenia.

Skin Effects

Metals are believed to develop antigenic properties and act as sensitizers by complexing with a protein, nucleic acid or polysaccharide to form a hapten—carrier conjugate. *Nickel* is probably the most common skin sensitizer, alloyed with other metals in jewellery, watch straps and fasteners. *Chromium* is another common sensitizer present in cements and used in the tanning of leather and in numerous household articles. A similar allergic dermatitis together with conjunctivitis can be produced by *cobalt* and by *platinum*. Skin sensitization to *beryllium* and to *zirconium* is associated with subcutaneous non-caseating granuloma formation.

Diagnosis of Heavy Metal Poisoning

The above account demonstrates the wide range of clinical effects observed in both acute and chronic poisoning by metallic compounds. There are only a few instances where a clear sequence of events or specific features occur which point to a specific form of metal poisoning. Amongst such specific features should be mentioned the garlic-like odour of the breath in poisoning by *selenium* or *tellurium compounds* and the raindrop pigmentation of the skin following exposure to *arsenic*.

History of Occupational Exposure

A history of exposure will more often provide the vital clue involved in a poisoning case. In an industrial situation this may be obtained from the patient, a relative, co-worker or employer, occupational hygienist, works medical officer or health and safety representative. The clinician should not fail to take a full and accurate occupational history. A history of exposure may not be obtained from any of the persons questioned, but may be inferred from a knowledge of the work processes involved, as in the example given on exposure to arsine gas in the section on haemopoietic effects. In the domestic environment, the need to collect and label pills, household chemicals, containers, vomit, etc., has already been described in Chapters 3 and 4. In the general environment, metal poisoning, especially if caused by long-term absorption of small amounts of a cumulative metal, can present a very difficult epidemiological problem. Methyl mercury poisoning in the fisher folk of Minamata Bay took more than five years to diagnose correctly (McAlpine and Araki 1958).

Laboratory Investigations

Toxicological and biochemical investigation should, of course, be performed along standard lines. Analysis of hair and of nail clippings may provide valuable evidence of exposure at a stage where examination of blood and urine samples is no longer helpful. It should be borne in mind that trace metal analysis of biological samples may be technically difficult and is best performed in special centres.

Treatment

The general principles for the management of the poisoned patient, such as prevention of further absorption of the poison, general supportive therapy and elimination of the absorbed poison have been considered in Chapter 4.

Chelating Agents

There are certain antidotes which have been specifically designed to compete for heavy metals with ligands essential for normal function (see Chapter 5). These heavy metal antagonists or chelating agents form a stable complex with the metal as a heterocyclic ring (Levine 1975). However, these agents are not without toxic effects themselves and they should not be administered where removal from further exposure or other simple measures would suffice to promote recovery.

Dimercaprol

This, the first of the chelating agents, is a dithiol compound which competes with sulphydryl groups for *arsenic compounds*, and for other heavy metals, particularly *inorganic mercury*. If given sufficiently early, it can be life-saving where a potentially lethal dose has been ingested. Dimercaprol is given by deep intramuscular injection on a body weight basis. In full dosage it may have unpleasant and even alarming side-effects.

Dimercaprol should *not* be given in chronic cadmium poisoning because of a nephrotoxic effect, or in organo-mercury poisoning where the uptake of organic mercury into the brain may even be enhanced. Dimercaprol may also be deleterious in selenium and tellurium poisoning.

Penicillamine

This is a particularly effective chelating agent for *copper, lead* and *mercury*, and is also effective in cases of poisoning with *iron* and *zinc*. Penicillamine is well absorbed from the gut and is normally given by mouth. It is rapidly excreted in the urine. It is a relatively non-toxic compound, although it demonstrates cross-sensitivity with penicillin and may also be nephrotoxic. It has been given for long periods in the treatment of Wilson's disease.

Desferrioxamine

This is the chelating agent of choice in the treatment of *iron* poisoning. Given by mouth it chelates and inactivates iron present in the gut, but is poorly absorbed and so has, in addition, to be given parenterally. It may be given intramuscularly or by slow intravenous infusion, when it rapidly complexes with available iron and is excreted in the urine. It should be used with caution where renal function is impaired, and hypersensitive and even anaphylactic reactions have occurred.

Calcium Disodium Edetate

This chelating agent is very effective in the treatment of *lead* poisoning, but may have toxic effects in the chelation of other metals. It is poorly absorbed from the GI tract and has to be given by intravenous infusion over a period of one to two hours. Its administration has to be monitored with care, particularly with regard to its possible nephotoxic effect.

Prussian Blue

Potassium ferric hexacyanoferrate (II) has been used successfully in the treatment of *thallium* poisoning. Following its administration by mouth, the potassium ion in the prussian blue molecule is replaced by thallium, thus rendering the metal inabsorbable and also increasing the movement of thallium into the gut. Constipation should be treated and potassium chloride should also be given intravenously with appropriate monitoring.

Diethyldithiocarbamate

This chelating agent has been used in the treatment of acute *nickel* poisoning and found to be of value.

Diethylenetriaminopentacetic Acid (DTPA)

This chelating agent appears to be effective in the chelation of *plutonium* and its subsequent excretion in the urine. One gram of DTPA given by slow intravenous infusion on alternate days for three weeks is effective.

References

Kazantzis G. Renal tubular dysfunction and abnormalities of calcium metabolism in cadmium workers. Environ Health Perspect 1979; 28:155–9.

Levine WG. Heavy metal antagonists. In: The Pharmacological Basis of Therapeutics. 5th edition: Goodman LS, Gilman A. Eds. New York: Macmillan, 1975; 912–45.

McAlpine D, Araki S. Minamata disease – an unusual neurological disorder caused by contaminated fish. Lancet 1958; ii:629–31.

Further Reading

Bair WJ, Thompson RC. Plutonium: biomedical research. Science 1974; 183:715–22.

Cavanagh JB, Fuller NH, Johnson HRM, Rudge P. The effects of thallium salts with particular reference to the nervous system changes. Q J Med 1974; 43:293–319.

Friberg L, Nordberg GF, Vouk VB, Eds. Handbook on the Toxicology of Metals. Amsterdam: Elsevier, 1979.

Goyer RA, Mehlman MA. Toxicology of Trace Elements. London: John Wiley & Sons, 1977.

Hunter D. The Diseases of Occupations. London: Hodder and Stoughton, 1978, 6th edition.

Chapter 27

T. J. Meredith and J. A. Vale

Iron Poisoning

Many different oral iron preparations are available on the market, and acute iron poisoning was once a common cause of death in young children. An increased awareness of the problem, changes in the forms of packaging and use of the chelating agent, desferrioxamine, have together resulted in a decline in the mortality from acute iron poisoning. Indeed, in the nine-year period, 1968 to 1976, only nine deaths were officially attributed to the ingestion of iron preparations by children under 15 years of age. Even so, iron poisoning is extremely dangerous, especially in young children, and particularly when more than 150 mg/kg body weight is ingested. Rapid necrosis of the gastrointestinal mucosa occurs, resulting in haemorrhage and fluid and electrolyte loss. The absorbed iron rapidly exceeds the binding capacity of transferrin and free serum iron builds up. Severe poisoning is indicated by serum iron levels in excess of 90 μmol/l (5 mg/l) in a child and 145 μmol/l (8 mg/l) in an adult. The clinical features of iron poisoning are described in the next section. In severe acute iron poisoning death may occur after only a few hours. If the patient survives and subsequently develops hepatic necrosis, death may occur at this stage also. The late development of pyloric stenosis has been described in a few patients following recovery from severe iron poisoning.

Clinical Features of Acute Iron Poisoning

Epigastric pain, nausea, vomiting and haematemesis may all occur within several hours of ingesting iron, accompanied by circulatory collapse if the haematemesis is severe. Subsequently black tarry stools may be passed and any one, or all, of the following complications may develop: acute encephalopathy (headache, confusion, convulsions, coma), cyanosis and pulmonary oedema, metabolic acidosis, acute renal failure, circulatory collapse and death. If the patient survives then hepatic necrosis may develop, sometimes proceeding to hepatic coma and death.

Treatment

Desferrioxamine mesylate (Desferal) (see page 35) should be given as follows in the treatment of acute iron poisoning. First 2 g of desferrioxamine (in 10 ml sterile water) should be injected intramuscularly. Gastric aspiration and lavage should then be performed using a solution of 2 g desferrioxamine in each litre of warm water; when this procedure has been completed 5 g of desferrioxamine (in 50 to 100 ml water) should be left in the stomach. Following this either a slow infusion of desferrioxamine should be administered at a rate not exceeding 15 mg/kg body weight/hr (maximum 80 mg/kg body weight in 24 hours) or further intramuscular injections (2 g in 10 ml sterile water) should be given at 12-hourly intervals.

The patient's progress should be checked with the aid of serial serum iron determinations. The effectiveness of treatment is dependent on an adequate urine output in order that the chelate, ferrioxamine, is excreted from the body. Therefore, if oliguria or anuria develop, peritoneal dialysis or haemodialysis may become necessary to remove the ferrioxamine complex.

Further Reading

Barr GDB, Fraser DKB. Acute iron poisoning in children: role of chelating agents. Br Med J 1968; 1:737–41.

Chisholm JJ. Poisoning due to heavy metals. Pediatr Clin North Am 1970; 17:591–615.

Greengard J. Iron poisoning in children. Clin Toxicol 1975; 8:575–97.

Haddad LM Iron poisoning. J Am Coll Emerg Phy 1976; 5:691–3.

Wallack MK, Winkelstein A. Acute iron intoxication in an adult. J Am Med Assoc 1974; 229:1333–4.

Westlin WF. Deferoxamine as a chelating agent. Clin Toxicol 1971; 4:597–60.

Whitten CF, Brough AJ. The pathophysiology of acute iron poisoning. Clin Toxicol 1971; 4:585–95.

Chapter 28

Donald Barltrop

Lead Poisoning

In contrast to many of the commonly encountered poisons, lead has a number of distinctive features. It is one of the elements which occurs naturally in the earth's crust, and has been extracted and used by mankind for at least 5000 years. Moreover, lead poisoning is a chronic and insidious process resulting from sustained or repeated exposures, which are usually inadvertent, and in which the hazard is unknown or unsuspected.

One of the earliest descriptions of lead poisoning was by Hippocrates in 300 BC, who reported a case of colic in a metal worker probably engaged in the extraction of lead. The hazard of occupational lead poisoning persists to the present day but it is non-occupational exposure, where the potential for lead poisoning may be suspected, that provides the greater risk. Many of the early records of lead poisoning are related to the contamination of beverages; poisoning due to the adulteration of wine with lead acetate (sugar of lead) was recognized in the Middle Ages. Massive outbreaks of lead poisoning due to the contamination of water supplies in Europe, rum in the Caribbean, and cider in SW England were reported in the eighteenth century when the use of lead piping and lead sheet became widespread.

The Industrial Revolution saw a proliferation of the use of lead and its compounds so that, at the turn of the century, lead poisoning was a common industrial disease with about 1000 cases per annum in the UK alone. Since then the picture has changed markedly. The progressive introduction of occupational health monitoring has reduced the exposure of workers in the lead industries and has eliminated fatalities. However, paradoxically the recognition of lead poisoning as a cause of illness and death in other members of the population, notably among children, has increased during the last few decades, perhaps reflecting an increased awareness of environmental hazards and improved laboratory methods for detection. Recently a new dimension has been added by claims that exposure to amounts of lead insufficient to cause clinically evident disease (sub-clinical lead poisoning) may have deleterious effects on the neurophysiological functions of infants and young children.

Lead Metabolism

Ingestion and Inhalation

All environments contain some lead, and varying amounts of this must inescapably be absorbed and contribute to the body burden. A knowledge of this 'background' exposure is necessary in order to interpret the significance of particular sources suspected of causing clinical poisoning. Lead can be detected in foodstuffs, beverages, water supplies, soils and dusts, and the atmosphere, in amounts which will vary according to the locality, so that only representative values can be given in this context. Inorganic lead can be absorbed only from the gut or from the lung. The contribution from all sources are summated in the body and cannot normally be distinguished from each other. It is thought that, on average, about 10 per cent of ingested lead is absorbed as opposed to about 30 per cent of inhaled lead, although there may be considerable individual and temporal variations·in these proportions.

If it is assumed that an adult ingests about 1 kg of food daily containing 0.1 p.p.m. lead (100 μg), and that his daily respiratory volume is 15 m^3 of an atmosphere containing 1 μg/m^3 lead, then the relevant

Table 28.1.	Lead intake and absorption by an adult.		
Source	Intake µg/dl	Uptake µg/dl	% Total uptake
Food	100	10	67
Air	15	5	33
Total	115	15	100

proportions of body lead contributed from these sources can be calculated (Table 28.1). It follows that about two-thirds of the body lead would be derived directly from the diet and about one-third from the atmosphere. However, it should be noted that no allowance has been made for the contribution from contaminated dusts or drinking water. Moreover, no assumptions have been made concerning the indirect contribution which atmospheric lead might make to the other sources.

Absorption

Lead not absorbed by the gut is excreted in the faeces so that faecal lead measurements provide a valuable index of ingested lead. Many factors may modify the absorption of lead including its chemical and physical form and, in the case of ingested lead, the composition of the diet and the nutritional status of the individual.

Binding to Erythrocytes and Bone

After absorption, lead enters the blood where it is rapidly taken up by the erythrocytes (ca. 97 per cent), only about 3 per cent remaining in the plasma. Although firmly bound to the erythrocytes with a half life of two to three weeks, the equilibrium is reversible and redistribution to other soft tissues takes place, notably to the liver and kidney. Ultimately soft tissue lead is either excreted in the urine or bile, or· deposited in the calcified tissues, i.e. the bones and teeth. Small amounts are shed with the hair, nails and other epidermal tissues.

The binding to bone takes place in two phases. First, an initial absorption occurs at the bone surface where lead remains exchangeable. Second, the lead is incorporated into the hydroxy-apatite crystal where it is less accessible. Accumulation in the calcified tissues is progressive and lifelong whereas soft tissue lead binding is transient and reversible. Lead sequestered in bone appears to be metabolically inert.

Blood Lead Levels

Circulating blood lead reflects a smoothed or integrated short-term index of the balance between absorption on the one hand and excretion plus deposition on the other. The blood lead concentration may take weeks or months to reach an equilibrium when intake is increased, and may take months or one to two years to return to normal after cessation of exposure.

Blood lead values in a given population have a log normal distribution and most individuals have blood lead values of less than 35 µg/dl (1.7 µmol/l) with values typically in the range 10 to 20 µg/dl (0.5 to 1.0 µmol/l). Children in the UK have blood lead concentrations a few µg/dl greater than those of adults living in the same environment and, in addition, show a seasonal variation of the same order with greater values in the summer months.

The Biochemical and Toxic Action of Lead

The precise mode of action of lead in the body is unknown and, although it is thought that its affinity for free sulphydryl groups is important, it is probably not the only mechanism involved. Not all of the signs and symptoms of lead poisoning can yet be explained in biochemical terms. For clinical purposes the interaction with porphyrin biosynthesis and with the nervous system are the most important.

Diagnosis of Lead Poisoning

Effects on Porphyrin Synthesis

Lead is known to interact with several steps in the porphyrin synthetic pathway, which culminates in the synthesis of heme, and many tests for the detection of lead poisoning have been based on this (Figure 28.1). Such tests depend on either the measurement of the activity of the enzyme catalysing a particular step or the measurement of the corresponding metabolite immediately preceding the enzyme affected. The tests vary greatly in their ability to detect the effects of lead and some are now of only historical significance. Guidelines as to the blood lead concentrations at which abnormal results might begin to be detected are as follows:

Test	Blood Lead µg/dl
Haemoglobin	80
Coproporphyrin	60
ALA Urine	40
FEP	20
ALAD	10

Anaemia is a late manifestation of lead poisoning and, similarly, coproporphyrin excretion is too insensitive to be of clinical value. Conversely ALAD is partly inhibited in even 'normally' exposed populations and is thus too sensitive for clinical use. For all practical purposes, therefore, measurements are now restricted to ALA in urine and to the concentration of free erythrocyte protoporphyrin (FEP) in the peripheral blood. However, neither of these tests is specific for lead exposure as ALA excretion in the urine may be increased after the ingestion of alcohol and erythrocyte protoporphyrin is increased as a result of iron deficiency.

Peripheral Blood Changes

Typically lead poisoning will give rise to a hypochromic anaemia in spite of normal values for serum iron and iron binding capacity, thus resembling a sidero-achrestic anaemia. There is some evidence that a haemolytic anaemia with reticulocytosis can also occur. In severe lead poisoning in adults (and to a certain extent in children), the persistence of nuclear material on the red cell membrane of the mature erythrocyte may give rise to a characteristic basophilic stippling. A confusing aspect is that iron deficiency is common among the underprivileged children in whom lead poisoning tends to occur, and may itself potentiate lead absorption from the gut.

Figure 28.1. *Sites of interference of heme synthesis by lead and tests for the detection of lead poisoning.*

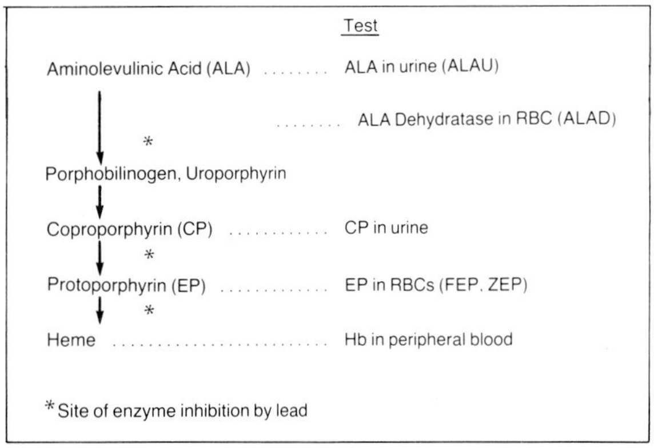

	Test
Aminolevulinic Acid (ALA)	ALA in urine (ALAU)
	.... ALA Dehydratase in RBC (ALAD)
↓ *	
Porphobilinogen, Uroporphyrin	
↓	
Coproporphyrin (CP)	CP in urine
↓ *	
Protoporphyrin (EP)	EP in RBCs (FEP, ZEP)
↓ *	
Heme	Hb in peripheral blood

* Site of enzyme inhibition by lead

Urine Analysis

The urine may contain excessive amounts of the porphyrin precursors, aminolevulinic acid and coproporphyrin, but it is doubtful whether these now have clinical value in the diagnosis of a suspected case of lead poisoning. These tests may, nevertheless, have an application in the monitoring of individuals with known and continuing exposure, e.g. in industry. Symptomatic lead poisoning is associated with impaired renal tubular function so that aminoaciduria, phosphaturia and glycosuria occur, thus resembling the Fanconi syndrome. In adults, impaired renal function may lead to hyperuricaemia and 'saturnine' gout. Urine lead determination is of limited value for diagnostic purposes.

Skeletal Changes

Recognisable skeletal changes due to lead poisoning are confined to children. They comprise characteristic dense metaphyseal bands at the growing ends of the long bones ('lead lines'), notably at the wrist and the knee. The lines are due to excessive deposition of bone mineral, presumably as a consequence of impaired bone resorption. These changes do not appear until several weeks after the onset of exposure and persist for months or years after its cessation, in a manner analogous to 'growth arrest' lines. Failure of remodelling of the femur can occur so that the distal end loses its characteristic shape, but this is nonspecific.

A plain film of the abdomen is mandatory in both adults and children suspected of having ingested metallic lead or other lead-containing materials such as flakes of lead-based paint. Although radio-opaque material in the gut is highly suggestive of lead ingestion, finely divided material may escape detection.

In young children with encephalopathy, x-ray of the skull may reveal signs of raised intracranial pressure with 'springing' of the sutures. Although rare, lead-containing foreign bodies, such as lead shot, may give rise to lead poisoning, particularly when lodged in close relation to synovial and mucosal surfaces.

Cerebrospinal Fluid Changes

Changes in the cerebrospinal fluid are a late manifestation of lead poisoning, and are indicative of actual or impending encephalopathy. The changes are nonspecific and can comprise increased protein content and some pleocytosis. They cannot be distinguished from the early stages of a viral meningoencephalitis with which lead encephalopathy can readily be confused.

Neurophysiological Effects

Involvement of both the central and peripheral nervous systems has been mentioned. EEG changes are late and non-specific, and are indistinguishable from other generalized encephalopathies. When compared with controls, diminution in peripheral nerve conduction time has been reported in groups of lead workers and in others with sustained exposure. However, although such comparisons reveal a statistically significant difference between the groups, the values seldom fall into the pathological range and are of limited value for diagnostic purposes.

Blood Lead Levels

The determination of the lead concentration in blood remains the only practical and definitive test for the confirmation of the diagnosis of lead poisoning.

The analysis requires an uncontaminated sample of whole blood collected with scrupulous care. Although this can be achieved with capillary samples by specially trained staff, venous blood samples are to be preferred. Commercially available tubes containing an anticoagulant are usually acceptable but the analyst concerned should be consulted before obtaining the specimen.

A variety of macro and microanalytical techniques may be used for the measurement of lead in blood and, of these, electrothermal (flameless) atomic absorption spectrophotometry is now predominant. Many laboratories in the UK participate in a National Quality Control Scheme in order to verify their performance and to maintain their analytical standards. Interpretation of the results should take into account the coefficient of variation for the analysis which, in most laboratories, is likely to be of the order of 5 to 10 per cent.

Clinical Picture of Lead Poisoning

Clinical Features

The clinical features of undue exposure to lead are non-specific in both adults and children. In the early stages of exposure blood lead values are increased and biochemical anomalies can be detected in the absence of any recognisable features in the individual. Subsequently symptoms such as lassitude, colicky abdominal pain and constipation may occur. Pallor, due to anaemia, is a relatively late feature. In severe sustained exposure, CNS involvement leads to impaired consciousness, seizures and other features of raised intracranial pressure. Blue lines at the gingival margins have been described in abnormally exposed adults, particularly in association with poor dental hygiene. However, these lines are now rare and virtually unknown in childhood. Peripheral nerve palsies, resulting in wrist drop and foot drop, were formerly encountered as complications of occupational exposure but are now rare. Insomnia and lack of concentration have been described but their significance is difficult to determine.

Grades of Exposure

Although the symptomatology is progressive with continuing exposure, assessment of the severity of the disorder must involve the determination of the blood lead concentration and, ideally, another index of the metabolic response to lead such as the erythrocyte protoporphyrin value. Four clinical grades of exposure can therefore be defined:

1. Grade I – 'normal' exposure.

2. Grade II – asymptomatic with early metabolic changes.

3. Grade III – symptomatic with marked biochemical changes, abdominal pain, constipation and lassitude.

4. Grade IV – neurological involvement – impaired consciousness, seizures and coma.

There is, however, considerable overlap in the blood lead values associated with these clinical grades and while Grade I is, by definition, associated with blood lead values in the range 0 to 40 μg/dl, the remaining grades are less clearly distinguished. In general, individuals with blood lead values of <60 μg/dl might be expected to be asymptomatic and those with blood lead concentrations of >100 μg/dl are at risk of encephalopathy. It should be noted, however, that occupational exposures resulting in blood lead concentrations of the order of 80 μg/dl are seldom associated with symptoms, whereas children with blood lead values in the 80 to 100 μg/dl range have occasionally developed a lead-induced encephalopathy.

It follows that the symptomatology cannot be predicted precisely from a particular blood lead value, and that the various clinical grades of exposure may be associated with wide and overlapping ranges of blood lead concentration. It is, however, important to note that, although it normally takes three to four months of exposure to develop severe lead poisoning, progression through the grades occurs at an accelerating rate. Thus, encephalopathy and death may supervene in a child with severe Grade III (symptomatic) poisoning even after admission to hospital in order to remove the child from the sources of lead.

Alternative Classification

An alternative approach to the classification of paediatric lead poisoning has been advocated by the United States Center for Disease Control in which four categories of lead poisoning are described on the basis of both lead and erythrocyte protoporphyrin measurements, namely:

1. Class I – normal.
2. Class II – minimal.
3. Class III – moderate.
4. Class IV – extreme.

The initial classification is on the basis of the blood lead concentration but is subsequently modified according to the erythrocyte protoporphyrin value. The scheme introduced two sub-groups, class Ia with a normal blood lead but raised erythrocyte protoporphyrin and class Ib with a raised blood lead but a normal erythrocyte protoporphyrin. This approach may have some merit for the interpretation of blood lead screening data, e.g. in an exposed population, but its validity as a guide to clinical management has yet to be established.

Coexistent iron deficiency, which is itself associated with increased erythrocyte protoporphyrin values, would result in the assignation of a more severe class than would otherwise be the case. Thus, class Ia 'lead poisoning' (blood lead <29 μg/dl, EP >59 μg/dl) represents iron deficiency in an individual not unduly exposed to lead. Nevertheless, in children, erythrocyte protoporphyrin values >60 μg/dl may be regarded as abnormal and values >200 μg/dl as markedly increased. In severe lead poisoning erythrocyte protoporphyrin values in excess of 1000 μg/dl have been encountered.

Subclinical Lead Poisoning

Recently a number of subclinical effects have been attributed to lead. These have included impaired intelligence, behavioural disturbance, poor educational attainment and minor defects of coordination.

While there is no doubt that many of these problems can be detected as sequelae of encephalopathy, opinion is divided as to whether they may arise as a result of low level exposures to lead. None of the anomalies is specific for lead poisoning so that it is difficult, or impossible, to ascribe them to this cause in individuals. Many of the studies in which these features have been described relate to the comparison of exposed with control populations which have not always been adequately matched.

Further research is in progress to test the hypothesis that blood lead values in the range of 40 to 80 μg/dl are deleterious to central or peripheral nervous function.

Management of Lead Poisoning

The three cardinal principles governing the clinical management of the individual with lead poisoning are as follows:

1. Provision of a safe environment.
2. Reduction of soft tissue lead burdens.
3. Identification and correction of the source.

The urgency and degree to which these principles are applied will depend on the severity of the exposure and the likelihood that it will be sustained.

Monitoring of Blood Lead Levels

In many industries adults subject to lead exposure are monitored by means of regular blood lead determinations at appropriate intervals. At present, in the UK, blood lead values of <80 μg/dl are considered acceptable for adult male workers and compatible with continuing employment. Workers with blood lead values of 80 to 100 μg/dl are permitted to continue in their occupations subject to more frequent blood lead determinations and stringent medical supervision. Employees with blood lead values of >100 μg/dl must be withdrawn from the workplace and either transferred to other duties or given leave until their blood lead values have returned to acceptable levels.

Individuals employed in small enterprises, and particularly those engaged in the cutting and recovery of scrap metals or in the preparation of metal structures for repainting, may escape medical supervision. Women of reproductive age should not be engaged in occupations involving exposure to lead which are likely to increase the blood lead concentrations to above 40 μg/dl.

Individuals who are not known to be occupationally exposed, but, nevertheless, are found to have markedly raised blood lead values of, say, greater than 60 μg/dl should be considered for admission to hospital as a means of preventing further exposure pending identification of the source. Temporary transfer of the place of residence is a less satisfactory alternative. Patients with blood lead values of >60 μg/dl may be followed on an outpatient basis, provided that close medical supervision is maintained and blood lead determinations are repeated at intervals of not more than two to three weeks.

Chelation Therapy

Diminution in the lead concentration of the blood and other soft tissues will occur in the absence of further exposure as a result of excretion and deposition in bone. However, the rate of decrease in blood lead values is slow, and months or even one to three years may elapse before normal values are attained. In the period immediately after cessation of ingestion the blood lead may, however, transiently increase. This is due to continued absorption of lead from residual material in the gut. Chelation therapy, although effective in reducing blood lead values, has some attendant risks (e.g. renal damage) so that it is a matter of judgement as to when these are outweighed by the benefits to be conferred.

Drugs Employed

Three drugs with metal binding properties have been used in the treatment of lead poisoning. D-penicillamine, calcium versenate (Ca-EDTA) and BAL (British Anti Lewisite) — see Chapter 5. The dosage regimes are given in Table 28.2.

In severe cases, i.e. acute encephalopathy, the EDTA and BAL therapy may be given simultaneously, divided into four-hourly doses by deep intramuscular injection at separate sites. The calcium EDTA injection may be painful and require the addition of procaine. BAL may induce vomiting. In less severe cases, Ca-EDTA or penicillamine alone are used according to the severity of the exposure.

Table 28.2. Daily dosage of chelating agents for lead poisoning in adults and children.

Chelating agent	Paediatric dosage (mg/m^2)	Adult dosage
D-penicillamine	600	250 mg–2 g orally
Dimercaprol	500	15–30 mg/kg i.m.
Calcium EDTA	1 500	50–75 mg/kg i.v. or i.m.

Treatment with BAL is discontinued after 48 hours if possible, but can be given for up to a maximum of five days. Ca-EDTA, whether alone or in combination with BAL, is normally given for five days in the first instance but a further five day course of Ca-EDTA alone can be repeated after an interval of one to two days. Oral penicillamine may be continued for several weeks, either as the initial treatment or following a course of treatment with the parenteral drugs.

Although blood lead values are rapidly reduced by chelating drugs, some rebound always occurs after the initial course. This is due to internal redistribution of lead from sites which are inaccessible to the chelating agent. The blood lead concentration should, therefore, always be rechecked several days after the chelating treatment has been discontinued.

Criteria for Use of Chelating Drugs

The criteria for the use of chelating drugs tend to be more stringent in paediatric as opposed to adult practice. While it is impossible to lay down rigid guidelines chelation of exposed children with penicillamine should be considered at pretreatment blood lead concentrations of 60 to 80 μg/dl and with Ca-EDTA at blood lead values of >80 μg/dl. Some authors advocate the addition of BAL, for a period of 48 to 72 hours, to Ca-EDTA therapy for children with blood lead values in the range 80 to 100 μg/dl, but others reserve the use of BAL for those with grossly elevated blood lead values or with actual or impending encephalopathy.

In adults the choice of chelation therapy is governed by similar considerations, but it is implemented at greater blood lead concentrations than are permitted in children. Thus, chelation treatment with penicillamine would be considered in a lead worker with a blood lead value of >100 μg/dl, although a lesser value would be reasonable in the non-occupationally exposed.

Non-Specific Measures

Other non-specific measures in addition to chelation may be required in acute encephalopathy, including the administration of diazepam or paraldehyde to control seizures and the use of mannitol to establish an adequate urine flow. Parenteral fluids, however, should be restricted to basal requirements. Surgical decompression procedures should be avoided.

All treated patients should be kept under regular review until the blood lead and erythrocyte proto-porphyrin values have returned to normal. The purpose of this continuing supervision is to ensure that further undue exposure does not recur when the patient is returned to his previous environment, and that the presumed source of lead has been correctly identified and eliminated. The margin of safety for any individual is reduced while the blood lead concentration remains increased.

Identification of Lead Source

An essential part of clinical management is the identification of the source of lead to which the patient was exposed. It is axiomatic that the poisoned individual should not be returned to his previous environment until it has been made safe.

Occupational Lead Poisoning

In the UK occupational lead poisoning is a notifiable disease and correction of the working environment is the responsibility of the Health and Safety Executive. Essential features in the control of industrial lead poisoning include a programme of continuing education of the work force, scrupulous attention to hygiene, the provision of industrial clothing and facilities for those to be laundered, and a double locker system and adequate washing and showering facilities in changing accommodation. The consumption of foodstuffs and tobacco products should be prohibited at the workplace and separate facilities for this made available. Where necessary, industrial respirators should be used. Nevertheless, individual workers may not always comply with the advice that is given or fully utilize the facilities which are available.

Domestic Lead Poisoning

The detection of a lead source for the non-occupationally exposed adult, and for children, requires careful investigation of the domestic environment and detailed knowledge of the individual's habits and activities.

In children, the most common source of lead poisoning is old lead-based paint in or around the home, particularly where this is flaking or poorly maintained. Samples for analysis should be obtained from all painted surfaces accessible to the child including windowsills, toys and nursery furniture. Special attention should be given to painted surfaces which show signs of damage or tooth marks attributable to the child.

Lead water pipes and storage tanks are a potent source of lead in areas with soft acidic water supplies which are plumbo-solvent, notably in parts of Scotland and Wales. Early morning 'first flush' samples of water should be obtained for analysis.

The use of electric motor car batteries for domestic fuel and the domestic manufacture of lead-containing articles such as fishing weights and certain types of jewellery should be excluded.

Asian families should be questioned as to the use of Surma and Hakim medicines, both of which may contain substantial amounts of lead.

A potent and frequently unsuspected source arises from the storage or fermentation of acidic foodstuffs and beverages in glazed ceramic or old pewter vessels.

A useful approach is the determination of blood lead values for all members of the family group. The profile thus obtained will indicate whether a specific source for one individual is involved or whether a more generalized source affecting the whole family is operative. For example, blood lead values with a gradient child>mother>father would suggest a domestic source such as contaminated foodstuff, whereas the reverse gradient would be compatible with contaminated industrial clothing brought to the home for laundering. A general elevation of blood lead values for the whole family would suggest an external source such as local industry, and would indicate the need for more extensive sampling of the local environment and other individuals in the locality.

Remedial Measures

The investigation of domestic sources of lead in the UK is the responsibility of the local environmental health department. However, remedial measures are not always readily achieved. The most common problem arises with the discovery of lead-based paint as a source of childhood lead poisoning. This requires the complete scraping and repainting of all surfaces accessible to the child with a paint of low lead content.

Extensive renovation of paint work, particularly where this involves burning or sanding, will itself release substantial amounts of lead-containing dust sufficient to provide an unacceptable lead burden for the child and other occupants of the house. Temporary or permanent rehousing should therefore be considered.

Further Reading

Chisolm JJ, Barltrop D. Recognition and management of children with increased lead absorption. Arch Dis Child 1979; 54:249—62.

Lead and Health. The Report of a DHSS Working Party on Lead in the Environment. HMSO, 1980.

Chapter 29

J. A. Vale and T. J. Meredith

Poisoning due to Miscellaneous Agents

Poisoning due to Antimuscarinic Drugs

The drugs described in this section inhibit the actions of acetylcholine on autonomic effectors innervated by postganglionic nerves, as well as on smooth muscles that lack cholinergic innervation, i.e., they antagonize the muscarinic actions of acetylcholine. The naturally occurring antimuscarinic drugs are the alkaloids of the belladonna plants. The most clinically important of these are atropine and scopolamine. Many semi-synthetic compounds, usually quaternary ammonium derivatives, have been developed. In addition, a large number of synthetic antimuscarinic compounds with structures unrelated to those of the naturally occurring belladonna alkaloids have been produced. Some of the above compounds, including atropine in high dosage, block transmission at autonomic ganglia and skeletal neuromuscular junctions. The ganglion blocking action is particularly marked with the quaternary ammonium compounds such as propantheline.

The belladonna alkaloids are absorbed rapidly from the GI tract, mucosal surfaces, and from parenteral sites.

Infants and young children are especially susceptible to the belladonna alkaloids and poisoning has occurred after conjunctival instillation; systemic absorption occurring from the nasal mucosa after the drug has traversed the nasolacrimal duct. In addition, serious poisoning may follow the accidental ingestion of berries or seeds containing belladonna alkaloids (Chapter 30 p 198). In recent years, asthma remedies containing stramonium have been abused for their hallucinatory effects.

Clinical Features

Dry mouth, nausea and vomiting.
Fixed dilated pupils, blurring of vision, photophobia.
Mental confusion, ataxia, excitement, hallucinations.
Tachycardia, cardiac arrhythmias, hyperpyrexia.
Urinary urgency and retention.

Note: The combination of parasympathetic blockade and central stimulation can produce a clinical syndrome described in the following mnemonic:

> Blind as a bat;
> Dry as a bone;
> Red as a beet;
> Hot as a hare;
> Mad as a hatter.

Treatment

1. Emesis or gastric lavage, if appropriate.

2. Supportive and symptomatic treatment.

3. Neostigmine 0.25 mg subcutaneously will reverse the peripheral effects.

4. Physostigmine 1 to 4 mg i.v. will antagonize the central effects but its action is short-lived.

In Lomotil (atropine + diphenoxylate) poisoning the initial clinical features are due to atropine; these are followed by those of diphenoxylate, i.e. cardio-respiratory depression and an impaired level of consciousness. Naloxone should be given to reverse the effects of diphenoxylate (Chapter 15 p 113).

Further Reading

Baker JP, Farley JD. Toxic psychosis following atropine eye drops. Br Med J 1958; 2:1390–2.

Beach GO, Fitzgerald RP, Holmes R. Phibbs B, Stuckenhoff H, Scopolamine poisoning. New Engl J Med 1964; 270:1354–5.

Blackburn WD, Spyker DA. Poisoning with homatropine. Va Med 1979; 106:689–91.

Boyd CE, Boyd EM. The acute toxicity of atropine sulfate. Can Med Assoc J 1961; 85:1241–4.

Carney MWP. Atropine poisoning. Br Med J 1974; 2:334.

Curtis JA, Goel KM. Lomotil poisoning in children. Arch Dis Child 1979; 54:222–25.

Duvoisin RC, Katz R. Reversal of central anticholinergic syndrome in man by physostigmine. J Am Med Assoc 1968; 206: 1963–5.

Mackenzie AL, Pigott JFG. Atropine overdose in three children. Br J Anaesth 1971; 43:1088–90.

Penfold D, Volans GN. Overdose from Lomotil. Br Med J 1977; 2:1401–2.

Welbourn RB, Buxton JD; Acute atopine poisoning: review of eight cases. Lancet 1948; ii:211–3.

Poisoning due to Hypoglycaemic Agents

Intentional overdose with hypoglycaemic agents is uncommon and is often difficult to recognise. Martin (1977) found 21 cases of suicidal insulin overdose in a review of the literature and reported an additional four cases of his own. In addition, two other cases have been reported in the forensic literature (Dickson et al. 1977; Sturner and Putman 1972). The overall mortality in these reports was 27 per cent. Most deliberate insulin overdoses are due to long-acting preparations. Despite the massive doses of insulin often associated with intentional poisoning, the degree of hypoglycaemia is sometimes surprisingly mild, though it may persist for several days.

Of 16 patients reported in the literature who deliberately ingested one of the sulphonylurea drugs, six died. Chlorpropamide has been the oral agent most commonly ingested and because of its long halflife it may, in overdose, induce hypoglycaemia for a considerable period.

In all cases of poisoning with hypoglycaemic agents, prompt diagnosis and treatment is essential if death or cerebral damage from neuroglycopenia is to be prevented.

Clinical Features

Nausea and vomiting.
Abdominal pain, rarely haematemesis and melaena.
Drowsiness, coma, twitching, convulsions.
Depressed limb reflexes with extensor plantar responses.
Hypernoea, acute pulmonary oedema.
Tachycardia, hypotension, circulatory failure.
Absence of sweating.
Hypoglycaemia, hyperkalaemia, metabolic (lactic) acidosis, leucocytosis.
(Late complication) Cholestatic jaundice following chlorpropamide.

Treatment

1. Emesis or gastric lavage, if appropriate.

2. Supportive treatment.

3. 50 ml of 50 per cent glucose intravenously to correct hypoglycaemia, repeated as necessary. Glucagon, 1 to 2 mg intravenously, should be given if glucose fails to maintain normoglycaemia.

4. Correct metabolic or electrolyte abnormalities.

References

Dickson SJ, Cairns ER, Blazey ND. The isolation and quantitation of insulin in postmortem specimens – a case report. Forensic Sci 1977; 9:37–42.

Martin FIR, Hansen N, Warne GL. Attempted suicide by insulin overdose in insulin requiring diabetics. Med J Aust 1977; 1:58–60.

Sturner WQ, Putnam RS. Suicidal insulin poisoning with nine day survival: recovering in bile at autopsy by radioimmunoassay. J Forensic Sci 1972; 17:514–21.

Further Reading

Bobzien WF. Suicidal overdoses with hypoglycaemic agents. J Am Coll Amerg Phy 1979; 8:467–70.

Cowan DL, Burtis B, Youmans J. Prolonged coma after acetohexamide ingestion. J Am Med Assoc 1967; 201: 141–2.

Davies DM, MacIntyre A, Millar EJ, Bell SM, Mehra SK. Need for glucagon in severe hypoglycaemia induced by sulfonylurea drugs. Lancet 1967; i:363–4.

Dowell RC, Imrie AH. Chlorpropamide poisoning in nondiabetics Scott Med J 1972; 17:305–9.

Forman BH, Feeney E, Boas L. Drug induced hypoglycaemia. J Am Med Assoc 1974; 229:522.

Forrest JAH. Chlorpropamide overdoses: delayed and prolonged hypoglycaemia. Clin Toxicol 1974; 7:19–24.

Frier BM, Stewart WK. Cholestatic jaundice following chlorpropamide self-poisoning. Clin Toxicol 1977; 11:13–7.

Greenberg B, Weihl C, Hug C. Chlorpropamide poisoning. Pediatrics 1968; 41:145–7.

Kullavanijaya P. Recovery from overdose of gibenclamide. Br Med J 1970; 4:53–4.

Selzer RS. Drug induced hypoglycaemia – a review based on 473 cases. Diabetes 1972; 21:955–66.

Poisoning due to Carbon Monoxide

Carbon monoxide is produced by the incomplete combustion of organic materials. It is endogenously produced in man from the α-methane carbon atom of the protoporphyrin ring during the catabolism of haemoglobin. The normal endogenous production of carbon monoxide is sufficient to maintain a resting carboxyhaemoglobin (COHb) saturation of 1 to 3 per cent.

Although the mortality due to carbon monoxide poisoning has fallen since the introduction of natural gas to the domestic supply, 1000 deaths still occur annually in England and Wales from this cause (Figure 29.1). Carbon monoxide is the main cause of death from poisoning in children. Common sources of carbon monoxide are the exhaust from automobiles, improperly maintained and ventilated heating systems, smoke from all types of fires and household gas (if supplies have not been converted to natural gas). Natural gas is not in itself toxic, except in very high concentrations when it may cause asphyxiation.

The affinity of haemoglobin for carbon monoxide is approximately 240 times greater than for oxygen and signs and symptoms following inhalation of carbon monoxide are primarily the result of tissue hypoxia. The amount of oxygen available to the tissues is further reduced by the inhibiting influence of COHb on the dissociation of any oxyhaemoglobin still remaining (see page 39).

The absorption of carbon monoxide and the resulting symptoms are closely dependent on the concentrations of carbon monoxide in the inspired air, the time of exposure and the general health of the individual (elderly patients or those with pre-existing cardiorespiratory disease are more 'at risk').

The severity of poisoning with carbon monoxide can be classified as shown in Table 29.2.

Clinical Features

Agitation, mental confusion, headache (usually frontal and band-like. sometimes occipital).

Nausea and vomiting, incontinence (occasionally), haematemesis and melaena.

Pink skin and mucosae (i.e. there is no sign of cyanosis) because of the carboxyhaemoglobin in the blood.

Decrease in light sensitivity and dark adaptation.

Hearing loss (central type).

Hyperventilation, pulmonary oedema, respiratory failure, Cheyne–Stokes respiration.

Bullous lesions.

Hyperpyrexia.

Loss of consciousness, hypertonia, hyper-reflexia,

Figure 29.1. *Deaths from carbon monoxide — England and Wales, 1956–1978.*

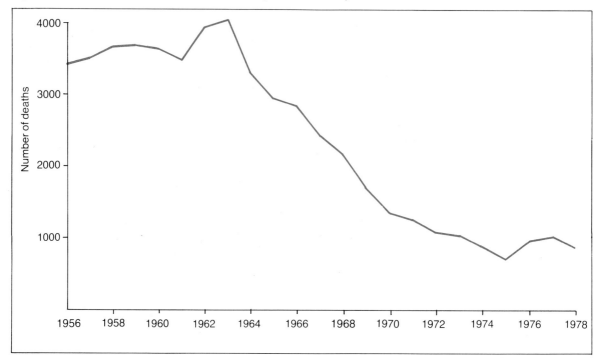

Plants
and
Fungi

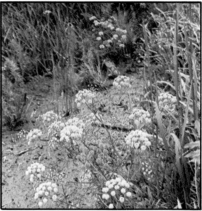

Plate 1. Tamus communis — *bright green berries turn red on ripening.*

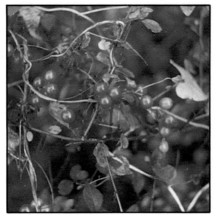

Plate 2. Cicuta virosa — *120 cm perennial found growing by lakes, ponds and ditches.*

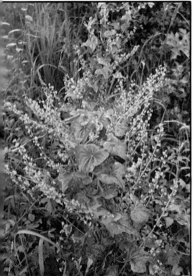

te **3.** Tamus communis — *perennial hedge- v plant, common in England.*

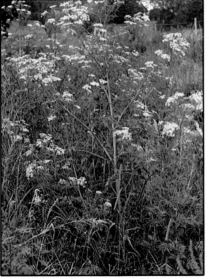

Plate 4. Conium maculatum — *150 cm high; biennial or perennial.*

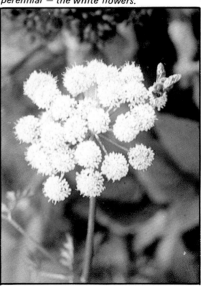

Plate 5. Oenanthe crocata — *150 cm high perennial — the white flowers.*

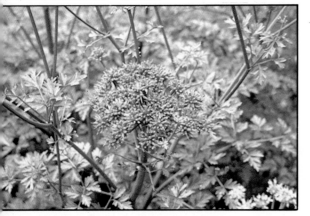

te **6.** Oenanthe crocata — *the fruit.*

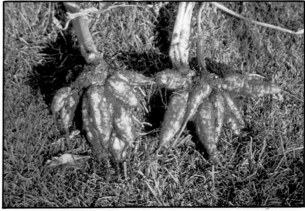

Plate 7. Oenanthe crocata — *the roots.*

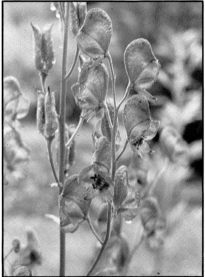

Plate 8. Aconitum napellus — *120 cm high herbaceous perennial with a black root, bright green leaves and helmet-shaped flowers.*

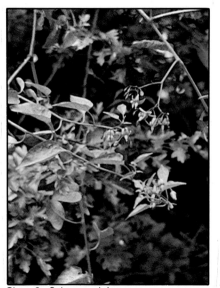

Plate 9. Solanum dulcamara — *a common climbing and trailing plant.*

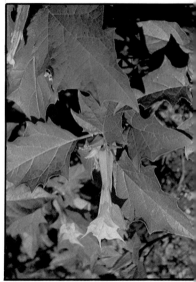

Plate 10. Datura stramonium — *100 cm h shrub with single white tubular flowers the centre of a forked branch.*

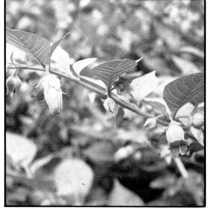

Plate 11. Atropa belladonna — *130 cm high herbaceous annual or biennial with berries; flower and unripe berries.*

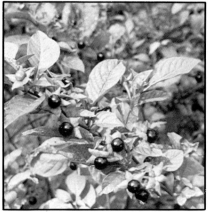

Plate 12. Atropa belladonna — *ripe berries.*

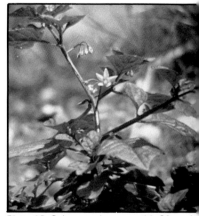

Plate 13. Solanum nigrum — *this 30 cm h herbaceous annual or biennial has sm white drooping flowers.*

Plate 14. Solanum dulcamara — *bearing shiny green or red berries.*

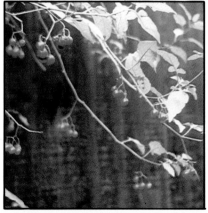

Plate 15. Amanita phalloides — *all parts of this fungus are poisonous; the cap is 9 cm in diameter.*

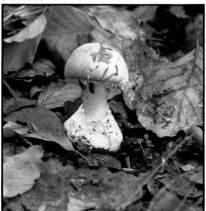

Plate 16. Amanita muscaria — *this fungu recognisable by its brilliant scarlet c which is about 12 cm in diameter.*

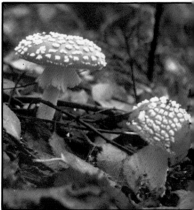

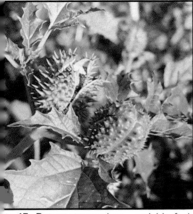

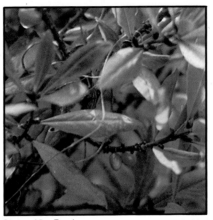

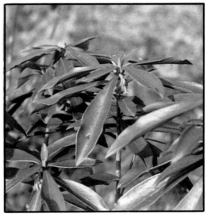

ate 17. Datura stramonium — *prickly fruit* *ntaining wrinkled black seeds.*

Plate 18. Daphne mezereum — *evergreen* *120 cm high shrub which is sparingly* *branched.*

Plate 19. Daphne laureola — *150 cm high* *shrub with blue-black, egg-shaped berries.*

ate 20. Arum maculatum — *30 cm high* *rennial.*

Plate 21. Bryonia dioica — *270 cm high* *perennial found in hedgerows.*

Plate 22. Bryonia dioica — *unripe and ripe* *berries.*

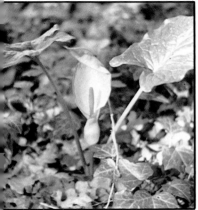

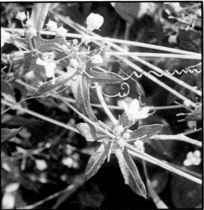

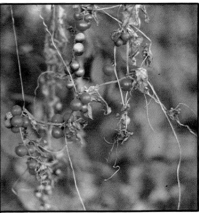

ate 23. Laburnum anagyroides — *the* *wers have five petals of unequal size and* *ng from branches in May and June.*

Plate 24. Laburnum anagyroides — *the fruit* *pod has up to eight kidney-shaped seeds,* *dark brown when ripe.*

Plate 25. Lupinus — *blue variety in flower.* *The fruit pod is covered with soft hairs and* *contains up to six seeds.*

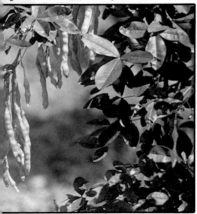

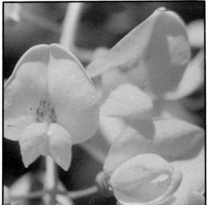

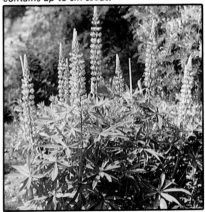

Poisonous Snakes

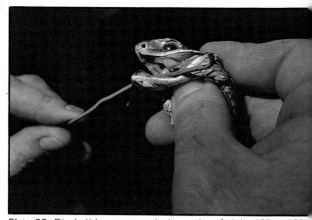

Plate 26. Dispholidus typus — *the boomslang (adults 120 to 180 ⸱ long), is an African 'back-fanged' colubrine tree snake (but m⸱ realistically should be called 'mid-fanged'). Freak fatal accider⸱ have occurred through handling this snake. Spontaneous bleed⸱ and non-clotting blood respond only to specific boomslang an⸱ venom.*

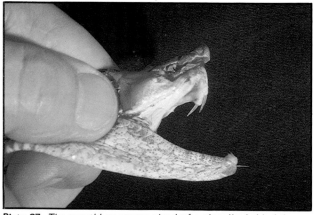

Plate 27. *The parotid or venom gland of a viper lies behind the eye (the skin over the gland has been removed) and connects by a duct along the upper gum to an opening at the top of the canalised fang which is long, mobile and easily seen when erected.*

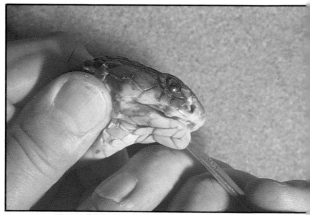

Plate 28. *Elapid (this is a cobra) fangs are short and hidden by gum-fold — the vagina dentis. They may therefore be difficult to s⸱*

Plate 29. Enhydrina schistosa — *the common seasnake, abounds in Asian—Pacific coastal waters. Adults grow up to 100 cm in length.*

Plate 30. Crotalus atrox — *the western diamondback rattlesna⸱ (adults up to 200 cm long), is the commonest cause of serio⸱ snake bit poisoning in North America. C. atrox occurs in southe⸱ states and Mexico.*

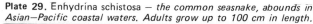
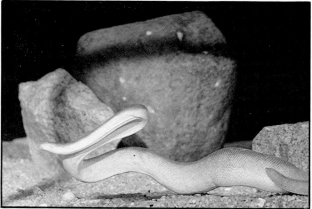

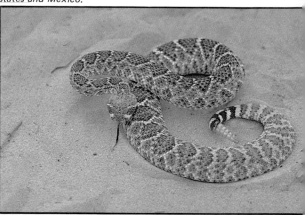

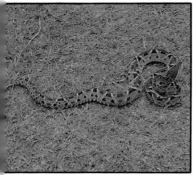

Plate 31. Bothrops atrox — *is often miscalled fer-de-lance (adults up to 180 cm long). probably causes more deaths in Central South America than any other snake.*

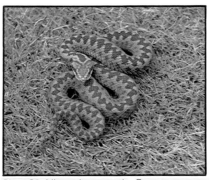

Plate 32. Vipera berus — *the European adder (adults 50 to 60 cm in length), is widely distributed throughout Britain, living in clearings, along the edges of woods, on moors and on mountains. In summer the adder prefers low-lying damp meadows.*

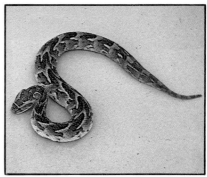

Plate 33. Bitis arietans — *the puff adder, grows to a length of 120 cm and is fat. It is a common cause of snake bite in Africa.*

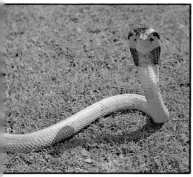

Plate 34. *Common cobras (mostly species of a) grow up to 150 cm in Africa and Asia. bra venom is neuro- and cardiotoxic but main effect in man of bites by Asian ras and the African spitting cobra, N. ricollis, is local necrosis.*

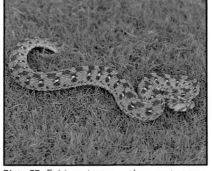

Plate 35. Echis carinatus — *the carpet or saw-scaled viper, is small (adults up to 50 cm long) but causes more deaths and serious poisoning than any other snake in the world. It is irritable and rubs its coils together when aroused, producing a rasping sound. Spontaneous haemorrhage (and non-clotting blood) is the most important clinical effect.*

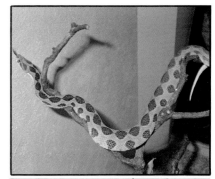

Plate 36. Vipera russelii — *(adults fat and up to 120 cm long) is common in parts of Asia, specially Burma, and causes haemorrhage — including pituitary haemorrhage — non-clotting blood and renal failure.*

Plate 37. Agkistrodon rhodostoma — *the Malayan pit viper (adults to 70 cm long), is a common cause of snake bite in south east a. Its venom is used to make ancrod, the defibrinating and anti-gulant drug.*

Plate 38. Acanthophis antarcticus — *the death adder (adults 60 to 80 cm long), is an Australian elapid despite its name and appearance. Venom is neurotoxic and, in contrast to some other Australian elapids, does not affect clotting in man.*

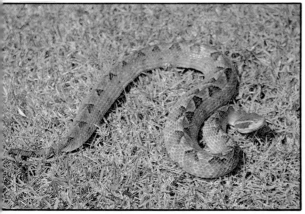

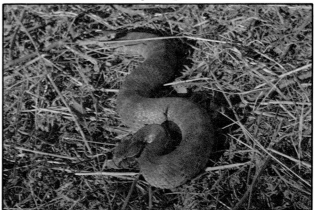

Snakebite, Tests and Treatment

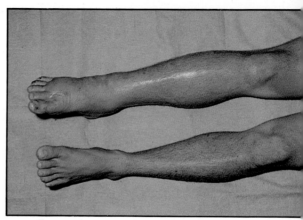

Plate 39. *Local swelling following a viper bite.*

Plate 40. *Blood-stained spit from the lungs is an early sign of systemic viper bite poisoning, and may be produced within 15 minutes of the bite if the patient is asked to cough hard enough.*

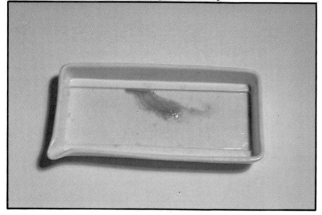

Plate 41. *Normal clot on left and 'speck' blood on right confirm defibrinogenation which is a useful bedside diagnostic sign* ~~bites by some (though not all) types of viper.~~

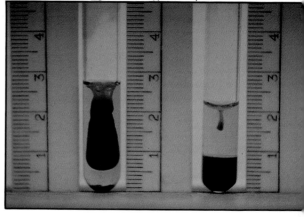

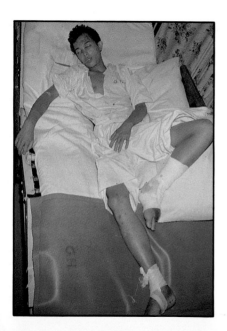

Plate 42. *Shock after viperine poisoning (and cobra bite poisoning) can be lethal but responds dramatically to intravenous anti-venom in adequate dosage (left).*

Plate 43. *Discoid ecchymoses on the left temple; another feature of systemic viper envenoming (right).*

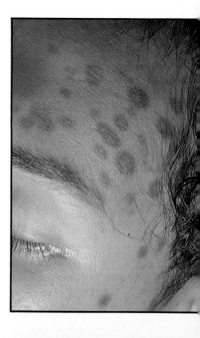

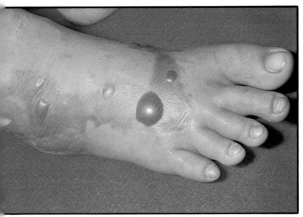

Plate 44. Blisters, skin darkening, and a putrid smell developing two [day]s after an Asian cobra bite confirm that local necrosis has [occ]urred.

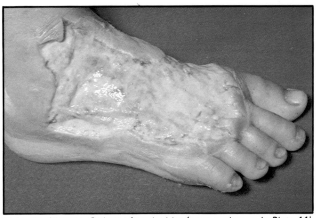

Plate 45. Necrosis 9 days after the bite (same patient as in Plate 44) is extensive but superficial. Conservative excision and skin grafting is indicated.

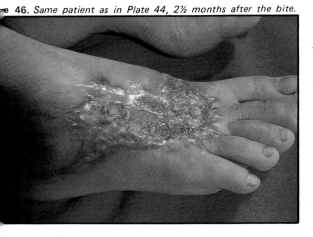

Plate 46. Same patient as in Plate 44, 2½ months after the bite.

Plate 47. Ptosis is an early sign of systemic elapid bite poisoning; antivenom is needed.

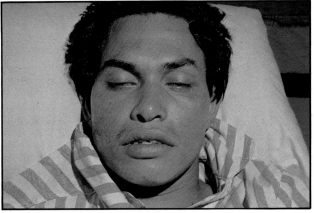

Plate 48. In seasnake bite poisoning, generalised myalgia (regardless [of t]he site of the bite) develops within an hour and is followed 3 to [ho]urs later by myoglobinuria.

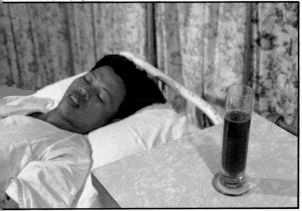

Plate 49. Before intravenous infusion of antivenom is started, adrenaline should be in the syringe to enable prompt intramuscular injection if serious immediate reactions occur.

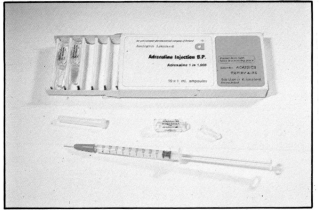

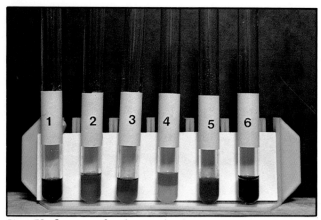

Plate 50. *Spot-tests for drugs and poison   1. salicylate; 2. pheno-thiazines; 3. paracetamol; 4. chloral hydrate; 5. ethchlorvynol; 6. paraquat.*

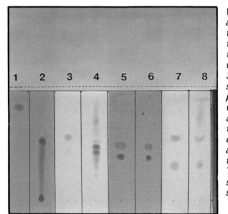

Plate 51. *Thin-layer chromatography c authentic drugs and sample extracts: 1. De: tropropoxyphene. 2. Extract of a urine sampl from a patient poisoned with Distalgesic. De: tropropoxyphene is degraded to metabolite which appear as a characteristic blue streak 3. Chlorpromazine. 4. Extract of a urin sample from a patient poisoned with chlo promazine. A range of metabolites givin various colour reactions is seen. 5. Morphin and methadone. 6. Extract of a urine sampl from a patient dependent on narcotics. Th deep blue spot is morphine. 7. Amitriptylin and nortriptyline. 8. Extract of a urine sampl from a patient poisoned with amitriptylin The major metabolite, nortriptyline, is th spot nearest the base-line. Other metabolit spots can be seen near the top of the plat*

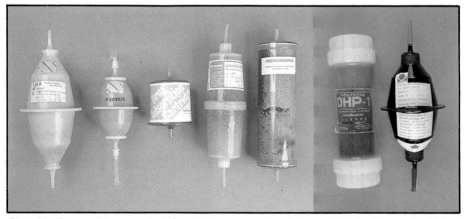

Plate 52. *Range of haemoperfusion columns now commercially available in Europe, the United States and Japan.*

Illustration acknowledgements

The publishers would like to thank Dr. H.A. Reid, Miss Pam North, The Pharmaceutical Society of Great Britain, Dr. B. Widc and the Editors for supplying the illustrations reproduced in t book.

Table 29.1.   Severity of poisoning.

COHb	10–30% – Mild poisoning
COHb	30–40% – Moderately severe poisoning
COHb	>40% – Very severe poisoning

extensor plantar responses, papilloedema, convulsions, monoplegia or hemiplegia, peripheral neuropathies. Cerebral, cerebellar and mid-brain damage (parkinsonism, akinetic mutism).

Myocardial ischaemia and infarction.

Arrhythmias (ECG changes: atrial fibrillation, prolonged P-R interval, A-V block, bundle branch block, ventricular extrasystoles, prolonged Q-T interval, ST depression).

Acute renal failure.

Muscle necrosis.

Thrombotic thrombocytopenia purpura.

Late neuropsychiatric sequelae.

Treatment

This is discussed in Chapter 5. Survival very much depends on how soon treatment is commenced. The administration of 100 per cent oxygen hastens the dissociation of COHb since the half-life of COHb in the blood varies inversely with the partial pressure of oxygen. The value of oxygen delivered at two to three atmospheres is discussed on page 40. Whatever oxygen source is to hand should be utilized with the least possible delay; removal of the patient to the fresh air will in itself result in improvement.

Further Reading

Anderson GK. Treatment of carbon monoxide poisoning with hyperbarbic oxygen. Milit Med 1978; 143:538–41.

Corya BC, Black MJ, McHenry PL. Echocardiographic findings after acute carbon monoxide poisoning. Br Heart J 1976; 38:712–7.

Finck PA. Exposure to carbon monoxide: review of the literature and 567 autopsies. Milit Med 1966; 131:1513–39.

Garland H, Pearce J. Neurological complications of carbon monoxide poisoning. Q J Med 1967; 36:445–55.

Gilbert GJ, Glaser GH. Neurological manifestations of chronic carbon monoxide poisoning. New Engl J Med 1959; 261: 1217–20.

Gordon EB. Carbon monoxide encephalopathy. Br Med J 1965; 1:1232.

Hopkinson JM, Pearce PJ, Oliver JS. Carbon monoxide poisoning mimicking gastro-enteritis. Br Med J 1980; 281: 214–5.

Jackson DL, Menges H. Accidental carbon monoxide poisoning. JAMA 1980; 243:772–4.

Jefferson JW. Subtle neuropsychiatric sequelae of carbon monoxide intoxication. Am J Psychiatry 1976; 133: 961–4.

Kelley JS, Sophocleus GJ. Retinal hemorrhages in subacute carbon monoxide poisoning J Am Med Assoc 1978; 239: 1515–7.

Long PI. Dermal changes associated with carbon monoxide intoxication. J Am Med Assoc 1968; 205:120–1.

Myers RAM, Linberg SE, Cowley RA. Carbon monoxide poisoning: the injury and its treatment. J Am Coll Emerg Phy 1979; 8:479–84.

Norman JN, Ledingham I McA. Carbon monoxide poisoning: investigations and treatment. Prog Brain Res 1976; 24: 101–22.

Radford EP, Levine MS. Occupational exposures to carbon monoxide in Baltimore firefighters. J Occup Med 1976; 18: 628–32.

Sammons JH, Coleman RL. Firefighters' occupational exposure to carbon monoxide. J Occup Med 1974; 16:543–6.

Sawada Y, Takahashi M, Ohashi N, Fusamato H, Maemura K, Kobayashi H, et al. Computerized tomography as an indication of long-term outcome after acute carbon monoxide poisoning. Lancet 1980; i:783–4.

Smith JS, Brandon S. Morbidity from acute carbon monoxide poisoning at three-year follow-up. Br Med J 1973; 1:318–21.

Sone S, Higashihara T, Kotake T, Morimoto S, Miura T, Ogawa M, et al. Pulmonary manifestations in acute carbon monoxide poisoning. Am J Roentgenol, Rad Therapy and Nuclear Med 1974; 120:865–71.

Stonesifer LD, Bone RC, Hiller FC. Thrombotic thrombocytopaenic purpura in carbon monoxide poisoning. Arch Int Med 1980; 140:104–5.

Winter PM, Miller JN. Carbon monoxide poisoning. J Am Med Assoc 1976; 236:1502–4.

Poisoning due to Chlorine

Chlorine gas is commonly used in industry as a reagent and for bleaching cloth and paper, as well as in water purification. It is also a common by-product in chemical plants. Exposure to the gas usually follows a leak from a storage tank and may, therefore, result in a large number of casualties.

The extent of injury from chlorine gas is proportional to the concentration of the gas, the duration of exposure and the water content of the tissue exposed. Cellular injury is due to the formation of hypochlorous and hydrochloric acid which, together with elemental chlorine and the potent oxidizing effect of nascent oxygen (produced when chlorine and water combine), react with sulphydryl groups and sulphur bonds in proteins. Chlorine gas has been reported to have a cellular toxicity of 10 to 30 times that of hydrochloric acid.

Clinical Features

Conjunctivitis, keratitis, pharyngitis.

Choking, coughing, burning chest pain, dyspnoea and haemoptysis (due to bronchiolar constriction and pulmonary oedema).

Nausea and vomiting.

Cardiac arrest secondary to hypoxia.

(Skin exposure) Partial and total thickness burns.

Treatment

1. Remove from contaminated environment. (A make-shift gas mask consisting of a water soaked cloth held to the face may minimize exposure during evacuation.)

2. Conjunctivitis and corneal defects. Irrigate eyes with copious amounts of saline after topical anaesthesia. Stain with fluorescein and refer to ophthalmologist if corneal abrasion is seen.

3. Cutaneous burns. Wash with saline. Apply topical burn cream and bandage.

4. Tracheobronchitis, pulmonary oedema. Humidified supplemental oxygen. Bronchodilators (salbutamol, terbutaline or aminophylline intravenously).

Mechanical ventilation, with positive end expiratory pressure (PEEP).

The use of steroids, diuretics and antibiotics seems to confer no advantage.

Further Reading

Decker WJ, Koch HF. Chlorine poisoning at the swimming pool: an overlooked hazard. Clin Toxicol 1978; 13:377–81.
Hedges JR, Morrissey WL. Acute chlorine gas exposure. J Am Coll Emerg Phy 1979; 8:59–63.
Kramer CG. Chlorine. J Occup Med 1967; 9:193–6.
National Institute of Occupational Safety and Health Criteria Document: Chlorine. Washington DC: US Department of Health, Education and Welfare, 1976.
Rafferty P. Voluntary chlorine inhalation: A new form of self-abuse? Br Med J 1980; 281:1178–79.

Poisoning due to Cyanide

Hydrocyanic acid (prussic acid) and its sodium and and potassium salts are present in some insecticides. rodenticides, metal polishes, electroplating solutions and in fumigant mixtures. In addition, cyanides are used in a variety of metallurgical processes.

Most deaths from cyanide have been due to suicide or homicide but some have arisen from accidental exposure in industry, the ingestion of apricot fruit seeds containing cyanogenic glycosides or the use of Laetrile as a non-approved anticancer agent. Chemically, Laetrile is a cyanogenic glycoside prepared from the seeds of apricots, prunes or peaches. Amygdalin is the major cyanogenic constituent which may be cleaved by the gastrointestinal flora to pro-

duce the disaccharide gentiobiose, benzaldehyde and hydrogen cyanide.

The ingestion of 50 mg hydrogen cyanide, or 200 to 500 mg of one of its salts, is likely to be fatal. The onset of poisoning is hastened by the presence of an empty stomach and high gastric acidity, but symptoms may be delayed for up to four hours if the poison is taken on a full stomach. Inhalation of hydrogen cyanide may produce symptoms within seconds and death within minutes.

Laboratory tests are seldom useful in determining either the prognosis or the treatment of cyanide poisoning and there is little information concerning the relationship between blood levels of cyanide and the ultimate outcome. However, specimens (including gastric contents) should be saved in case there is a subsequent legal need for chemical analysis.

Clinical Features

Acute Poisoning

The symptoms of poisoning appear within a few seconds to minutes after the ingestion or inhalation of cyanide and include:

Dizziness, headache, palpitations, anxiety, a feeling of constriction in the chest.

Dyspsnoea, pulmonary oedema.

Confusion, vertigo, ataxia, coma, paralysis.

Cardiovascular collapse and respiratory arrest.

Metabolic acidosis.

Note 1. Cyanosis is not present; the skin colour may be 'brick-red'.

2. There is sometimes an odour of bitter almonds on the breath.

Chronic Poisoning

Ataxia, peripheral neuropathies, optic atrophy, nerve deafness, dermatitis.

Toxic amblyopia associated with heavy cigarette smoking has also been attributed to the cyanide content of tobacco.

Treatment

The rationale for the use of specific antidotes in cyanide poisoning is discussed in detail in Chapter 5.

1. Dicobalt edetate (Kelocyanor)
Inject 300–600 mg i.v. over one minute with a

further 300 mg if recovery does not occur wihin one minute.

(**Note**: Dicobalt edetate may cause hypotension, tachycardia and chest pain).

2. If there is no response to dicobalt edetate, give intravenously 10 ml of a 3 per cent sodium nitrite solution followed by 25 ml of a 50 per cent sodium thiosulphate solution (See Chapter 5, p 37).

3. Supportive measures including mechanical ventilation.

Further Reading

Bryson DD. Cyanide Poisoning. Lancet 1979; i:92.

Carter JH, McLafferty MA, Goldman P. Role of the gastro-intestinal microflora in amygdalin (Laetrile)-induced cyanide toxicity. Biochem Pharmacol 1980; 29:301–4.

Editorial. Which antidote for cyanide? Lancet 1977; ii:1167.

Editorial. Chronic cyanide neurotoxicity. Lancet 1969; ii: 942–3.

El Ghawabi SH, Gaafar MA, El-Saharti AA, Ahmed SH, Malash KK, Fares R. Chronic cyanide exposure: a clinical, radioisotope and laboratory study. Br J Ind Med 1975; 32: 215–9.

Graham DL, Laman D, Theodore J, Robin ED. Acute cyanide poisoning complicated by lactic acidosis and pulmonary oedema. Arch Intern Med 1977; 137:1051–5.

Herbert V. Laetrile: the cult of cyanide. Am J Clin Nutr 1979; 32:1121–58.

Lee-Jones M, Bennett MA, Sherwell JM. Cyanide self-poisoning. Br Med J 1970; 4:780–1.

Naughton M. Acute cyanide poisoning. Anaesth Intensive Care 1974; 4:351–6.

Peterson RD, Rumack BH. Laetrile and pregnancy. Clin Toxicol 1979; 15:181–4.

Sayre JW, Kaymakcalen S. Cyanide poisoning from apricot seeds among children in central Turkey. New Engl J Med 1964; 270:1113–5.

Winek CL, Fusia E, Collom WD, Shanor SP. Cyanide poisoning as a mode of suicide. Forensic Sci 1978; 11:51–5.

Metoclopramide Poisoning

Metoclopramide is a chlorbenzamide derivative that is used as an antiemetic. Extrapyramidal side-effects have been reported in children receiving the 'recommended dose' and in those who have taken the drug in excess.

Clinical Features

Drowsiness, tachycardia, nausea, constipation or diarrhoea, fever.
Opisthotonos, torticollis, increased muscle tone, occulogyric crisis, facial grimacing, conjugate deviation of the eyes, diplopia, trismus, nystagmus, rhythmic protrusion of the tongue.
Agitation, anxiety, oedema of the tongue, periorbital oedema.

Treatment

Emesis or gastric lavage, if appropriate.
Benztropine, 1–2 mg intravenously, if extrapyramidal features are present.

Further Reading

Casteels–Van Daele M, Jacken J, Van der Schueren P, Zimmerman A, Van den Bon P. Dystonic reaction in children caused by metoclopramide. Arch Dis Child 1970; 45:130–3.

Fournier A, Pavli A, Duronlombier H, Cousins J. Effets du surdosage en metoclopramide chez l'enfant: a propos de 9 observations cliniques. Pediatrie 1969; 24:799–805.

Low LCK, Goel KM. Metoclopramide poisoning in children. Arch Dis Child 1980; 55:310–2.

Melmed S, Bank H. Metoclopramide and facial dyskenesia. Br Med J 1975; 1:331.

Robinson OPW. Metoclopramide – side-effects and safety. Postgrad Med J 1973; 49:Suppl. 4. 77–80.

Phencyclidine Poisoning

Phenycyclidine was synthesized in 1957 and made available as a general anaesthetic in 1958 (Sernyl). During the clinical trial period adverse psychotic reactions such as agitation, disorientation, delusions and hallucinations developed in many postoperative patients. As a result, use of this drug in humans was discontinued though, since 1967, it has been available as a veterinary product (Sernylan).

The illicit use of phencyclidine was first reported in 1967, though major abuse of 'Angel dust' in the USA did not occur until more recently. Phencyclidine abuse has not been reported in the UK.

Phencyclidine may be 'snorted' (nasal inhalation), smoked with parsley or marijuana, ingested or injected.

Clinical Features

Agitation or drowsiness, confusion, ataxia, stupor, blurred vision, nystagmus, tremors, hyper-reflexia, muscle rigidity, opisthotonos, acute dystonia, hallucinations, convulsions, coma.

Hypertension, cardiac arrhythmias.
Increased bronchial and salivary secretions.
Rhabdomyolysis.
Acute renal failure.

Treatment

1. Gastric lavage, if appropriate. Oral charcoal adsorbs phencyclidine.
2. Supportive measures.
3. Prevent self-injury.
4. Forced acid diuresis (Chapter 8).

Further Reading

Burns RS, Lerner SE. Perspectives: acute phencyclidine intoxication. Clin Toxicol 1976; 9:477−501.

Cogen FC, Rigg G, Simmons JL, Domino EF. Phencyclidine-associated acute rhabdomyolysis. Annals Intern Med 1978; 88:210−2.

Eastman JW, Cohen SN. Hypertensive crisis and death associated with phencyclidine poisoning. J Am Med Assoc 1975; 231:1270−1.

Editorial. Phencyclidine: the new American street drug. Br Med J 1980; 281:1511−12.

Hoogwerf B, Kern J, Bullock M, Comty CM. Phencyclidine-induced rhabdomyolysis and acute renal failure. Clin Toxicol 1979; 14:47−53.

Liden CB, Lovejoy Jnr FH, Costello CE. Phencyclidine: nine cases of poisoning. J Am Med Assoc 1975; 234:513−6.

Picchioni AL, Consroe PF. Activated charcoal − a phencyclidine antidote, or hog in dogs, N Engl J Med 1979; 300:202.

Sioris LJ, Krenzelok EP. Phencyclidine intoxication: a literature review. Am J Hosp Pharm 1978; 35:1362−7.

Showalter CB, Thornton WE. Clinical pharmacology of phencyclidine toxicity. Am J Psychiatry 1977; 134:1234−8.

Yesavage JA, Freman AM. Acute phencyclidine (PCP) intoxication: psychopathology and prognosis. J Clin Psychiatry 1978; 39:664−6.

Phenylbutazone Poisoning

Phenybutazone, a non-steroidal anti-inflammatory agent, is rarely taken in overdose. It is highly protein-bound and extensively metabolized. Hepatic damage may be due to a toxic metabolite.

Clinical Features

Upper abdominal pain, nausea, vomiting, haematemesis, diarrhoea.
Hyperventilation, dizziness, coma and convulsions.
Hepatic and renal damage.

Sodium and water retention.
Possible depression of bone marrow.

Treatment

Emesis or gastric lavage, if appropriate.
Supportive measures.
Treat convulsions with diazepam 5−10 mg i.v.
Cimetidine 200 mg 4−6 hourly i.v. for GI bleeding.
Forced alkaline diuresis, dialysis and haemoperfusion are unlikely to enhance excretion significantly.

Further Reading

Prescott LF, Critchley JAJH, Balali-Mood M. Phenylbutazone overdosage: abnormal metabolism associated with hepatic and renal damage. Br Med J 1980; 281:1106−7.

Rifampicin Poisoning

Overdose of rifampicin results in the 'red man syndrome', which may be fatal.

Clinical Features

Yellow/orange discoloration of the skin and subsequently the sclera (discoloration of the skin may be removed by washing).
Nausea, vomiting, abdominal pain.
Pruritus.
Cardio-respiratory arrest.

Treatment

1. Emesis or gastric lavage, if appropriate.
2. Supportive and symptomatic treatment.

Further Reading

Broadwell RO, Broadwell SD, Comer PB. Suicide by rifampicin overdose. J Am Med Ass 1978; 240:2283−84.

Jack DB, Knepil J, McLay WDS, Fergie R. Fatal rifampicin-ethambutol overdosage. Lancet 1978; ii:1107−8.

Newton RW, Forrest ARW. Rifampicin overdose − 'the red man syndrome'. Scott Med J 1975; 20:55−56.

Chapter 30

J. A. Vale and T. J. Meredith

Poisonous Plants and Fungi

The colour plates cited in this chapter are to be found between pages 188 and 189.

*"My heart aches and a drowsy numbness pains
My sense, as though of hemlock I had drunk."*

*John Keats
Medical Student, Guy's Hospital, 1815–16*

In his poem 'Ode to a Nightingale' Keats was describing the use of an alkaloid containing extract of hemlock which at the time was still in use as a narcotic and sedative. Its dangers were well known — it is thought, for example, that it was responsible for the death of Socrates.

It is popularly assumed that poisonous plants, if not abounding, certainly exist in Great Britain to a significant extent. The walls of many casualty departments and doctors' waiting rooms are covered by coloured posters ominously depicting a variety of poisonous plants. The impression is given that any child simply touching, let alone chewing, some plant or other would be in immediate peril.

Yet experience suggests otherwise. During the 16 years that the National Poisons Information Service (NPIS) has been in existence in the UK, some 20,000 enquiries have been received about 'poisonous plants' at the five centres (London, Edinburgh, Cardiff, Belfast and Dublin). However, only two people in the UK are known to have died from plant poisoning in the past 15 years and that was due respectively to *Amanita phalloides* and *Laburnum spp.* Most inquiries concern inquisitive children, although adults are occasionally poisoned when, for example, they ingest daffodil bulbs in mistake for onions and deadly nightshade berries instead of blueberries.

The plants which most frequently give cause for concern are either those which are widely distributed or those with a reputation for being 'poisonous' (Table 30.1).

Several plants shown in Table 30.1 — cotoneaster, mountain ash, honeysuckle, firethorn, hawthorn and berberis — are of low or doubtful toxicity and may be regarded as non-poisonous in the quantities eaten by children, and, following ingestion, no treatment need be given. The other plants in the list, which is arranged alphabetically rather than in order of toxicity, are possibly more dangerous and merit more detailed consideration.

Black Bryony (*Tamus communis*)

The bright scarlet berries of the black bryony (Plates 1 and 3) contain an unidentified irritant which causes blistering of the skin. When ingested, there may be burning and blistering in the mouth followed by vomiting and diarrhoea. It has been asserted that death following ingestion of the berries may be rapid but, in Britain, no serious cases have been encountered in recent years and treatment can usually be restricted to simple symptomatic measures.

Broom (*Cytisus spp.*)

Although the various species of broom are related to the laburnum and contain toxic alkaloids, the latter are present in only small quantities and symptoms other than vomiting are seldom reported. The ingestion of this plant should give cause neither for anxiety nor for energetic therapy.

Table 30.1.   Plants commonly ingested in the UK.

Common name(s)	Parts usually ingested
Berberis	Berries
Black bryony	Berries
Broom	Seeds and pods
Bulbs — many varieties	Bulbs
Cotoneaster	Berries
Firethorn	Berries
Hawthorn	Berries
Hemlock	Leaves and seeds
Hemlock water dropwort	Roots
Water hemlock, cowbane	Roots
Holly	Seeds
Honeysuckle	Berries
Laburnum	Seeds and pods
Lupin	Seeds
Mistletoe	Berries
Monkshood, aconite, wolfsbane	Leaves, flowers, seeds
Mountain ash, rowan	Berries
Mushrooms or toadstools	—
Nightshade — Black (garden)	Berries
— Deadly	Berries
— Woody (bittersweet)	Berries
Oak tree — acorns	Acorns
Spurge laurel	Berries
Spurge olive, mezereon	Berries
Dwarf bay tree	Berries
Thornapple, jimson weed	Seeds
Wild arum, lords and ladies, cuckoo pint	Berries
Winter cherry	Berries
Jerusalem cherry	Berries
White bryony	Berries
Yew	Berries

Bulbs

Bulbs from the daffodil, narcissus and related plants may cause GI disturbance with vomiting, abdominal colic and diarrhoea. Rarely the ingestion of large numbers of bulbs has resulted in collapse and convulsions.

Treatment is symptomatic unless a dozen or more bulbs have been ingested, when a gastric lavage should be undertaken and supportive measures adopted.

The Hemlock Family

Three members of the family Umbelliferae are highly poisonous.

Hemlock (Conium maculatum)

Hemlock (Plate 4) is found throughout Britain and grows on wasteland, hedgebanks, road verges and near streams. It may be distinguished from other members of the Umbelliferae family by the smooth, spotted stem and the distinct odour of mice which each part of the plant emits when bruised or crushed.

Toxicity

All parts of the hemlock are poisonous due to the presence of the alkaloids coniine, cohydrine, N-methyconiine and coniceine. In the young plant the leaves are the most poisonous part, but the toxic alkaloids pass to the fruits or 'seeds' as they form and these are in their most dangerous state when still green but fully formed, i.e. about three-quarters ripe. Fatal cases of accidental hemlock poisoning may be due to a failure to distinguish the leaves from those of parsley and the fruits from those of anise.

Clinical Features

Poisoning with hemlock can cause vomiting, diarrhoea, tachycardia, depressed respiration, dilatation of the pupils, muscular weakness (particularly of the limbs), hypothermia, mental confusion, coma, convulsions and death from respiratory paralysis.

Treatment

Syrup of ipecacuanha, 10 to 15 ml, should be given or a stomach washout performed. As no specific antidote is available, appropriate supportive measures should be instituted.

Hemlock Water Dropwort (Oenanthe crocata)

The leaves are similar to those of celery and, indeed, have a similar aroma, making them attractive to children. The stem is hollow and grooved, also rather like celery. The white flowers (Plate 5) have a wine-like scent, hence the generic name. The roots (Plate 7), which are the most poisonous part of the plant, resemble the tubers of dahlias and are said to have a pleasant taste, rather like parsnip.

Toxicity

Hemlock water dropwort is probably the most poisonous plant in Britain. The active toxin is oenanthotoxin which is present in the roots in highest concentration in the winter and early spring. This century, 14 people (11 of them children) have been reported to have been poisoned following the ingestion of the tubers; nine of them died.

Clinical Features

The initial and almost invariable symptom is vomiting which may continue for several hours and, when convulsions supervene, may lead to aspiration of gastric contents. Hyperventilation, and hence a respiratory alkalosis, hypersalivation, limb weakness and tonic or clonic muscle spasms accompanied by trismus have been described. A transient elevation in the serum concentration of unconjugated bilirubin has been noted.

Treatment

The few cases reported to date suggest that the short-acting barbiturates are the drugs of choice in the treatment of convulsions.

Water Hemlock — Cowbane (*Cicuta virosa* — Plate 2)

Water hemlock is rare and confined to a few parts of Britain. It is found particularly near marshy areas, banks and ditches.

Clinical Features

The toxic principle, circutoxin, is very similar to oenanthotoxin with, as a result, similar presenting symptoms. In addition, circutoxin appears to produce muscle tenderness with associated high creatine phosphokinase levels.

Treatment

Treatment is as for hemlock water dropwort.

Holly(*Ilex aquifolium*)

Like mistletoe, holly is so familiar that a detailed description is unnecessary. Although holly berries have an emetic and purgative effect if eaten in quantities of more than about 20, children seldom complain of symptoms and therefore usually need no treatment.

Laburnum (*Laburnum anagyroides Plates 23 and 24*)

This attractive ornamental tree is seldom seen growing wild.

Toxicity

All parts of the tree contain the toxic alkaloid cytisine. In summer and autumn, the miniature 'pea-pods' containing the small kidney-shaped seeds are often eaten by children at play and are the most common cause of plant poisoning in this country.

Clinical Features

The commonest symptoms of laburnum poisoning are vomiting and restlessness. Rarely, abdominal pain, dizziness, drowsiness, incoordination, delirium and twitching have occurred. All these symptoms occur within 12 hours.

Treatment

If more than 20 seeds (10 in a child) have been ingested then a stomach washout should be performed and appropriate supportive and symptomatic measures instituted.

A recent adult case is worth noting. A 23-year-old male claimed to have ingested 300 laburnum seeds three-and-a-quarter hours before attending a casualty department. He had already vomited, was drowsy and complained of abdominal pain. Stomach washout returned about 60 seeds. He vomited once more some hours later but otherwise suffered no further symptoms and made a complete recovery.

Lupins (*Lupinus spp.*)

Lupins are common garden perennials, related to laburnum; the fruits are also like tiny pea-pods and contain the same type of poisonous alkaloid. When eaten in quantity, the seeds can rarely cause respiratory depression, bradycardia, paralysis and convulsions. The toxicity of this plant seems to vary considerably under different conditions and in different seasons. As a precaution, syrup of ipecacuanha, 10 to 15 ml, should be given or gastric lavage performed in those who have eaten a considerable number of seeds (Plate 25).

Mistletoe (*Phoradendron flavescens; Viscum album*)

Inquiries about poisoning by mistletoe berries occur almost exclusively in December and January, since the plant grows wild as a parasite high up in trees but is brought within easy reach of children during the festive season, just when the shiny pearly berries are ripe and most desirable.

Toxicity

Toxicity is due to the berries which contain tyramine and β-phenylethylamine.

Clinical Features

These consist of gastroenteritis and bradycardia. The reported cases of poisoning have usually involved no more than three or four berries and have resulted in very mild symptoms.

Treatment

The only treatment usually required is to give plenty to drink. A stomach washout is only necessary if very large numbers of berries have been swallowed.

Monkshood (*Aconitum napellus*)

The popular name for this plant (Plate 8) is taken from the dark blue helmet-shaped flowers. The native British species is found growing wild on river banks and in most shady places in western counties of England and in South Wales. The cultivated forms are to be found throughout the British Isles and are as toxic as the wild plant.

Toxicity

The toxicity is chiefly due to aconitine, one of the narcotic alkaloids. The tuberous roots have sometimes been mistaken for horseradish or celery and the leaves for parsley.

Clinical Features

Symptoms occur within a few minutes of ingestion and include tingling of the mouth, stomach and skin, restlessness, bradycardia, respiratory distress, muscular incoordination and weakness, vomiting and diarrhoea. Convulsions and death from cardiorespiratory failure can occur within a few hours.

Treatment

Treatment may include gastric lavage (or syrup of ipecacuanha, 10 to 15 ml, if more appropriate), symptomatic and supportive measures.

Mushrooms

Many poisonous mushrooms can be confused with edible species and eaten by mistake. Serious poisoning is fortunately rare in Britain. The best-known poisonous mushroom is the Death Cap (*Amanita phalloides* – Plate 15), but other mushrooms are a more common cause of poisoning. Many mushroom toxins are unidentified, heat-labile substances that cause gastrointestinal upset or excoriation of the lips and tongue when the mushrooms are eaten raw. Some fungi contain alkaloids resembling muscarine, atropine or ergot, others contain psychoactive substances such as bufotoxin, psilocin and mescaline.

Poisoning due to Mushrooms other than the Death Cap

Fly Agaric (*Amanita muscaria* – Plate 16) is now known to contain little or no muscarine but does contain hallucinogenic substances. The Liberty Cap (*Psilocybe semilanceate*) and *Panaeolus foenisecii* contain psilocybin and have been taken deliberately for their hallucinogenic effects. The Ink Cap (*Coprinus atramentarius*) contains a dehydrogenase inhibitor with a disulfiram (antabuse)-like effect – that is, vomiting will occur if alcohol is also ingested.

Clinical Features

Most patients have a violent but self-limiting attack of abdominal colic, diarrhoea, thirst, nausea and vomiting which occurs about two hours after eating the fungus.

The main danger is fluid and electrolyte loss, which should be corrected. A delayed onset of the symptoms (six to eight hours) usually indicates much more serious poisoning. Rarely the symptoms and signs are those of excessive cholinergic stimulation (bronchospasm, bradycardia, constricted pupils, sweating and collapse); these should be treated with atropine sulphate, 0.6 to 2 mg, parenterally in an adult. Atropine should be avoided, however, if the patient is excited, disorientated or hallucinated; chlorpromazine should then be given.

Treatment

Patients suspected of having eaten poisonous mushrooms other than *Amanita phalloides* should either be given syrup of ipecacuanha, 10 to 15 mg, to induce vomiting, or gastric lavage may be performed.

Poisoning due to the Death Cap

Amanita phalloides (Plate 15) contains two types of toxin: the phallotoxins (phalloidin, phalloin and phallolysin), which act rapidly and cause violent gastroenteritis four to eight hours after ingestion, and the amatoxins (α, β and γ amanitin), which have a more delayed effect and destroy cells primarily in the renal tubules and in the liver. Recent reports suggest that the amatoxins may also cause early gastrointestinal symptoms. Both types of toxins are strongly bound to plasma albumin and are extremely active in this state. Their toxicity can be reduced by displacing them from albumin, probably because more unbound toxin is then excreted by the kidneys.

Clinical Features

After ingestion the symptoms may be divided into the following four clinical stages:

1. An asymptomatic period which may last for up to a day (usually four to eight hours).
2. A period of severe vomiting, diarrhoea and abdominal cramps.
3. The clinical course can be complicated by jaundice, hypoglycaemia and hyponatraemia, hypokalaemia, thrombocytopenia and coagulation abnormalities, sepsis and acidosis.
4. In some cases hepatocellular failure occurs.

Diagnosis

A radioimmunoassay for amatoxins has been developed recently (Kleine Mitteilungen 1980).

Treatment

Gastric aspiration and lavage should be performed and intravenous fluids given. Renal impairment and liver damage follow a few days later. The use of penicillin or sulphamethoxazole to displace the toxin from plasma albumin, together with early haemodialysis, is a logical treatment, and even haemodialysis alone seems to have improved mortality. Haemodialysis may also be required for renal failure.

Nightshades

Three wild plants are commonly known as nightshade in Great Britain. They are often inaccurately named by those inquiring about possible causes of poisoning, although they are, in fact, relatively easy to identify.

Black Nightshade *(Solanum nigrum)*

This is a common garden weed with white flowers (not purple, as in woody nightshade) – Plate 13.

Toxicity

The berries are black when ripe, and are quite attractive to children because they look like blackcurrants. They contain an alkaloid, solanine, the amount of which varies with soil, season and district.

Clinical Features

Symptoms include nausea, vomiting, abdominal pain, diarrhoea, trembling, paralysis, coma and, very rarely, death.

Treatment

Treatment consists of symptomatic and supportive measures following gastric lavage, or after emesis has been induced with 10 to 15 ml of syrup of ipecacuanha.

Deadly Nightshade *(Atropa belladonna – Plates 11 and 12)*

This plant is found mainly in the South of England. It has erect stems, large, oval leaves and single drooping flowers of a dull, faded purple which give rise to single black, cherry-sized berries.

Toxicity

The berries contain the alkaloids hyoscyamine, atropine and hyoscine, which are all potentially extremely toxic. A single berry may give rise to symptoms and, according to some reports, children have died from as few as three berries, although no fatalities have been recorded in the last decade.

Clinical Features

The symptoms are due to the anticholinergic effects of the alkaloids and include dry mouth, dry, hot skin, dilated pupils, blurred vision, tachycardia, excitement and delirium, followed by drowsiness, hallucinations and coma.

Treatment

All patients should be referred to hospital where the treatment should include immediate stomach washout and symptomatic measures. In very severe cases it may be necessary to use anticonvulsants, sedatives or, occasionally, physostigmine to counteract the anticholinergic effects. Children generally show a remarkable resilience to the effects of ingested belladonna alkaloids.

Woody Nightshade (*Solanum dulcamara*) **or bittersweet** (*Plates 9 and 14*)

This is a common, climbing, trailing plant found on damp wasteland and in shady hedges. In late summer and autumn the plant bears shiny green or red berries which children often eat as 'currants'.

Toxicity

The toxic alkaloid solanine is found in all parts of the plant. The symptoms and treatment are as for black nightshade.

Oak Tree—Acorns (*Quercus*)

Both the leaves and the acorns contain tannic acid which is thought to be responsible for their ill effects.

The toxicity varies from species to species. Usually only two or three acorns are eaten, the symptoms are limited to abdominal pain and no treatment, therefore, is necessary.

Spurge Laurel and Olive (*Daphne laureola* and *mezereum*)

Spurge olive (Plate 18), a shrub cultivated for its attractive sweet-smelling purple flowers, and its relative spurge laurel, which has sweet-smelling greenish flowers, grow wild only in chalky woodland in the South of England.

Toxicity

In summer, spurge laurel (Plate 19) has blue-black, egg-shaped berries, which contain the toxic glycoside aglycone dihydroxycoumarin. Children usually only eat two or three of the berries, often in mistake for currants.

Clinical Features

If more than 10 berries are ingested, burning and swelling of the lips, mouth and tongue, abdominal pain, vomiting, bloody diarrhoea and muscular twitching may occur.

Treatment

Treatment includes the induction of vomiting by giving syrup of ipecacuanha, 10 to 15 ml, or stomach washout followed by appropriate supportive measures.

Thornapple (*Datura stramonium*)

This plant (Plates 10 and 17) grows up to one metre high in Southern England on cultivated ground and rubbish heaps. The flowers are white or purple in colour and are usually seen during July and August. The fruit is covered with long, sharp spines and contains many dark-coloured seeds.

Toxicity

All parts of the plant, particularly the seeds, are poisonous and contain a number of alkaloids including atropine, hyoscine and hyoscyamine.

Clinical Features

If a patient is severely poisoned, symptoms may include headache, nausea, vomiting, dizziness, thirst, dry and burning sensations on the skin, visual disturbances, flushing, nervous twitching, delirium and tachycardia. Rarely these may be followed by convulsions, coma and death. In non-fatal cases some symptoms may continue for several days.

Treatment

The treatment is as for deadly nightshade.

In recent years datura intoxication has become commoner in the USA, Australia and England as a result of the discovery that the leaves of datura trees (*D. sanguinea*, *D. suveolens*, *D. cornigera* and *D. aurea*), and certain asthma remedies (in Britain) can yield a legal and readily available hallucinogen.

Wild Arum (*Arum maculatum*)

Wild arum (Plate 20), a plant commonly found in hedges, banks and ditches, has shiny, spotted, arrow-shaped leaves and a bunch of shiny, red or green berries on a leafless stem from July onwards.

Toxicity

Children find these berries very attractive, but rarely eat many of them because of the acrid irritant juice which they contain.

Clinical Features

Symptoms include a burning sensation in the mouth, vomiting and diarrhoea.

Treatment

Syrup of ipecacuanha, 10 to 15 ml, should be given, or a stomach washout performed if more than 10 berries have been eaten. Otherwise, liberal fluids should be given.

Winter Cherry (*Solanum pseudocapsicum*)

Winter or Jerusalem cherry is a common pot plant, prized for its bright red berries, which are probably toxic, and are seen particularly at Christmas time. Several alkaloids have been isolated from the plant but there is no record of fatalities and, therefore, no treatment is required.

White Bryony (*Bryonia dioica*)

This is one of the best known hedge-climbers of the English countryside (Plates 21 and 22). Its red berries are up to 8 mm in diameter and contain several large, yellow/black, mottled, flattened seeds. The berries are attractive to children and the roots have been eaten in mistake for parsnips. The toxic substance is probably a glycoside and it has been suggested that about 15 berries might be fatal in a child. Symptoms include vomiting, abdominal pain and severe diarrhoea. Treatment consists of symptomatic and supportive measures.

Yew (*Taxus baccata*)

Toxicity

The leaves and seeds of the yew tree (though not the flesh of the yew berry) are poisonous due to the presence of an alkaloid which is not destroyed by drying or storage.

Clinical Features

Symptoms include vomiting, diarrhoea, abdominal pain, delirium, convulsions, bradycardia and coma. Although the ripe berry is attractive to children and the seed itself is highly toxic, poisoning is rare, possibly due to the fact that the toxicity is well known and parents warn their children of the danger.

Treatment

Treatment is symptomatic and supportive. In severe cases gastric lavage or emesis needs to be performed soon after ingestion to be effective as the alkaloid is rapidly absorbed from the intestine.

'Greened' Potatoes (*Solanum tuberosum*)

Toxicity

Potato stems and leaves contain a series of alkaloidal glycosides, including α-solanine and α-chaconine which are highly toxic. The normal tuber contains only small amounts of solanines in the peel and none in the flesh. Although poisoning due to feeding the leaves and stems to domestic animals is well recognized, the main hazard in humans comes from eating 'greened' potatoes.

Greening and sprouting occur when potato tubers are exposed to light or are stored in adverse conditions, and these processes are associated with the production of the solanine alkaloids. Except in times of food shortages, few people cook greened or sprouted potatoes because they have a bitter, unpleasant taste. Occasionally, however, outbreaks of solanine poisoning have occurred due to catering errors.

Clinical Features

An outbreak has been recently described (McMillan and Thompson 1979), in which 78 schoolboys developed vomiting, diarrhoea and abdominal pain between 4 and 14 hours after ingestion. Slight fever occurred in some patients and depression of the central nervous system (coma and convulsions) occurred in the more serious cases, as did peripheral circulatory collapse, even when dehydration was only slight. All of the boys recovered in this outbreak, though some were confused and hallucinated for several days. Death has, however, occurred in previous outbreaks, usually within 24 hours.

Treatment

Treatment consists of supportive measures (replacement of fluid and electrolyte losses and the use of anticonvulsants if needed), following a diagnosis made on the basis of the history and symptoms. Subsequently the clinical diagnosis can be confirmed by examining the remaining potatoes and potato waste for solanine alkaloids.

Conclusion

The fears of poisoning from plants and fungi in Britain are more imagined than real, often due to disproportionate and sensational reporting. There is seldom occasion for alarm or, medically, for more than mild symptomatic and reassuring measures.

In the event of doubt about the consequences of inappropriately swallowed plants, the guidance of the National Poisons Information Service may be sought, though prior identification is a pre-requisite. In Britain, serious reactions from poisonous plants are rare indeed and it is nearly always sufficient just to treat the symptoms.

Acknowledgements

The authors gratefully acknowledge the generosity of the Pharmaceutical Society of Great Britain and Miss Pamela North in allowing the reproduction of the photographs in the colour section.

References

Solanine Poisoning

McMillan M, Thompson JC. An outbreak of suspected solanine poisoning in schoolboys: examination of criteria of solanine poisoning. Q J Med 1979; 48:227–43.

Further Reading

General

Forsyth AA. British Poisonous Plants. London: HMSO, 1968.
Hardin JW, Arena JM. Human Poisoning from Native and Cultivated Plants. North Carolina: Duke University Press, 1974.
Kingsbury JM. Poisonous Plants of the US and Canada. New York: Prentice Hall, 1964.
Lampe KF, Fagerstrom R. Plant Toxicity and Dermatitis: A Manual for Physicians. Baltimore: Williams and Wilkins and Co, 1968.
North PM. Poisonous Plants and Fungi. Poole: Blandford Press, 1967.
Poisonous Plants of Florida. J Fla Med Assoc 1978; 65:No 3.

Hemlock Poisoning

Applefield JJ, Caplan ES. A case of water hemlock poisoning. J Am Coll Emerg Phy 1979; 8:401–3.
Carlton BE, Tufts E, Girard DE. Water hemlock poisoning complicated by rhabdomyolysis and renal failure. Clin Toxicol 1979; 14:87–92.
Mitchell MI, Routledge PA. Hemlock water dropwort poisoning – a review. Clin Toxicol 1978; 12:417–26.
Robson R. Water hemlock poisoning. Lancet 1965; 2:1274–5.
Starreveld E. Cicutoxin poisoning (water hemlock). Neurology 1975; 25:730–4.

Laburnum Poisoning

Richards HGH, Stephens A. A fatal case of laburnum seed poisoning. Med Sci Law 1970; 10:260–6.

Mushroom Poisoning

Benjamin C. Persistent psychiatric symptoms after eating psilocybin mushrooms. Br Med J 1979; 1:1319–20.

Bertelli A, Fournier E, Frimmer M, Gorini S. Clinical and Experimental Aspects of Fungal Poisoning. Bern: Hans Huber, 1977.

Bertelli A, et al. Clinical and experimental aspects of fungal poisoning. Curr Probl Clin Biochem 1977; 7:1–207.

Cooles P. Abuse of the mushroom *Paneolus foenisecii*. Br Med J 1980; 280:446–7.

Editorial. Mushroom poisoning. Lancet 1980; 2:351–2.

Hyde C, Glancy G, Omerod P, Hall D, Taylor GS. Abuse of indigenous psilocybin mushrooms: a new fashion and some psychiatric complications. Br J Psychiatry 1978; 132:602–4.

Kleine Mitteilungen. Knollenbläterpilzvergiftung – Diagnose in 2 Stunden. Dtsch Med Wochensher 1980; 25:906.

Lincoff G, Mitchell DH. Toxic and Hallucinogenic Mushroom Poisoning. New York: Van Nostrand Reinhold, 1977.

McCormick DJ, Avbel AJ, Gibbons RB. Non-lethal mushroom poisoning. Ann Intern Med 1979; 90:332–35.

Paaso B, Harrison DC. A new look at an old problem: mushroom poisoning. Am J Med 1975; 58:505–9.

Rumack BH, Salzman E. Mushroom Poisoning: Diagnosis and Treatment. Florida: CRC Press, 1978.

Wauters JP, Roussel C, Farquet JJ. *Amanita phalloides* poisoning treated by early charcoal haemoperfusion. Br Med J 1975; 2:1465.

Datura Poisoning

Belton PA, Gibbons DO. Datura intoxication in West Cornwall. Br Med 1979; 1:585–6.

Hall RCW, Popkin MK, McHenry LE. Angel's trumpet psychosis: a central nervous system anticholinergic syndrome. Am J Psychiatry 1977; 134:312–4.

Screiber W. Jimson seed intoxication: recognition and therapy. Milit Med 1979; 144:329–32.

Taxus Baccata Poisoning

Schulte T. Lethal intoxicatson with leaves of the yew tree. Arch Toxicol 1975; 34:153–8.

Chapter 31

H. Alistair Reid

Poisoning due to Snake Bite

The colour plates cited in this chapter are to be found between pages 188 and 189.

Medically important snakes have fangs at the front of their mouths which enable them to inject venom secreted by the parotid glands (Plate 27). These are the 'poisonous' snakes of which there are three families — elapids (neurotoxic), seasnakes (myotoxic) and vipers (vasculotoxic). Elapids are landsnakes with short fixed fangs (Plate 28). Seasnakes have very short fixed fangs and characteristic flat tails. (Plate 29). Vipers have long erectile fangs (Plate 27), triangular heads and, usually, short fat bodies. Vipers are subdivided into crotaline or pit vipers, having a thermosensitive pit between eye and nose, and viperine vipers, without pits. The pit detects warm-blooded prey in the dark.

Throughout the world, viper bites of man are much more common than elapid bites, except in the Pacific–Australian area where vipers do not occur naturally. Seasnake bites are common among fishing folk of Asian and Western Pacific coastal areas. Land-snakes known to be medically important include the western diamondback rattlesnake (*Crotalus atrox;* Plate 30), *C.adamanteus* and *C.viridis* in North America; *Bothrops atrox* (Plate 31), *B.jararaca* and the tropical rattlesnake *(C.durissus* or *C.terrificus)* in Central and South America; the European adder (*Vipera berus;* Plate 32), the only native venomous snake in Britain, and the long-nosed viper *(V.ammodytes)* in Europe; the night adder (*Causus* species), the puff adder (*Bitis arietans;* Plate 33), and mambas (four species of *Dendroaspis*) in Africa. Cobras (mostly *Naja* species; Plate 34) and the saw-scaled viper (*Echis carinatus;* Plate 35) are common both in Africa and in Asia; in parts of Asia, Russell's viper (*V.russelii;* Plate 36), the Malayan pit viper (*Agkistrodon rhodostoma;* Plate 37), the sharp-nosed pit viper (*A.acutus*), the mamushi pit viper (*A. halys*), the habu viper (*Trimeresurus flavoviridis*), and kraits (*Bungarus coeruleus* and *B.multicinctus*) are important. The

tiger snake (*Notechis scutatus*), death adder (*Acanthophis antarcticus;* Plate 38), the taipan (*Oxyuranus scutellatus*), and the Papuan black snake (*Pseudechis papuanus*) are important in the Pacific–Australian area.

Some colubrine snakes have fangs at the back of the mouth but, though technically venomous, their bites are usually harmless to man, with the rare exception of the boomslang (*Dispholidus typus;* Plate 26) and the vine snake (*Thelotornis capensis*) in Africa, and the keel-back (*Rhabdophis* species) in Asia.

Epidemiology of Snake Bite

Snake bite is mainly a rural and occupational hazard and, as such, affects men more than women; farmers, landworkers, and fishermen are at greatest risk. Most bites occur in the daytime when more people are around, and involve the foot, toe or lower leg as a result of accidentally disturbing the snake. In temperate regions most bites are avoidable as the victim deliberately handles the snake and is bitten on the fingers or hands.

Unfortunately there are few statistics which reliably indicate the incidence, morbidity and mortality of snake bite. Available statistics are misleading because they are based largely on hospital cases, yet in the rural tropics, where snake bite is common, victims rarely go to hospital, preferring treatment from traditional healers. In Nigeria, for example, one such healer treats several hundred snake bite patients each year, his house being just a mile from the university teaching hospital which records only about five cases during the same period. A survey of fishing villages in

Asia, where sea snakes are a scourge, revealed that less than 15 per cent of those bitten sought treatment from the government medical services. Even outside the tropics snake bite victims often do not go to hospital. However, recent work has established that enzyme-linked immunosorbent assay can reliably identify and sensitively quantify both venom and venom-antibody in body fluids. Application of this technique will greatly advance epidemiological as well as clinical and forensic studies of venomous bites and stings.

Reliable observations confirm that at least half of all those sustaining snake bites escape with little or no poisoning because little or no venom is injected. On the other hand, in serious poisoning mortality can be high when adequate medical treatment is not given – it can be as high as 50 per cent in seasnake bite poisoning (which occurs in 20 per cent of all seasnake bites). Snake bite in its early stages is very unpredictable and all victims should be observed closely for at least 12 hours, to assess the severity of poisoning and to ensure rational treatment.

Pathophysiology of Snake Bite Poisoning

Envenoming in man involves multiple toxic reactions occurring simultaneously or sequentially. Furthermore autopharmacological substances may be released by activation of the kinin system, complement system, etc.

Swelling

Most viper venoms are predominantly vasculotoxic in man causing a rapidly developing swelling of the bitten part. This swelling is often misinterpreted as being due to venous thrombosis or to inflammation (or both), but necropsy in such cases has revealed patent veins and no evidence of inflammation. The swelling is presumably due to venom diffusing through the subcutaneous tissues and affecting vascular permeability from the outside.

Local Necrosis

Local necrosis in viper bites is mainly ischaemic, thrombosis blocking local blood vessels and causing slowly developing 'dry gangrene' (which almost inevitably becomes infected later). Local necrosis in cobra bites is clinically different, more like 'wet gangrene', developing rapidly within a few days and with a characteristic putrid smell; presumably it is due mainly to direct cytolytic venom action.

Shock

Systemic absorption of venom and its products is usually through the lymphatics, although venous absorption can occur with low molecular weight venoms such as cobra venom. Early shock is common with some viper bites, especially those of *V.berus*. Within a few minutes of the bite, vomiting, abdominal pain, explosive diarrhoea, and collapse with unrecordable blood pressue can occur, but usually resolve spontaneously within half an hour to an hour. This early collapse may be due to activation of the kinin system followed by inhibition of the bradykinin released.

Shock which persists or starts later (some hours after the bite) is a main cause of death in viper bites. It appears to be multifactorial – with hypovolaemia from loss of plasma and blood into the swollen limb, cardiac effects as evidenced by changes in the electrocardiogram and serum enzymes, and damage to vascular endothelium (pulmonary oedema may be severe).

Spontaneous Haemorrhage

Spontaneous haemorrhage into a vital organ, especially the brain, is the usual cause of death in viper envenoming. This lethal capillary oozing, often delayed until several days after the bite, is *not* necessarily related to the coagulation defect which also results with certain viper venoms. Spontaneous bleeding is caused mainly by direct damage to capillary endothelium by a venom component ('haemorrhagin'), which does not affect coagulation.

Effects on Blood Clotting

Some of the crotaline venoms (certain species of *Crotalus, Bothrops* and *Agkistrodon*) have a direct thrombin-like effect on fibrinogen, splitting off fibrinopeptide A (but not B). This activity is not affected by heparin. Some viperine venoms, such as *E. carinatus* and *V. russelii*, exert an indirect effect on fibrinogen by activating prothrombin or Factor X; this action is inhibited by heparin. These venom effects constitute in vitro 'procoagulant' activity. In vivo, if the dose of venom is large, as for example when the viper attacks prey for food, massive intravascular clotting stops the circulation and causes very rapid death. With small doses of venom, however, such as those injected into human victims, there is a continual action on fibrinogen to produce a fibrin more susceptible to lysis than natural fibrin. The venom thus eliminates fibrinogen as quickly as the liver provides it, and although these venoms are 'procoagulant', by in vitro and by intravenous animal tests, the effect in human victims is non-clotting or poorly clotting blood because of absent or very low fibrinogen. The latter is not the primary cause of spontaneous bleeding. However, it can aggravate bleeding from blood vessels damaged by 'haemorrhagins', and even more so from vessels damaged by local incisions, fasciotomy and so on.

Most of the venoms affecting coagulation in man are strongly 'procoagulant' and, therefore, non-clotting blood is a simple and very sensitive bedside test of systemic envenoming, giving warning of abnormal bleeding to follow. On the other hand, a few venoms are only weakly 'procoagulant' (e.g. juvenile *C.atrox*) and in these cases non-clotting blood indicates a high, potentially lethal venom dose. Non-clotting blood can also differentiate envenoming by one type of viper from that of another (e.g., *E.carinatus* envenoming in Africa causes non-clotting blood whereas *B.arietans* does not). This can facilitate choice of appropriate antivenom and can be used to monitor response to antivenom.

By in vitro tests it has been found that venoms often have anticoagulant and haemolytic activities, and effects on platelets, but these are usually of no clinical importance in man.

Neurotoxic Effects

Most elapid venoms are principally neurotoxic, producing a selective neuromuscular block affecting mainly the muscles of the eyes, tongue, throat and chest, and leading to respiratory failure in severe poisoning.

Myotoxic Effects

Although seasnake venoms appear to be neurotoxic in animal experiments, producing a myoneural block, the effects in humans are primarily myotoxic. Clinical and pathological findings are typical of generalized myopathic lesions in skeletal muscle.

Cardiac Effects

Cardiovascular depression with hypotension and electrocardiographic changes (usually in ST segments and T-waves) are observed in severe cobra (*Naja naja*) and some viper bites — *V.berus* for example. Raised serum creatine phosphokinase in such cases suggests a direct cardiotoxic effect.

Renal Failure

Acute renal failure may follow serious poisoning by all three types of venomous snake — viper, elapid and seasnake. As with shock, the pathogenesis is probably multifactorial, and can include decreased renal blood flow (due in turn to several factors), haemoglobinuria, myoglobinuria, and probably a direct nephrotoxic effect of venom.

Exceptions to the Rule

Finally although the effects of snake envenoming in man may be conveniently, though arbitrarily, classified into vasculotoxic for vipers, neurotoxic for elapids, and myotoxic for seasnakes, there are notable exceptions to such a classification. Thus, some vipers such as *C.durissus* have mainly neurotoxic, not haemorrhagic, effects. The African spitting cobra, *N.nigricollis*, causes local necrosis and neurotoxic signs have not been observed. Some Pacific—Australian elapids are myotoxic rather than neurotoxic; others can cause significant haemorrhage and non-clotting blood in addition to neurotoxic effects. Also, as related above, many viper venoms, such as *B.arietans, Causus* species, and *B.gabonica* in Africa, do not affect clotting in human victims.

Clinical Features of Snake Bite Poisoning

These are summarized in Table 31.1. The most common symptom is fright, producing collapse with feeble pulse within minutes; collapse due to envenoming rarely appearing until half an hour to an hour after the bite. However, early collapse with hypotension is sometimes due to venom effects and not to fright (e.g. in bites by the adder, *V. berus*). In such cases the early shock usually resolves spontaneously within half an hour to an hour.

Early Features of Envenoming

Local Swelling

Local swelling (Plate 39) starts within a few minutes of a viper bite if venom is injected. It is a very valuable clinical sign because, if swelling is absent and one knows the biting snake was a viper, then poisoning can be excluded immediately. Local swelling is also a feature of poisoning in bites by Asian cobras and the African spitting cobra, *N.nigricollis*, though it may not appear for one to two hours. Bites by other elapids (non-spitting African cobras, mambas, kraits, coral snakes and seasnakes) do not usually cause swelling (although a tourniquet may do so). Local pain and fang marks are extremely variable and of no help in diagnosis.

Early Signs of Systemic Envenoming

Nonspecific Signs

There are three important nonspecific early signs of systemic envenoming:

1. Vomiting (sometimes of emotional origin but more often denotes systemic poisoning).
2. Hypotension (elapid and viper bites, but not sea-snake bites).
3. Polymorph leucocytosis.

Specific Signs

More specific early signs of systemic poisoning may develop within 15 minutes of the bite but, on the other hand, their onset may be delayed by up to 10 hours after an elapid bite (hence the great importance of careful observation of all patients with snake bite). These specific signs are as follows:

1. Viper — abnormal bleeding in the spit (Plate 40), from bite, injection sites, or the gums, in vomit or stool; discoid ecchymoses (Plate 43) and positive Hess test may start within 20 minutes of the bite; later non-clotting blood (Plate 41).
2. Elapid — ptosis (Plate 47), glossopharyngeal palsy.
3. Seasnake — generalized myalgia, 3 to 5 hours later myoglobinuria (Plate 48).

Later Features of Envenoming

Increased Local Swelling

The local swelling of viperine poisoning can increase both in extent, to involve the whole limb and trunk, and in amount, over 48 to 72 hours after the bite, depending on the dose of venom injected. The swelling is tense and can be massive; it may or may not be accompanied by discoloration due to escape of erythrocytes as well as the plasma. Discoloration then goes through the stages of a bruise.

Blisters

Blisters around the site of the bite are common in cobra and viper envenoming, and blisters extending up the limb (Plate 44) suggests a large dose of venom and often precede necrosis.

Local Necrosis

Local necrosis is characteristic of poisoning from Asian and African spitting cobra bites and some viper bites. It becomes evident a few days after the bite and is shown by a darkening of the skin (Plate 44), together with an offensive 'putrid' smell, which is particularly marked in cobra bite necrosis. Necrosis can be extensive (Plate 45), but it is usually superficial; involvement of tendons, muscle, and bones is exceptional. Bacterial infection follows necrosis and, in late neglected cases, may spread to joints. But in the absence of necrosis or meddlesome local measures such as incision, application of dressings, etc., bacterial infection virtually never occurs.

Haemorrhage

Haemorrhage into a vital organ, especially the brain, can be delayed until at least a week after a viper bite if effective antivenom is not given. It is often, though not inevitably, fatal.

Shock

Shock in viper (Plate 42) and in cobra bite envenoming is shown by prostration, sweating, cold extremities, tachycardia, hypotension, and sometimes electrocardiographic and serum enzyme abnormalities.

Respiratory Failure

In severe advanced elapid poisoning the patient is unable to speak, cough, swallow, protrude his tongue, or move the lower jaw. Respiratory failure is shown by confusion and stupor, shallow breathing, rise in pulse, respiration rate and blood pressure, increased sweating, and cyanosis of finger tips. At any time during this phase of respiratory failure obstruction by inhaled vomitus or secretions can result in sudden death. Otherwise, deepening coma, nonreactive dilated pupils, twitchings and convulsions presage death.

Venom Allergy

Occasionally victims exhibit reactions such as urticaria and fever in the absence of antivenom or other allergenic medications. Presumably these symptoms are caused by venom allergy.

Seasnake Bite

In seasnake bite poisoning, true paresis of a peripheral type may ensue after some hours and, later still, tendon reflexes become depressed and then absent. Respiratory failure from muscle weakness may supervene within a few hours of the bite, or as long as 60 hours after the bite. Other patients succumb from hyperkalaemic cardiac arrest or (later) from acute renal failure.

Diagnosis and Prognosis

The diagnostic importance of local swelling and non-clotting blood in viperine poisoning has already been stressed. The swelling may become massive but this is not a cause for alarm. It will resolve (completely as a rule) within a few weeks, provided there is no underlying necrosis. Local necrosis often entails prolonged, even permanent, disability.

The early signs of systemic poisoning have also been noted. Usually the majority of victims who receive a venom dose large enough to cause systemic poisoning will already have signs of this by the time they see a doctor. In the rare cases seen soon after the bite, within the latent period between bite and possible onset of systemic symptoms (one or two hours

generally, but up to 10 hours with some elapids), the patient should be given a placebo injection and then carefully observed every 30 minutes for these early systemic signs. Differentiation of viperine from elapid systemic poisoning is usually obvious from simple clinical evaluation.

Severe Poisoning

Viperine poisoning is severe if, within one to two hours of the bite, swelling is above the knee or elbow, shock is evident, or haemorrhagic signs besides haemoptysis develop (gum bleeding, ecchymoses, positive tourniquet test, etc., do not usually appear for four to five hours). Elapid poisoning is severe if neurotoxic signs start within one hour or less of the bite and rapidly progress to respiratory failure. Mental confusion strongly suggests respiratory failure, though ptosis and glossopharyngeal palsy can make assessment of mental awareness difficult. Shock may also be a feature of severe elapid poisoning. Severe seasnake poisoning is shown by myoglobuniuria as early as one to two hours after the bite, and by the development, within a few hours, of respiratory failure.

Severe Systemic Poisoning

In severe systemic poisoning, following either elapid or viper bites, the electrocardiogram may show T-wave inversion and deviation of the ST segment. In seasnake bites, an electrocardiogram is specially valuable in detecting hyperkalaemia which can result from generalized muscle damage. Tall peaked T-waves in chest leads may appear within a few hours of the bite and give early warning of impending death or of acute renal failure.

Mortality

Considering the lethal potential of most venomous snakes, the natural mortality of snake bite is surprisingly low. Generally speaking, deaths occur most rapidly after elapid bites, especially cobra bites (average mortality time is about five hours after the bite), and are most protracted after viper bites (average two to three days after the bite). Death in seasnake bite (usually 12 to 24 hours after the bite) and in elapid bite is due mainly to respiratory failure. Shock and haemorrhage into vital organs are the main causes of death in viper bites. Later deaths can occur from acute renal failure.

Hospital Treatment

It is very important neither to panic (there is usually abundant time to administer antivenom if indicated) nor to dismiss a case of snake bite as trivial without proper observation. Adequate reassurance is most important, so tetanus toxoid or a placebo injection should be given promptly unless antivenom is already indicated. Except in cases in which significant poisoning can be excluded, the patient should be admitted and carefully observed, preferably in an intensive care unit, at least until the next day. Fatalities have occurred because patients, on admission, were judged to have only slight poisoning. The following should be monitored and charted:

1. Hourly blood pressure, pulse and respiration rate.
2. Electrocardiogram, white blood cell count, serum bicarbonate, and creatine phosphokinase (CPK) twice daily (more often if hypotension persists).
3. Urine output, specific gravity, blood urea.
4. Local necrosis if relevant (extent of blisters and skin darkening, putrid smell).

Additionally, in viper bites: abnormal bleeding (injection sites, gums, etc.), blood clottability (positive or negative), haemoglobin and swelling (circumferences compared with unbitten limb). In elapid bites: ptosis, difficulty in talking and swallowing, vomiting and breathing. In seasnake bites: myalgic pains, myoglobinuria, ptosis, difficulty in talking, swallowing, vomiting and breathing, CPK (reflecting skeletal muscle, not cardiac, damage) raised.

General Measures

Tourniquets should be released. After cleansing (if necessary), the site of the bite should be left alone as interference often causes infection. Cryotherapy can aggravate local necrosis and heparin can aggravate bleeding, so both are contraindicated. Antibiotics are not indicated unless, or until, there is clinical evidence of local necrosis.

Local dressings should not be applied at this stage as they enhance secondary bacterial infection. For the same reason, blisters should be left strictly alone; they will then break spontaneously and will quickly heal without infection provided there is no underlying necrosis. But as soon as local necrosis is obvious sloughs should be excised. At this stage, systemic antibiotics and tetanus antiserum (in the tropics) may be helpful, and skin grafting should be carried out early rather than late, even if infection is still evident. Results are usually very satisfactory (Plate 46).

Blood Transfusion

Blood transfusion helps in viperine shock, especially if the victim was anaemic before the bite, but specific antivenom is usually dramatically successful in viperine shock if given in adequate dosage. A controlled trial of steroids in viper bite poisoning showed that prednisone benefited neither local nor systemic poisoning, although steroids are useful for delayed antivenom reactions. Steroids may delay the appearance of local necrosis in cobra bites, but do not lessen the final severity.

'Spitting' Cobra Venom

Some cobra species in Africa and Asia are able to 'spit' from the fang tips whose venom-duct exits are directed forwards instead of downwards. These cobras can eject venom up to two metres and venom may enter the eyes of the victims. If the eyes are promptly bathed with water only mild inflammation results.

Dysphagia

Patients with dysphagia (elapid bites) should be nursed in the prone position to minimize the risk of inhaling vomit. Respiratory and renal failure may need supportive treatment.

Antivenom

Indications for Use

The main indication for antivenom therapy is systemic envenoming. If used correctly antivenom can effectively reverse systemic poisoning, although it is not given until hours or even days after the bite. One should therefore wait for clear clinical evidence of systemic poisoning (Table 31.1) before giving antivenom. Antivenom should not be given as a routine measure in all cases of snake bite because severe immediate reactions occur in about one per cent of patients and, on very rare occasions, have been fatal. (For a list of some institutes which make antivenom see Appendix 1).

Table 31.1.   Main clinical features of snake bite.

| Snake | No poisoning | Effects of poisoning | | Natural mortality approximate | Average death time |
		Local	Systemic		
Elapids	50%	Slow swelling then necrosis by Asian cobras, African spitting cobras. Usually no local effects with other elapids.	Neurotoxic effects — ptosis, glosso-pharyngeal palsy. Respiratory paresis. Cardiac effects.	10%	5 to 20 hours
Seasnakes	80%	None	Myotoxic effects. Myalgia on moving. Paresis. Myoglobinuria. Hyperkalaemia.	10%	15 hours
Vipers	30%	Rapid swelling. Necrosis in 5 to 10% (some vipers only).	Vasculotoxic effects. Abnormal bleeding. Non-clotting blood (some vipers only). Shock	1—15%	2 days

Prevention of Local Effects

Provided the patient presents within a reasonable time after the bite, antivenom may prevent or mini-mize local effects, especially necrosis, in bites by snakes such as Asian cobras, African spitting cobras, puff adders and rattlesnakes. In adder bites Zagreb antivenom can prevent or minimize prolonged local painful swelling in adult patients (local necrosis does not follow *V. berus* bites, and local effects in chil-dren are rarely serious). In such cases, antivenom should be considered if the patient presents within four hours of the bite and has clear signs of local envenoming, such as swelling already spreading beyond the wrist or ankle.

Serum Sensitivity Test

A serum sensitivity test is not advisable when anti-venom is indicated. Results of such tests in several hundred patients were confusing. Reactions some-times occurred when antivenom was infused, despite negative test results, and, in some patients with a positive reaction, intravenous antivenom was subse-quently infused without any reaction.

Allergic History

A known allergic history contraindicates the use of antivenom unless the risk of death from envenoming is high. Such cases are rare, but if antivenom adminis-tration is undertaken two intravenous drips of isotonic saline should be set up, one containing the antivenom and one containing adrenaline. Small amounts of the adrenaline are infused first, followed by antivenom. The patient must be watched closely for anaphylaxis and, according to progress, alternate amounts of anti-venom increased and adrenaline decreased.

Administration of Antivenom

Intravenous Infusion

Clear antivenom is fully effective: check that there are no opacities which precede loss of potency. Anti-venom should always be given by intravenous in-fusion, the safest and most effective route. Depending on the severity of poisoning and the potency of the antivenom, 20 to 50 ml, sometimes 100 ml in bites by foreign snakes, are diluted in two to three volumes of isotonic (normal) saline. These dosages are required by all age groups.

Use of Adrenaline

The intravenous drip is started slowly at 15 drops a minute. If a reaction occurs the drip should be stopped temporarily and 0.5 ml adrenaline (1:1000 solution) injected intramuscularly. If adrenaline is injected at the first sign of anaphylaxis (Plate 49), it is quickly effective and the drip can be restarted cautiously. In some cases several injections of adrenaline may be needed.

Speed

The speed of administration is increased progressively so that the infusion is completed within about one hour. If, by then, there has been little significant improvement, further antivenom should be given. This is specially important in neurotoxic poisoning because antivenoms are usually less potent against elapid venoms than viper venoms.

Monitoring

Monitoring and charting as detailed above should continue at increasing intervals until all evidence of poisoning has resolved.

Appendix

The following are some institutes making antivenom:

1. *Algeria:* Institute Pasteur d'Algeria, Rue Docteur Laveran, Algiers.

2. *Australia:* Commonwealth Serum Laboratories, Parkville, Melbourne.

3. *Brazil:* Instituto Butantan, Caixa Postal 65, Sao Paulo.

4. *Costa Rica:* Instituto Clodomiro Picado, San Jose.

5. *France:* Institut Pasteur, Service de Serotherapie, 36 Rue du Docteur Roux, Paris XV.

6. *Germany:* Behringwerke AG, Postfachliessfach 167, 355 Marburg.

7. *India:* (a) Central Research Institute, Kasauli, R.I., Punjab. (b) Haffkind Institute, Parel, Bombay 12.

8. *Indonesia:* Perusahaan Negara Bio Farma, 9 Djalan Pasteur, Bandung.

9. *Iran:* Institut d'Etat des Serums et Vaccins Razi, Boite Postale 656, Teheran.

10. *Japan:* Institute for Infectious Diseases, University of Tokyo, Shiba Shirokane-daimachi, Minato-Ku, Tokyo.

11. *South Africa:* South African Institute for Medical Research, P.O. Box 1038, Johannesburg.

12. *Taiwan:* Taiwan Serum Vaccine Laboratory, 130 Fuh-lin Road, Shiling, Taipei.

13. *Thailand:* Queen Saovabha Memorial Institute, Bangkok.

14. *United States:* Wyeth Inc., Box 8299, Philadelphia, 1, Pa.

Scorpion antivenoms are made at institutes 1, 3 and 11; spider antivenoms at institutes 2, 3 and 11; jelly-fish (sea-wasp) antivenom at 2.

Doctors who need supplies of antivenom for use in various geographical areas may find the following most useful:

Americas: polyvalent viper antivenom from 4 or 14; coral snake antivenom from 3, 4, or 14.

North Africa: viper antivenom from 1, 5 or 6.

Mid-Africa: polyvalent antivenom from 5, 6, or 11.

South Africa: polyvalent antivenom from 11.

Middle East: viper–cobra antivenom from 5, 6 or 9.

Asia: (seasnake bite) seasnake or tiger snake antivenom from 2.

Burma, India, and Pakistan: cobra–krait–viper antivenom from 7(a) or 7(b).

Cambodia, Laos, Malaysia, Vietnam, Thailand: viper and cobra antivenom from 13.

Indonesia: cobra–krait–viper antivenom from 8.

Japan: viper antivenom from 10.

Philippines and Taiwan: cobra–krait–viper antivenom from 12.

Sources of Information

Primary Sources of Information

Texts on General Pharmacology and Adverse Drug Reactions

American Pharmaceutical Association. Evaluation of drug interactions. 2nd Ed. and supplement. Washington DC: Am Pharm Assoc 1976; (Suppl. 1978).

Avery GS. Drug Treatment. 2nd Ed. Sydney: Adis Press; Edinburgh: Churchill Livingstone, 1980.

Briggs M, Briggs M. The Chemistry and Metabolism of Drugs and Toxins. London: Heineman, 1974.

D'Arcy PF, Griffin JP. 2nd Ed. Iatrogenic Diseases. Oxford: Oxford University Press. 1979.

D'Arcy PF, Griffin JP. A Manual of Adverse Drug Interactions. 2nd Ed. Bristol: John Wright 1979.

Davies DM (Ed). Textbook of Adverse Drug Reactions. Oxford: Oxford University Press, 1977.

Dukes MNG (Ed). Side Effects of Drugs: Annual 4. Amsterdam: Excerpta Medica, 1980.

Dukes MNG (Ed). Meyler's Side Effects of Drugs Vol 9. Amsterdam: Excerpta Medica, 1980.

Gilman GA, Goodman LS, Gilman A (Eds). The Pharmacological Basis of Therapeutics. 6th Ed. New York: Macmillan 1980.

Griffin JP, D'Arcy PF. Drug Induced Emergencies. Bristol: John Wright, 1980.

Hansten PD. Drug Interactions. 4th Ed. Philadelphia: Lea and Febiger, 1979.

Ladu BN, Mandell HG, Way EL. Fundamentals of Drug Metabolism and Drug Disposition. Baltimore: Williams and Wilkins, 1971.

Laurence DR, Bennett PN. Clinical Pharmacology. 5th Ed. Edinburgh: Churchill Livingstone, 1980.

Melmon KL, Morrelli HF (Eds). Clinical Pharmacology, 2nd Ed. New York: Macmillan, 1978.

Wade A, Reynolds JEF (Eds). Martindale's Extra Pharmacopoeia. 27th Ed. London: Pharmaceutical Press, 1977.

Windholz M. Merck Index. 9th Ed. Rahway, New Jersey: Merck & Co. Inc., 1976.

Texts on Clinical Toxicology

(See also the references in each chapter)

Ansell G. Radiology in Clinical Toxicology. London: Butterworth, 1974.

Arena JM. Poisoning: Toxicology, Symptoms, Treatments. 4th Ed. Springfield, Illinois: Charles C. Thomas 1978.

Boyland E, Goulding R. Modern Trends in Toxicology − 2. London: Butterworth, 1974.

Casarett and Doull: Toxicology − The Basic Science of poisons. Doull J, Klaassen CD, Amdur MO (Eds). 2nd Ed. New York: Macmillan, 1980.

Clayton GD, Clayton FE (Eds). Patty's Industrial Hygiene and Toxicology. 3rd Revised Ed. Vol. 1 − General Principles. New York: John Wiley & Sons, 1978.

Cralley LV, Cralley LJ (Eds). Patty's Industrial Hygiene and Toxicology. 3rd Revised Ed. Vol. III − Theory and Rationale of Industrial Hygiene Practice. New York: John Wiley & Sons, 1979.

Dreisbach RH. Handbook of Poisoning. 10th Ed. Los Altos, California: Lange Medical Publications, 1980.

Fassett DW, Irish DD. Patty's Industrial Hygiene and Toxicology. 2nd Revised Ed. Vol. II − Toxicology. New York: John Wiley & Sons, 1963.

Gosselin RE, Hodge HC, Smith RP, Gleason MN. Clinical Toxicology of Commercial Products. 4th Ed. Baltimore Md: Williams and Wilkins, 1976.

Grant W. Toxicology of the Eye. 2nd Ed. Springfield Illinois: Charles C. Thomas, 1974.

Hamilton A, Hardy HL. Industrial Toxicology. 3rd Ed. Acton, Mass: Publishing Sciences Group, 1974.

Matthew H, Lawson AAH. Treatment of Common Acute Poisonings. 4th Ed. Edinburgh: Churchill Livingstone, 1979.

Moeschlin S. Poisoning: Diagnosis and Treatment. New York: Grune and Stratton, 1965.

Procter NH, Hughes JP. Chemical Hazards of the Workplace. Philadelphia: JB Lippincott, 1978.

Sax NI. Dangerous Properties of Industrial Materials. 5th Ed. New York: Van Nostrand Reinhold, 1979.

Sittig M. Hazardous and Toxic Effects of Industrial Chemicals. Park Ridge, New Jersey: Noyes Data Corporation, 1979.

Periodicals

Most general and specialist medical journals publish original articles, reviews and correspondence concerned with drug treatment and its complications. The following journals publish the results of original research or reviews of pharmacology and toxicology.

Adverse Drug Reaction Bulletin (Shotley Bridge General Hospital, Consett, Co. Durham, England).

Archives of Toxicology (Springer-Verlag).

British Journal of Clinical Pharmacology (Macmillan Journals).

British Journal of Pharmacology (Macmillan Journals).

Clinical Pharmacology and Therapeutics (St. Louis: CV Mosby).

Clinical Toxicology (Marcel Dekker Journals).

Developmental Pharmacology and Therapeutics (Basel: S Karger).

Drugs (Sydney: ADIS Press).

Drug and Chemical Toxicity (Marcel Dekker Journals).

Drug and Therapeutics Bulletin (Caxton Hill, Hertford, England: Consumers Association).

European Journal of Clinical Pharmacology (Springer-Verlag).

European Journal of Pharmacology (Amsterdam: Elsevier/North Holland Publishing Co.).

European Journal of Toxicology (Paris: 49 Rue St. Andre-des-Arts 75006).

Journal of Clinical Pharmacology (Box 842, Stamford, Ct 06904: Hall Associates).

Journal of Pharmacology and Experimental Therapeutics (Baltimore, Md: Williams and Wilkins).

Journal of Pharmacy and Pharmacology (London: Pharmaceutical Press).

Journal of Toxicology and Environmental Health (Washington, DC: Hemisphere Publishing Corporation)

Medical Letter (New Rochelle, NY 10801).

Prescribers Journal (London: DHSS).

Toxicology (Amsterdam: Elsevier/North Holland Publishing Co.).

Toxicology and Applied Pharmacology (Academic Press).

Veterinary and Human Toxicology (Manhattan KS 66505: Kansas State University).

Xenobiotica (London: Taylor and Francis).

Secondary Sources of Information

Abstracts and Bibliographies

Adverse Reactions Titles. Amsterdam: Excerpta Medica.

Bulletin of the National Clearinghouse for Poison Control Centers. Maryland: US Department of Health, Education and Welfare.

Clin-Alert. Louisville, Kentucky: Science Editors Inc.

Drug Literature Index. Amsterdam: Excerpta Medica.

Index Medicus. Bethesda, Maryland: National Library of Medicine.

Pharmacology and Toxicology. Amsterdam: Excerpta Medica.

Reactions. Sydney: ADIS Press.

Toxicology Abstracts. London: Information Retrieval Ltd.

Microfiche Information

Drugdex. Colorado: Micromedex Inc.

IOWA. Iowa: Iowa Drug Information Service, University of Iowa.

Poisindex. Colorado: Micromedex Inc.

Computer Services

Computer searches of the drug literature either 'on line' (carried out by subscribers themselves by means of remote computer terminals) or 'off line' (those carried out by the organisation for subscribers) are provided by:

Index Medicus (Medline, Toxline).

Excerpta Medica (Embase).

Micromedex (Drugdex, Poisindex).

Iowa Drug Information Service (IOWA).

Biological Information Service of Biological Abstracts (BIOSIS).

Chemical Abstracts Service (CACON/CASIA).

International Occupational Safety and Health Information Centre (CIS Abstracts).

Index